Clinical Ophthalmic Oncology

AF877508

Jacob Pe'er • Bertil E. Damato • Arun D. Singh
Editors

Clinical Ophthalmic Oncology

Conjunctival Tumors

Fourth Edition 2024

Springer

Editors
Jacob Pe'er
Ocular Onocology Service and Ophthalmic Pathology Laboratory
Department of Ophthalmology, Hadassah - Hebrew University Medical Center
Jerusalem, Israel

Bertil E. Damato
Moorfields Eye Hospital
University of Oxford
City Rd, London, UK

Arun D. Singh
Cole Eye Institute
Cleveland Clinic
Cleveland, OH, USA

ISBN 978-3-031-72445-9 ISBN 978-3-031-72443-5 (eBook)
https://doi.org/10.1007/978-3-031-72443-5

© The Editor(s) (if applicable) and The Author(s), under exclusive license to Springer Nature Switzerland AG 2019, 2024
This work is subject to copyright. All rights are solely and exclusively licensed by the Publisher, whether the whole or part of the material is concerned, specifically the rights of translation, reprinting, reuse of illustrations, recitation, broadcasting, reproduction on microfilms or in any other physical way, and transmission or information storage and retrieval, electronic adaptation, computer software, or by similar or dissimilar methodology now known or hereafter developed.
The use of general descriptive names, registered names, trademarks, service marks, etc. in this publication does not imply, even in the absence of a specific statement, that such names are exempt from the relevant protective laws and regulations and therefore free for general use.
The publisher, the authors and the editors are safe to assume that the advice and information in this book are believed to be true and accurate at the date of publication. Neither the publisher nor the authors or the editors give a warranty, expressed or implied, with respect to the material contained herein or for any errors or omissions that may have been made. The publisher remains neutral with regard to jurisdictional claims in published maps and institutional affiliations.

This Springer imprint is published by the registered company Springer Nature Switzerland AG
The registered company address is: Gewerbestrasse 11, 6330 Cham, Switzerland

If disposing of this product, please recycle the paper.

Contents

Conjunctival Tumors: Examination Techniques

1

Jacob Pe'er and Shahar Frenkel

1.1 Introduction

The conjunctiva is a transparent, vascular, mucous membrane [1]. It comprises: the bulbar conjunctiva, including the corneo-conjunctival limbus, which covers the sclera in the anterior part of the eyeball; the superior, inferior, and lateral conjunctival fornices; the palpebral conjunctiva, which covers the posterior surface of the upper and lower eyelids and which extends to the mucocutaneous junction at the eyelid margin; the plica semilunaris; and the caruncle.

Conjunctival and corneo-conjunctival tumors are usually detected and diagnosed at a relatively early stage. Because these tumors tend to have characteristic clinical features, the correct diagnosis can usually be made by slit-lamp examination performed by an experienced ophthalmologist.

1.2 External Examination

Inspection (under good light conditions) should include the face as well as the eyes, comparing both sides to detect conditions such as anisocoria, iris heterochromia, and nevus of Ota. When malignancy is suspected, it is important to palpate the preauricular (parotid), retro-auricular, and submandibular areas for enlarged lymph nodes to detect any regional metastases.

J. Pe'er (✉) · S. Frenkel
Ocular Oncology Service and Ophthalmic Pathology Laboratory, Department of Ophthalmology, Hadassah—Hebrew University Medical Center, Jerusalem, Israel
e-mail: peer@hadassah.org.il

1.3 Slit-Lamp Examination and Photography

It is essential to examine the entire conjunctiva, including the upper and lower fornices, the palpebral conjunctiva, the plica semilunaris, and the caruncle. The superior fornix can be visualized by double eversion, using a Desmarres retractor, or by gently pinching the skin of the upper eyelid and pulling the eyelid away from the globe while inspecting the fornix with a loupe or 20D lens. The bulbar conjunctiva can be gently pushed sideways with a cotton-tipped applicator to determine whether it moves freely or whether it is tethered to the sclera as a result of fibrosis or scleral invasion by a tumor.

The tumor should be described according to the location of anterior and posterior margins (e.g., cornea to bulbar conjunctiva), circumferential spread (e.g., 5–20 clock minutes), thickness, pigmentation, internal features (e.g., vascularity, clear cysts), surface features (e.g., leukoplakia, ulceration), and secondary effects (e.g., feeder vessels). The location and extent of the conjunctival and corneal involvement by any tumor should be accurately defined by slit-lamp examination, with respect both to nodular and flat components of the disease. This is particularly important if surgery is planned since it may be difficult to evaluate conjunctival lesions under the diffuse lighting of an operating microscope. Documentation of tumor dimensions and extent is important also for staging according to the AJCC TNM staging system, which is based on the tumor's size (in the case of squamous tumors), circumferential extent, and involvement of non-bulbar structures (i.e., plica, caruncle, globe, eyelid, orbit, and sinuses).

Fluorescein, rose bengal, and lissamine green stains can be used to define abnormal epithelium and tumor margins, especially with diffuse lesions. Rose bengal and lissamine green have similar staining patterns, and the latter is better tolerated by patients [2]. Toluidine blue drops provide a stippled stain with most pre-malignant and all malignant conjunctival epithelial lesions at 1–0.05% concentrations with a high sensitivity but moderate specificity [3, 4]. The lesion

© The Author(s), under exclusive license to Springer Nature Switzerland AG 2024
J. Pe'er et al. (eds.), *Clinical Ophthalmic Oncology*, https://doi.org/10.1007/978-3-031-72443-5_1

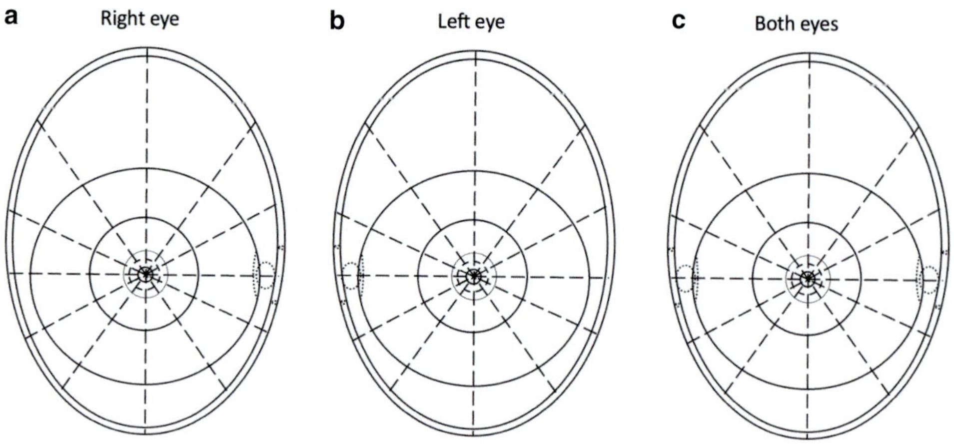

Fig. 1.1 A system for clinically mapping conjunctival tumor location and extent. Right eye (**a**), left eye (**b**), and for both eyes (**c**). Courtesy Prof. Bertil Damato, London, UK

should be drawn. Photography is useful for documenting the clinical features and extent. A system for clinically mapping conjunctival tumor location and extent has been described for staging purposes (Fig. 1.1) [5].

Assessment of patients for iatrogenic ocular morbidity caused by radiotherapy, topical chemotherapy, and/or surgical tumor excision should include history taking, tear-film breakup time, corneal staining, tear film meniscus, Schirmer test, corneal esthesiomtery, and assessment of meibomian gland function by identifying blockage of meibomian gland orifices; documenting any lid margin irregularity, vascular engorgement, and mucocutaneous junction abnormality, as well as meibomian quality in terms of viscosity and quality. Some also perform infrared meibography, which reveals more about the structure of the meibomian glands than slit-lamp examination alone.

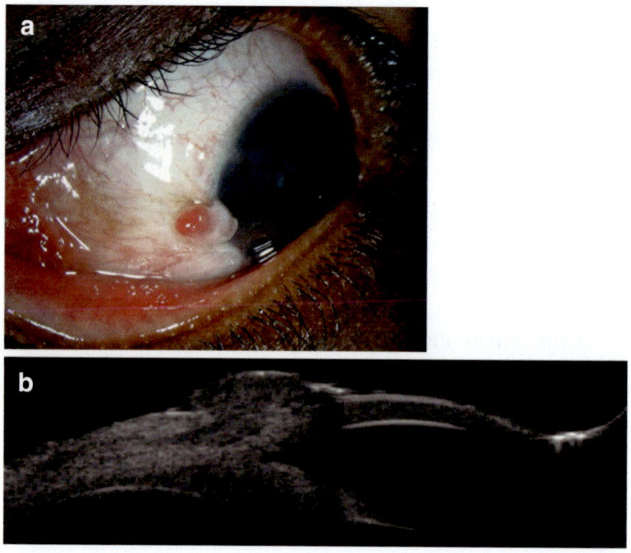

Fig. 1.2 Recurrent amelanotic melanoma. Clinical photograph (**a**). UBM showing partial thickness scleral extension (**b**)

1.4 Ancillary Studies

Anterior-segment imaging with high-frequency ultrasonography [25–80 MHz, also known as ultrasound biomicroscopy (UBM)], anterior-segment OCT, and confocal microscopy can be useful for measuring tumor thickness, evaluating invasion of adjacent structures and perhaps aiding diagnosis.

1.4.1 Ultrasound Biomicroscopy

Conjunctival lesions can be assessed by high-frequency ultrasonography to determine the tumor thickness and its extension into the sclera and cornea or, rarely, intraocularly [6–9] (Fig. 1.2). Low-frequency (10–20 MHz), posterior segment ultrasonography may define advanced intraocular and/or orbital invasion.

1.4.2 Anterior-Segment OCT

Superficial, amelanotic, conjunctival, and corneal tumors can be readily identified with high-resolution, anterior-segment OCT (AS-OCT), which can provide useful information about the tumors' size, extension, shape, and internal features [10–15]. Preliminary observations suggest that OCT findings may even assist in differentiating ocular surface squamous neoplasia (Fig. 1.3) from pingueculum (Fig. 1.4) and pterygium (Fig. 1.5). A recent study found that AS-OCT defines tumor margins similarly to toluidine blue staining [16]. The use of AS-OCT has been found useful also with stromal conjunctival tumors [17]. In recent years, AS-OCT angiography has been used to display the vascularity of conjunctival lesions and differentiate benign from malignant tumors [18–20].

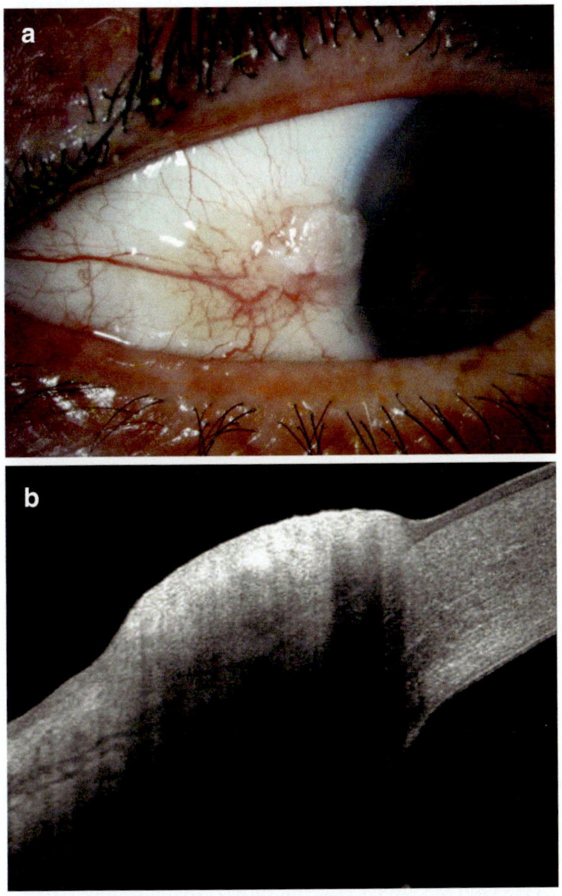

Fig. 1.3 Conjunctival intraepithelial neoplasia. Clinical photograph (**a**) and optical coherence tomography (**b**). Note a hyper-reflective and thickened epithelium with an abrupt transition zone from abnormal to normal epithelium, consistent with ocular surface squamous neoplasia

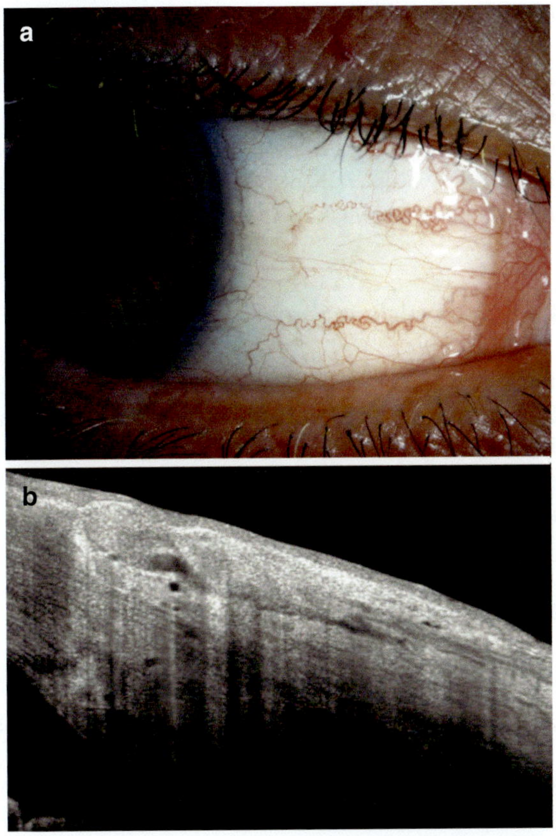

Fig. 1.4 Pinguecula. Clinical photograph (**a**) and optical coherence tomography (**b**). Note a normal surface epithelium with underlying hyper-reflective, subepithelial mass, consistent with pinguecula

Fig. 1.5 Pterygium. Clinical photograph (**a**) and optical coherence tomography (**b**). Note a normal surface epithelium with underlying hyper-reflective, subepithelial mass

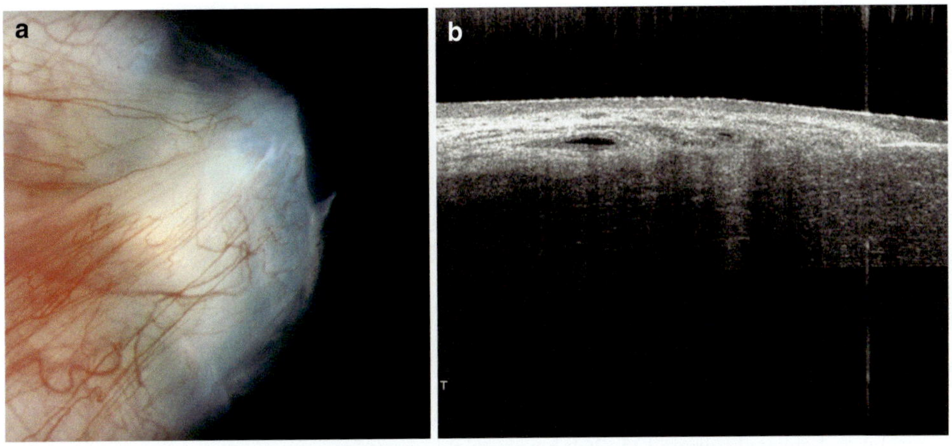

1.4.3 Confocal Microscopy

In vivo confocal microscopy can be a useful tool for structural and cellular analysis of nonpigmented and pigmented conjunctival and corneal tumors. It is a noninvasive technique for in vivo assessment of tissue features and shows good correlation with histological findings [12, 21–24].

1.4.4 Systemic Imaging

Other imaging methods, such as computed tomography (CT), magnetic resonance imaging (MRI), and positron emission tomography /CT (PET-CT), may be necessary to assess extensive local invasion, including orbital involvement, nodal disease, and systemic spread.

1.4.5 Biopsy

Histopathological examination provides a definitive diagnosis of conjunctival and corneal tumors. Nevertheless, benign, asymptomatic tumors, such as nevi with cysts, are often managed by observation, so that biopsy is performed only if there is evidence of tumor growth or malignant change. If a small tumor does require biopsy, it is preferable to completely excise the lesion, using a no-touch technique, to avoid seeding of tumor cells if the tumor proves to be malignant. When complete excision of a diffuse lesion (e.g., primary acquired melanosis) may cause severe morbidity or when it is impossible to perform such extensive surgery, it may be appropriate to perform an incisional biopsy, sampling the tumor by wedge biopsy or punch biopsy. Such biopsy is also appropriate with tumors that are preferably treated by methods other than excision (e.g., radiotherapy, cryotherapy, and topical chemotherapy).

There are two main surgical approaches for excisional biopsies. With the no-touch technique, the tumor is excised with wide (3 mm) margins, and cryotherapy is applied to the surgical bed and margins. With the "adjuvant approach," excision is performed with minimal (0.5 mm) safety margins and, once the surgical wound has healed, adjuvant treatment is administered, consisting of topical chemotherapy or immunotherapy, or radiotherapy (e.g., plaque brachytherapy).

Exfoliative cytology has been used for diagnosing conjunctival and corneal tumors [25, 26]; however, this samples only the superficial layers of the lesion and does reveal whether the tumor is invasive. This is important for management planning. With diffuse tumors, such as sebaceous adenocarcinomas, conjunctival map biopsies may be performed to determine the extent of the disease [27, 28].

Immunohistochemistry is routine when examining conjunctival tumor biopsies. Advanced techniques such as fluorescence in situ hybridization (FISH) and ex vivo fluorescence confocal microscopy have also been used [29, 30]. Investigation may now include genetic tests, such as analysis of multiple DNA copy number alterations, genome-wide analysis, microRNA expression profile, and whole-exome profiling [31–34].

Sentinel lymph node biopsy (SLNB) is performed in some ophthalmic oncology centers, especially in patients with conjunctival melanoma. This procedure is safe, with minimal morbidity; however, the relation between SLNB and patient survival and tumor recurrence requires further investigation (Volume 2, Chap. 12) [35–37].

References

1. Pepperl JE, Ghuman T, Gill KS, et al. Conjunctiva. In: Tasman W, Jaeger EA, Duane's Foundations of Clinical Ophthalmology, editors. Ocular anatomy, embryology and teratology, vol. 1. Philadelphia: Lippincott Williams & Wilkins; 2004. p. 1–30.
2. Machado LM, Castro RS, Fontes BM. Staining patterns in dry eye syndrome: rose Bengal versus lissamine green. Cornea. 2009;28:732–4.
3. Romero IL, Barros Jde N, Martins MC, Ballalai PL. The use of 1% toluidine blue eye drops in the diagnosis of ocular surface squamous neoplasia. Cornea. 2013;32(1):36–9.
4. Gichuhi S, Macharia E, Kabiru J, Zindamoyen AM, Rono H, Ollando E, Wanyonyi L, Wachira J, Munene R, Onyuma T, Jaoko WG, Sagoo MS, Weiss HA, Burton MJ. Toluidine blue 0.05% vital staining for the diagnosis of ocular surface squamous neoplasia in Kenya. JAMA Ophthalmol. 2015;133(11):1314–21.
5. Damato B, Coupland SE. Clinical mapping of conjunctival melanomas. Br J Opthalmol. 2008;92:1545–9.
6. Conway RM, Chew T, Golchet P, Desai K, Lin S, O'Brien J. Ultrasound biomicroscopy: role in diagnosis and management in 130 consecutive patients evaluated for anterior segment tumours. Br J Ophthalmol. 2005;89:950–5.
7. Ho VH, Prager TC, Diwan H, Prieto V, Esmaeli B. Ultrasound biomicroscopy for estimation of tumor thickness for conjunctival melanoma. J Clin Ultrasound. 2007;35:533–7.
8. Bianciotto C, Shields CL, Guzman JM, et al. Assessment of anterior segment tumors with ultrasound biomicroscopy versus anterior segment optical coherence tomography in 200 cases. Ophthalmology. 2011;118:1297–302.
9. Lauwers N, Janssens K, Mertens M, et al. Anterior segment optical coherent tomography and ultrasound biomicroscopy for measuring thickness of corneal and bulbar conjunctival tumours. Br J Ophthalmol. 2022;106:760–4.
10. Kieval JZ, Karp CL, Abou Shousha M, et al. Ultra-high resolution optical coherence tomography for differentiation of ocular surface squamous neoplasia and pterygia. Ophthalmology. 2012;119(3):481–6.
11. Thomas BJ, Galor A, Nanji AA, et al. Ultra high-resolution anterior segment optical coherence tomography in the diagnosis and management of ocular surface squamous neoplasia. Ocul Surf. 2014;12:46–58.
12. Janssens K, Mertens M, Lauwers N, de Keizer RJ, Mathysen DG, De Groot V. To study and determine the role of anterior segment optical coherence tomography and ultrasound biomicroscopy in corneal and conjunctival tumors. J Opthalmol. 2016;2016:1048760.

13. Karp CL, Mercado C, Venkateswaran N, et al. Use of high-resolution optical coherent tomography in the surgical management of ocular surface squamous neoplasia: a pilot study. Am J Ophthalmol. 2019;206:17–31.
14. Stevens SM, Reyes-Capo DP, Patel U, et al. Clinical and optical coherence tomography comparison between ocular surface squamous neoplasia and squamous metaplasia. Cornea. 2023;42:429–34.
15. Aboumourad AJ, Galor A, Karp CL. Case series: high-resolution optical coherence tomography as an optical biopsy in ocular surface squamous neoplasia. Optom Vis Sci. 2021;98:450–5.
16. Ferraz FB, Castelo Branco AMP, da Cruz LGI, Fernandes BF, Morales MC, Neto RB. Fernandes AG toluidine blue 1% eye drop versus optical coherence tomography for margin delimitation of ocular surface squamous neoplasia. Eur J Ophthalmol. 2023;34:859.
17. Das J, Basak SK, Das N. Conjunctival stromal tumour (COST): anterior OCT findings. BMJ Case Rep. 2019;21:12.
18. Nampei K, Oie Y, Kiritoshi S, et al. Comparison of ocular surface squamous neoplasia and pterygium using anterior segment optical coherence tomography angiography. Am J Ophthalmol Case Rep. 2020;20:100902.
19. Brouwer NJ, Marinkovic M, Bleeker JC, et al. Anterior segment OCTA of melanocytic lesions of the conjunctiva and iris. Am J Ophthalmol. 2021;222:137–47.
20. Theotoka D, Liu Z, Wall S, et al. Optical coherence tomography angiography in the evaluation of vascular patterns of ocular surface squamour neoplasia during topical medical treatment. Ocul Surf. 2022;25:8–18.
21. Messmer EM, Mackert MJ, Zapp DM, Kampik A. In vivo confocal microscopy of pigmented conjunctival tumors. Graefes Arch Clin Exp Ophthalmol. 2006;244:1437–45.
22. Alomar TS, Nubile M, Lowe J, Dua HS. Corneal intraepithelial neoplasia: in vivo confocal microscopic study with histopathologic correlation. Am J Opthalmol. 2011;151:238–47.
23. Xu Y, Zhou Z, Xu Y, Wang M, Liu F, Qu H, Hong J. The clinical value of in vivo confocal microscopy for diagnosis of ocular surface squamous neoplasia. Eye (Lond). 2012;26(6):781–7.
24. Cinotti E, Singer A, Labeille B, et al. Handheld in vivo reflectance confocal microscopy for the diagnosis of eyelid margin and conjunctival tumors. JAMA Opthalmol. 2017;135:845–51.
25. Semenova EA, Milman T, Finger PT, Natesh S, Kurli M, Schneider S, Iacob CE, McCormick SA. The diagnostic value of exfoliative cytology vs histopathology for ocular surface squamous neoplasia. Am J Ophthalmol. 2009;148(5):772–8.
26. Kayat KV, Correa Dantas PE, Felberg S, Galvão MA, Saieg MA. Exfoliative cytology in the diagnosis of ocular surface squamous neoplasms. Cornea. 2017;36:127–30.
27. Putterman AM. Conjunctival map biopsy to determine pagetoid spread. Am J Ophthalmol. 1986;102:87–90.
28. McConnell LK, Syed NA, Zimmerman MB, et al. An analysis of conjunctival map biopsies in sebaceous carcinoma. Ophthalmic Plast Reconstr Surg. 2017;33:17–21.
29. Mudhar HS, Smith K, Talley P, Whitworth A, Atkey N, Rennie IG. Fluorescence in situ hybridisation (FISH) in histologically challenging conjunctival melanocytic lesions. Br J Ophthalmol. 2013;97:40–6.
30. Iovieno A, Longo C, De Luca M, Piana S, Fontana L, Ragazzi M. Fluorescence confocal microscopy for ex vivo diagnosis of conjunctival tumors: a pilot study. Am J Ophthalmol. 2016;168:207–16.
31. Asnaghi L, Alkatan H, Mahale A, et al. Identification of multiple DNA copy number alterations including frequent 8p11.22 amplification in conjunctival squamous cell carcinoma. Invest Opthalmol Vis Sci. 2014;55:8604–13.
32. Takahashi H, Usui Y, Ueda S, et al. Genome-wide analysis of ocular adnexal lymphoproliferative disorders using high-resolution single nucleotide polymorphism Array. Invest Opthalmol Vis Sci. 2015;56:4156–65.
33. Larsen AC, Mikkelsen LH, Borup R, et al. MicroRNA expression profile in conjunctival melanoma. Invest Ophthalmol Vis Sci. 2016;57:4205–12.
34. Galor A, Karp CL, Sant D, et al. Whole exome profiling of ocular surface squamous neoplasia. Ophthalmology. 2016;123:216–7.
35. Maalouf TJ, Dolivet G, Angioi KS, Leroux A, Genin P, George JL. Sentinel lymph node biopsy in patients with conjunctival and eyelid cancers: experience in 17 patients. Ophthal Plast Reconst Surg. 2012;28:30–4.
36. Cohen VM, Tsimpida M, Hungerford JL, Jan H, Cerio R, Moir G. Prospective study of sentinel lymph node biopsy for conjunctival melanoma. Br J Ophthalmol. 2013;97:1525–9.
37. Pfeiffer ML, Ozgur OK, Myers JN, et al. Sentinel lymph node biopsy for ocular adnexal melanoma. Acta Ophthalmol. 2017;95:e323–8.

Conjunctival Tumors: Classification and Differential Diagnosis

2

Jacob Pe'er and Shahar Frenkel

2.1 Introduction

Many different types of tumors can arise in the conjunctiva, which is composed of a wide variety of cells that form the epithelium and the substantia propria. The bulbar conjunctiva that lies within the palpebral fissure is exposed to sunlight, which may be a factor in the development of some of the tumors. The entire conjunctiva may be affected by a wide variety of chemical, physical, and biological insults that may influence the development of some of the tumors. Most of the conjunctival and corneal tumors are detected early because they are readily visible.

Epithelial nonmelanocytic and melanocytic tumors of the cornea are very rare and are usually the result of involvement of the cornea in conjunctival tumors. Corneal stromal tumors are almost nonexistent.

The conjunctiva may be invaded by tumors from its surrounding structures—the eyeball, eyelid, and orbit—and may develop metastases from distant organs.

2.2 Anatomical Features

2.2.1 Epithelium

The conjunctival epithelium extends from the limbus, where it is continuous with the corneal epithelium, to the mucocutaneous junction, where it is continuous with the eyelid skin epidermis. It is a non-keratinized stratified squamous epithelium. The epithelial cells are stratified columnar in the fornix and tend to be cuboidal elsewhere. Goblet cells are present in the middle and superficial layers of the epithelium and most numerous in the lower fornix and close to the plica semilunaris, being almost completely absent in the limbal areas. Melanocytes are scattered in the basal layer of the epithelium.

2.2.2 Stroma

The conjunctival stroma is composed of fibrovascular connective tissue that is thicker in the fornix and thinner over the globe and the posterior surface of the eyelids. It contains collagenous and elastic tissue; vessels including arteries, veins, and lymphatics; nerves; and accessory lacrimal glands of Krause and Wolfring. Like other mucous membranes, the conjunctiva contains associated lymphoid tissue. Numerous lymphocytes, plasma cells, mast cells, and neutrophils are present in the conjunctival stroma. Lymphocytes may be aggregated into nodules but without the formation of follicles.

2.2.3 Specialized Regions

2.2.3.1 Plica Semilunaris

The plica semilunaris is a vertical fold of conjunctiva lying lateral to the caruncle. There are 8–10 layers of epithelial cells containing many goblet cells. The loose, highly vascular stroma may have some nonstriated muscle fibers supplied by sympathetic nerves and may contain fatty tissue. This tissue resembles the third (horizontal) transparent eyelids in some animals to allow wetting of the ocular surface while maintaining vision.

2.2.3.2 Caruncle

The caruncle is a fleshy prominence located in the medial canthus. It contains both conjunctival and cutaneous structures. It is covered by nonkeratinized stratified squamous epithelium with many goblet cells and contains hair, fat, and glands: sebaceous, sweat, and accessory lacrimal glands. Its blood and nerve supplies are abundant. Tumors of the caruncle can be of both mucosal and cutaneous origin.

J. Pe'er (✉) · S. Frenkel
Ocular Oncology Service and Ophthalmic Pathology Laboratory, Department of Ophthalmology, Hadassah—Hebrew University Medical Center, Jerusalem, Israel
e-mail: peer@hadassah.org.il

© The Author(s), under exclusive license to Springer Nature Switzerland AG 2024
J. Pe'er et al. (eds.), *Clinical Ophthalmic Oncology*, https://doi.org/10.1007/978-3-031-72443-5_2

2.3 Classification of Conjunctival and Corneal Tumors

The classification of conjunctival tumors, like tumors of other parts of the body, is made according to two major lines: the tissue or cell of origin of the tumor and its being benign or malignant. In groups of tumors, there may be subtypes of tumors that, due to special histological structures, features, and location of the tumor cells, can appear or behave differently despite being of the same cell of origin.

Most conjunctival tumors are of epithelial and melanocytic origin. The remainders arise from various elements of the conjunctival stroma and include vascular, fibrous, neural, histiocytic, myogenic, myxoid, lipomatous, and lymphoproliferative tumors. Three unique groups of conjunctival tumors are developmental (hamartomas and choristomas), caruncular, and metastatic and secondary tumors.

The classification of conjunctival and corneal tumors that appear in this section is based primarily on the second edition of the World Health Organization (WHO) International Histological Classification of Tumors, in its volume on histological typing of tumors of the eye and its adnexa [1]. Since this classification does not include all conjunctival tumors, the list has been completed by using some other major series of conjunctival and corneal tumors [2–4]. The following list of tumors (Tables 2.1, 2.2, and 2.3) includes both common and rare, sometimes very rare, tumors so as to familiarize the reader with the current terminology.

Table 2.1 Major types of conjunctival tumor

Epithelial	Nonmelanocytic
	Melanocytic
Stromal	Vascular
	Neural
	Myxoid
	Lipomatous
	Melanocytic
	Fibrous tissue
	Histiocytic
	Myogenic
	Lymphoproliferative
Congenital	Hamartoma
	Choristoma
Caruncular	
Metastatic	
Secondary	
Simulating lesions	

Table 2.2 Classification of epidermal tumors of the conjunctiva

Types		Subtypes
Nonmelanocytic	Benign	Squamous papilloma
		Keratotic plaque
		Keratoacanthoma
		Reactive hyperplasia (pseudoepitheliomatous hyperplasia)
		Inverted follicular keratosis
		Hereditary intraepithelial dyskeratosis
		Oncocytoma
		Dacryoadenoma
		Epithelial cysts
	Premalignant and malignant	Actinic (solar) keratosis
		Conjunctival intraepithelial neoplasia (CIN)
		Xeroderma pigmentosum
		Squamous cell carcinoma
		Mucoepidermoid carcinoma
		Spindle cell carcinoma
		Sebaceous gland carcinoma (pagetoid spread)
		Basal cell carcinoma
Melanocytic	Benign	Junctional nevus
		Compound nevus
		Spitz nevus
		Blue nevus
		PAM without atypia
		Congenital melanosis
		Complexion melanosis
	Premalignant and malignant	PAM with atypia
		Melanoma arising from nevi
		Melanoma arising in PAM
		Melanoma arising de novo

Table 2.3 Classification of stromal tumors of the conjunctiva

Types	Subtypes
Vascular	Pyogenic granuloma
	Capillary hemangioma
	Varix
	Hemangiopericytoma
	Kaposi's sarcoma
	Malignant hemangioendothelioma
	Cavernous hemangioma
	Racemose malformation
	Lymphangiectasia
	Lymphangioma
	Nodular fasciitis
Fibrous	Benign fibrous histiocytoma
	Fibroma
	Malignant fibrous histiocytoma
Neural	Neurofibroma (localized)
	Schwannoma (neurilemmoma)
	Neurofibroma (diffuse)
	Granular cell tumor
Histiocytic	Xanthoma
	Reticulohistiocytoma
	Juvenile xanthogranuloma
Myxoid	Myxoma
Myogenic	Rhabdomyosarcoma
Lipomatous	Lipoma
	Liposarcoma
	Herniated orbital fat
Lymphoproliferative	Benign reactive lymphoid hyperplasia
	Leukemic infiltrates
	Lymphoma

2.4 Differential Diagnosis

Most conjunctival tumors are benign; malignant tumors are relatively rare. When considering the differential diagnosis, it is important to take into account the patient's general health as well as the clinical features of the lesion. The more important diagnostic clues are the color of the lesion (i.e., pigmented, nonpigmented, red, pink, blue, white, or yellow); consistency (i.e., hard, soft, rubbery, gelatinous); solid or cystic nature; size; number (i.e., solitary or multiple); surface (i.e., smooth, irregular, granular, papillary, ulcerated or umbilicated, with or without keratin); shape (i.e., flat or raised, pedunculated, papillary); thickness; location (i.e., bulbar, palpebral, forniceal, caruncular); layer (i.e., epithelial or stromal); growth rate; and adherence to underlying structures, such as the sclera. Other diagnostic clues include the patient's race, age, and sex; as well as any present or previous systemic diseases, such as metabolic disease or malignancy, particularly in adjacent tissues (e.g., lacrimal drainage system, eyelids, globe, orbit).

2.4.1 Epithelial

Epithelial tumors are usually classified into melanocytic and nonmelanocytic tumors based on the clinical presence or absence of brown-black pigmentation and histological evidence of melanocytes. However, nonmelanocytic tumors (e.g., squamous cell carcinoma) can rarely also be pigmented.

2.4.1.1 Melanocytic Lesions

Melanocytic lesions include nevi, primary acquired melanosis (PAM) without or with atypia, and melanomas. While melanosis is purely epithelial, nevi and melanomas also involve the stroma. While bulbar conjunctival melanosis is movable with the conjunctiva, scleral melanocytosis is not. Melanoma, may be fixed to the underlying sclera. Staging of conjunctival melanoma can be found in the *AJCC Cancer Staging Manual* [5].

2.4.1.2 Nonmelanocytic Lesions

Nonmelanocytic lesions are usually epithelial. Epithelial tumors, such as papilloma and carcinoma, usually have irregular, granular, or papillary surfaces, and may be leukoplakic (because they are covered by keratin). Sometimes, they may be gelatinous in appearance. They may be superficial and thin or thick and fleshy. Conjunctival carcinoma can invade the orbit, eyelid, and the globe. The staging of conjunctival carcinoma can be found in the *AJCC Cancer Staging Manual* [6].

2.4.2 Stromal Tumors

Stromal tumors, including secondary tumors and metastasis, have a smooth surface due to their location under the conjunctival surface. The color of the tumor can be very helpful in the diagnosis. Most vascular tumors are red, pink, or sometimes blue. Fibrous tumors are white but may be pink. Neural, histiocytic, and lipomatous tumors are yellow, and lymphoid tumors and leukemic infiltrates are pink, similar to smoked salmon, and thus are termed "salmon patch" (see Chaps. 8 and 9).

2.4.3 Congenital Tumors

Congenital tumors diagnosed in infancy and childhood are usually hamartomatous or choristomatous lesions (see Chap. 11).

2.4.4 Caruncular Tumors

Caruncular tumors present a special challenge of differential diagnosis of both conjunctival and cutaneous tumors (see Chap. 10).

2.4.5 Metastatic and Secondary Tumors

In the case of metastatic tumors, there is usually a history of primary malignancy elsewhere in the body. In secondary involvement of the conjunctiva by tumors in surrounding structures, the primary tumor is usually well known, except for many cases of pagetoid spread of sebaceous gland carcinoma of the eyelid in which the presentation of the malignancy can be in the conjunctiva. An important secondary tumor is extraocular extension of uveal melanoma.

2.4.6 Simulating Lesions

It is interesting to note that the WHO histological classification of conjunctival tumors includes lesions that simulate tumors such as pinguecula and pterygium. These most common conjunctival lesions are not real neoplasms but sometimes can be confused with real tumors when they are covered by a keratin plaque or have a gelatinous appearance. Keloid is also included in this classification. Among conditions that may simulate pigmented conjunctival tumors, we have to consider drug and metallic deposits, mascara deposits, foreign body, post-inflammatory melanosis, and systemic conditions with flat pigmentary patches, such as in Addison's disease [7]. Inflammatory and infectious lesions such as lepromatous and sarcoidal nodules and, more commonly, allergic and granulomatous nodules should be included in the differential diagnosis of conjunctival tumors.

References

1. Campbell RJ, Sobin LH. Tumors of the conjunctiva and caruncle. In: World Health Organization International Histological Classification of Tumours, editor. Histological typing of tumours of the eye and its adnexa. 2nd ed. Berlin: Springer; 1998. p. 9–15.
2. Shields CL, Shields JA. Tumors of the conjunctiva and cornea. Surv Ophthalmol. 2004;49:3–24.
3. Grossniklaus HE, Green WR, Luckenbach M, Chan CC. Conjunctival lesions in adults. A clinical and histopathologic review. Cornea. 1987;6:78–116.
4. Elsas FJ, Green WR. Epibulbar tumors in childhood. Am J Ophthalmol. 1975;79:1001–7.
5. Conway RM, Graue GF, Pelayes D, et al. Conjunctival carcinoma. In: Amin MB, et al., editors. AJCC cancer staging manual. 8th ed. Cham: Springer; 2017. p. 787–93.
6. Coupland SE, Barnhill R, Rm C, et al. Conjunctival melanoma. In: Amin MB, et al., editors. AJCC cancer staging manual. 8th ed. Cham: Springer; 2017. p. 795–803.
7. Folberg R, Jakobiec FA, Bernardino VB, Iwamoto T. Benign conjunctival melanocytic lesions. Clinicopathologic features. Ophthalmology. 1989;96:436–501.

Conjunctival Tumors: Benign Epithelial Tumors

3

Maya Eiger-Moscovich, Shahar Frenkel, and Jacob Pe'er

3.1 Introduction

Abnormal cellular proliferation and differentiation that is confined to the conjunctival epithelium may cause thickening (acanthosis), papillary or nodular focal elevation of the conjunctiva, and sometimes white, plaque-like opacification (leukoplakia). Such lesions rarely progress to malignancy.

3.1.1 Squamous Papilloma

Conjunctival squamous papilloma is an acquired benign and common epithelial tumor that can be seen at almost any age, although it more commonly occurs in children and young adults [1–4]. More males than females develop conjunctival papilloma [4]. Conjunctival squamous papillomas are often located in the inferior fornix or bulbar conjunctiva but may appear in any part of the conjunctiva, including the palpebral conjunctiva, lid margin, caruncle, and plica semilunaris. According to one study, most of the papillomas are located medially and inferiorly, which is explained by the direction of the tear flow [4]. Although it is a benign tumor, which tends to progress slowly, papillomas can grow significantly [5]. Many papillomas recur, more with multiple lesions and less with cryotherapy treatment [6], and some undergo malignant transformation, more in elderly patients and in lesions that demonstrate corneal limbus or corneal involvement [6]. In one study, a recurrence after surgical excision was associated with epithelial atypia [7].

3.1.1.1 Clinical Features

Childhood Papilloma

In children, the papillomas have been documented to be associated with human papilloma virus (HPV) (mostly types 6, 11, and 16) infection of the conjunctiva, which might be transmitted from the mother's vagina to a newborn's conjunctiva while passing in the birth canal [8]. The papilloma appears as sessile or pedunculated pink/red fleshy fronds of tissue or finger-like projections with an irregular surface that sometimes resembles a cauliflower (Fig. 3.1a). They are often asymptomatic, without associated inflammatory reactions. However, large and more pedunculated lesions are usually symptomatic and may cause foreign body sensation, mucous secretion, hemorrhagic tears, incomplete eyelid closure, and poor cosmetic appearance. They are usually solitary but can be bilateral and multiple and may become confluent.

Adulthood Papilloma

In adults, conjunctival squamous papilloma usually appears as a single and unilateral lesion, commonly arising close to the limbal area or bulbar conjunctiva. They are usually flat with a broad base, may be large and cover a large area of the conjunctiva, and may cover the cornea and interfere with vision. Papillomas should be freely mobile over the sclera, with the body of the papilloma forming a mushroom shape over a pedicle attached to the conjunctiva [9].

Sometimes, it may be difficult to differentiate them clinically from squamous cell carcinoma, and anterior-segment OCT can help make the correct diagnosis. According to one study, papilloma presented in anterior-segment OCT with an overhanging edge on the top of an underlying normal epithelium. Corrugated epithelial surface, intrinsic spaces, and posterior shadowing are other features more common in papilloma compared to ocular surface squamous neoplasia [10].

M. Eiger-Moscovich · S. Frenkel · J. Pe'er (✉)
Ocular Oncology Service and Ophthalmic Pathology Laboratory, Department of Ophthalmology, Hadassah—Hebrew University Medical Center, Jerusalem, Israel
e-mail: peer@hadassah.org.il

© The Author(s), under exclusive license to Springer Nature Switzerland AG 2024
J. Pe'er et al. (eds.), *Clinical Ophthalmic Oncology*, https://doi.org/10.1007/978-3-031-72443-5_3

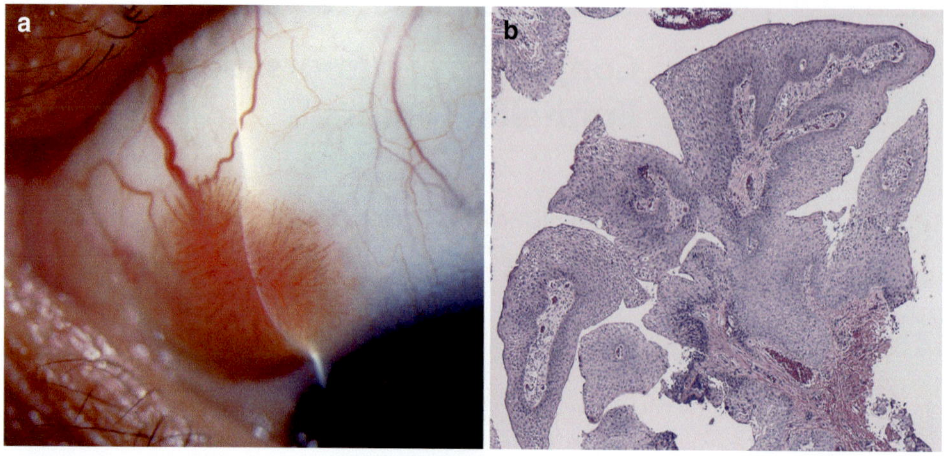

Fig. 3.1 Solitary sessile squamous papilloma of the bulbar conjunctiva. (**a**) Clinical appearance. (**b**) Histopathology shows papillomatous fronds of acanthotic nonkeratinized squamous epithelium with central fibrovascular cores (hematoxylin and eosin, original magnification ×4)

3.1.1.2 Histopathological Features

Histologically, the squamous papilloma of childhood is composed of epithelial projections covered by nonkeratinized acanthotic stratified squamous epithelium, which may have goblet cells, and a fibrovascular core in which acute and chronic inflammatory cells are often found (Fig. 3.1b). The basement membrane is always intact. Various types of HPV, the most common are HPV-6 and HPV-11, have been demonstrated in these papillomas by various immunohistochemical and molecular techniques [11–13]. In one study, low-risk HPV types were detected in 83% of conjunctival papillomas by RNA or DNA probes, more in lesions that demonstrated reactive atypia and dysplasia [14]. Some clinical and histopathological features, such as extralimbal location and the presence of goblet cells, were more frequently associated with HPV infection [13].

In adults, the squamous papilloma usually has a broader base, and its acanthotic epithelium may show varying degrees of epithelial pleomorphism, and even dysplasia can occur, albeit generally mild. Although the lesions are usually nonkeratinized, moderate keratinization may be present. The basement membrane is typically intact.

3.1.1.3 Treatment

Small papillomas in children can be observed as there usually is a slow spontaneous resolution. However, larger papillomas should be treated by complete surgical excision, where some prefer the use of the "no-touch technique" to avoid spreading the papilloma-related virus [3]. Others find that this spread has already occurred through the tears and through hemorrhage at the time of the surgery and, therefore, do not use this technique and opt for adjuvant topical chemotherapy if needed. Cryotherapy is often used in conjunction with the "no-touch" surgical technique, either to the conjunctiva around the excised lesion or to the lesion itself that is then excised in a frozen state. Sometimes cryotherapy may be performed without excision, letting the lesion slough off the conjunctival surface later.

Conjunctival papillomas tend to recur often, usually when multiple lesions are caused by papillomavirus. Such lesions may be treated by adjuvant interferon alpha-2b locally (topically and/or intralesional) [9] or systemically [15–17], topical 0.02% mitomycin C [18], or topical 5-fluorouracil [19]. Others have used carbon dioxide laser vaporization [20], photodynamic therapy [21], scanning laser photocoagulation [22], oral cimetidine [21, 23], subconjunctival bevacizumab [24], and even HPV vaccine (Gardasil-9 vaccine) [25, 26]. In a comparison between surgical excision (with cryotherapy and when needed with adjuvant topical interferon alpha-2b) and medical treatment with topical interferon alpha-2b or 5-fluorouracil, papilloma resolution was faster with surgical excision, but there were more recurrences (11% vs. 0, albeit not statistically significant) [19].

3.1.2 Inverted Papilloma (Inverted Follicular Keratosis)

The lesions derive their name from the propensity to invaginate inward into the underlying conjunctival substantia propria instead of growing in an exophytic manner outward like the other conjunctival papillomas. Some of the lesions may show a mixed inverted-exophytic papilloma [27].

3.1.2.1 Clinical Features

These are rare lesions that appear as solid or cystic solitary nodules in the conjunctiva, although they may present as papillary sessile lesions [27, 28]. They have been reported to appear in the limbal area, plica semilunaris, and tarsal conjunctiva.

3.1.2.2 Histopathological Features

Lobules of proliferating epithelium without keratinization or inflammation invaginate the underlying connective tissue. Mucus-producing goblet cells are scattered throughout the lesions, and mucoid material, when it exists, is found in the wall of the cyst. Lesions without goblet cells at all [7] and inverted mucoepidermoid papilloma [29] were also reported.

Unlike inverted papillomas in other sites, such as the nose, paranasal sinuses, and lacrimal sac, conjunctival inverted papillomas usually do not exhibit locally aggressive behavior, do not involve extensive segments of the conjunctival epithelium, and do not display diffuse spread or multicentricity. Therefore, it is suggested that a clear distinction is made between inverted squamous papillomas of the conjunctiva and the nasal cavity and sinuses [30]. Nevertheless, a lesion with high-risk HPV [31] and a lesion that underwent carcinomatous transformation were described [32]. Therefore, complete removal of these lesions is recommended.

3.1.3 Seborrheic Keratosis

Seborrheic keratosis of the conjunctiva is extremely rare, and only a very few case reports are found in the medical literature [33, 34]. They mostly appear as a pigmented conjunctival lesion and may be misdiagnosed clinically as conjunctival melanoma or pigmented ocular surface squamous neoplasia [35]. There can also be an inflammatory reaction [35]. The typical basaloid cell acanthosis and keratin-filled pseudocysts confirm the diagnosis.

3.1.4 Reactive Epithelial Hyperplasia (Pseudoepitheliomatous Hyperplasia and Pseudocarcinomatous Hyperplasia)

This conjunctival lesion is secondary to irritation by concurrent or preexisting stromal inflammation [1–3].

3.1.4.1 Clinical Features

It appears as an elevated leukoplakic pink lesion in the limbal area. Anterior-segment OCT shows homogeneous, low-medium reflective subepithelial lesions with smooth borders, and dot-like infiltrates, which are more hyperreflective compared to lymphoma [36].

3.1.4.2 Histopathological Features

Acanthosis, hyperkeratosis, parakeratosis, and subepithelial inflammation are observed. Mitotic figures may be present, but cytologic atypia is generally lacking. Due to the possible clinical and histological difficulty in differentiating such lesions from conjunctival squamous cell carcinoma, it should be completely excised, and additional cryotherapy, or topical adjuvant therapy with either chemotherapy (mitomycin C or 5-fluorouracil) or immunotherapy (interferon α2b or α2a) should be considered.

3.1.5 Keratoacanthoma

This is a benign conjunctival reactive inflammatory lesion that grows rapidly and then can stabilize or undergo spontaneous regression [1, 3, 37, 38]. It can simulate carcinoma.

3.1.5.1 Clinical Features

Keratoacanthoma appears as a benign, solitary, gelatinous, or leukoplakic rapidly growing nodule on the bulbar conjunctiva surrounded by dilated blood vessels [1, 3, 37, 39]. In some cases, an umbilicated center is observed (Fig. 3.2a). Malignant transformation is uncommon [40].

3.1.5.2 Histopathological Features

The lesion shows marked invasive acanthotic epithelium with keratin-filled pseudocysts, hyperkeratosis, and parakeratosis (Fig. 3.2b). Usually there is minimal cytologic atypia. In cases with a marked degree of atypia, it may be difficult to distinguish the lesion from well-differentiated squamous cell carcinoma.

3.1.5.3 Treatment

Conjunctival keratoacanthoma should be treated by complete excision, and additional topical adjuvant treatment should be considered either with cryotherapy, chemotherapy (mitomycin C or 5-fluorouracil), or immunotherapy (interferon α2b or α2a).

3.1.6 Hereditary Benign Intraepithelial Dyskeratosis (HBID)

HBID is an autosomal-dominant disorder with a high degree of penetrance occurring in descendants of an inbred isolate of European, African American, and Native American (Haliwa Indian) origin in northeastern North Carolina. HBID has been subsequently detected in other parts of the United States. Using genetic linkage analysis, the HBID gene was localized to chromosome 4 (4q35) [41].

3.1.6.1 Clinical Features

HBID is characterized by bilateral elevated fleshy plaques on the nasal or temporal perilimbal bulbar conjunctiva, with dilated conjunctival vessels around it, causing the eye to appear red [1, 3] (Fig. 3.3a). In mild cases, the patients are asymptomatic, but in severe cases, most of the bulbar conjunctiva and cornea are involved, causing corneal opacification and vascularization, leading to loss of vision. Patients may complain of foreign body sensations, photophobia, and tearing, especially in the spring. Similar lesions may occur in the buccal mucosa.

3.1.6.2 Histopathological Features

The lesions are characterized by acanthosis, prominent dyskeratosis in the surface and deep epithelium, and severe chronic inflammation in the stroma (Fig. 3.3b). The basement membrane is intact. The lesions do not have malignant potential.

3.1.6.3 Treatment

HBID usually does not require aggressive treatment. Mild cases can be treated by ocular lubricants and, if needed, by topical corticosteroids. Nevertheless, larger lesions are usually treated by local excision, and most tend to recur, and

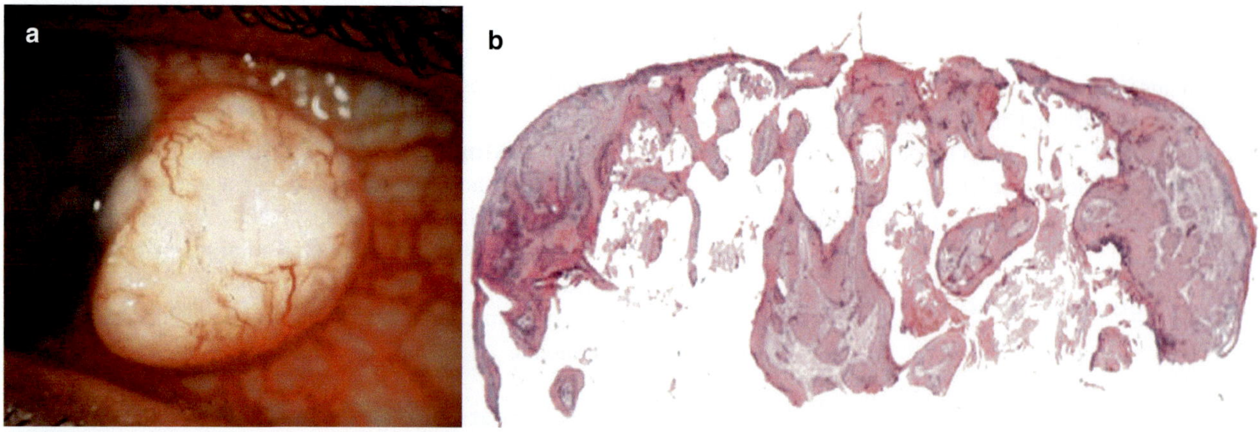

Fig. 3.2 A rapidly growing keratoacanthoma of the bulbar conjunctiva at the limbus. (**a**) Clinical appearance. (**b**) Histopathology of the lesion demonstrates squamous epithelium with invasive acanthosis and hyperkeratosis (hematoxylin and eosin, original magnification ×2). (Reprinted from Munro S, Brownstein S, Liddy B. Conjunctival keratoacanthoma. Am J Ophthalmol. 1993;116:654–5. With permission from Elsevier)

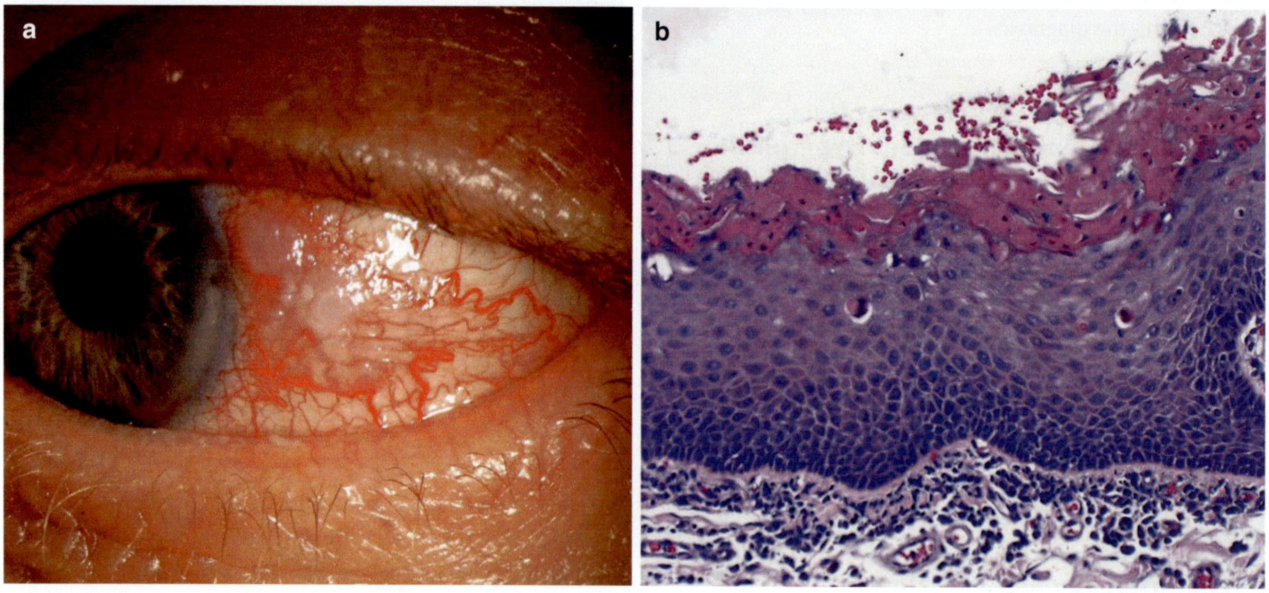

Fig. 3.3 Hereditary benign intraepithelial dyskeratosis. (**a**) A typical clinical appearance is of a white lesion of the temporal conjunctiva with dilated conjunctival vessels around it. (**b**) Histopathology showing acanthosis, hyperkeratosis, dyskeratosis, and marked chronic inflammation in the stroma beneath the intact basement membrane (hematoxylin and eosin, original magnification ×20). (Courtesy of Gordon Klintworth, MD)

can require keratectomy with mucous membrane grafting or even keratoprosthesis [42]. A case of HBID recurrence involving a Boston keratoprosthesis was described [43].

3.1.7 Lacrimal Gland Hamartoma (Dacryoadenoma)

Dacryoadenoma is a rare conjunctival tumor that occurs in children and young adults. It appears as a translucent pink lesion in the bulbar, forniceal, or palpebral conjunctiva [3]. It is uncertain whether the lesion is congenital or acquired, but it possibly originated from precursor cellular elements indigenous to the conjunctiva that grew into disorganized lacrimal gland tissue [44]. Histologically it is a benign epithelioid cell proliferation forming glandular lobules, similar to the lacrimal gland, but differs from it morphologically and immunohistochemically [44]. In one reported case, scattered myoepithelial cells were associated with acinar-type epithelium, and goblet cells were intermixed [45]. The lesions are treated by simple excision.

3.1.8 Oncocytoma

Oncocytoma, also known as oxyphilic cell adenoma, is a rather common lesion of the lacrimal gland. It often arises in the caruncle or adjacent plica semilunaris and canthal conjunctiva as a slowly growing benign yellow-tan or reddish lesion in older individuals, with higher prevalence in women [2, 46–48]. Histologically, large cells with eosinophilic granular cytoplasm are arranged in nests, cords, or sheets and may form glandular or ductal structures. Ultrastructurally, the cytoplasm is laden with mitochondria. The lesion is treated by simple excision. Rarely, the tumor may undergo malignant transformation.

3.1.9 Epithelial Cysts

Conjunctival cysts are common and may be congenital or acquired. The acquired cysts are more common and are mostly epithelial inclusion cysts that can occur spontaneously or following surgical or nonsurgical trauma [1, 3, 49] (Fig. 3.4). Other common cysts are ductal cysts, usually of accessory lacrimal gland origin (Fig. 3.5).

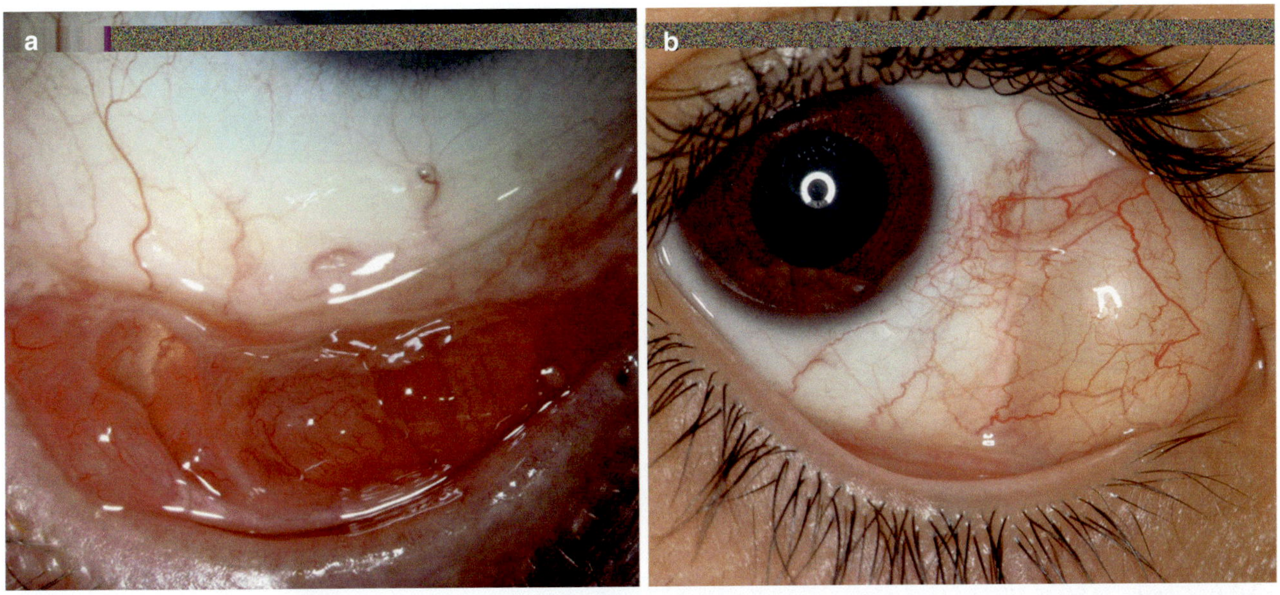

Fig. 3.4 Epithelial inclusion cyst. (**a**) Multiple cysts in the inferior fornix. (**b**) A large conjunctival cyst in the nasal bulbar conjunctiva that occurred after strabismus surgery

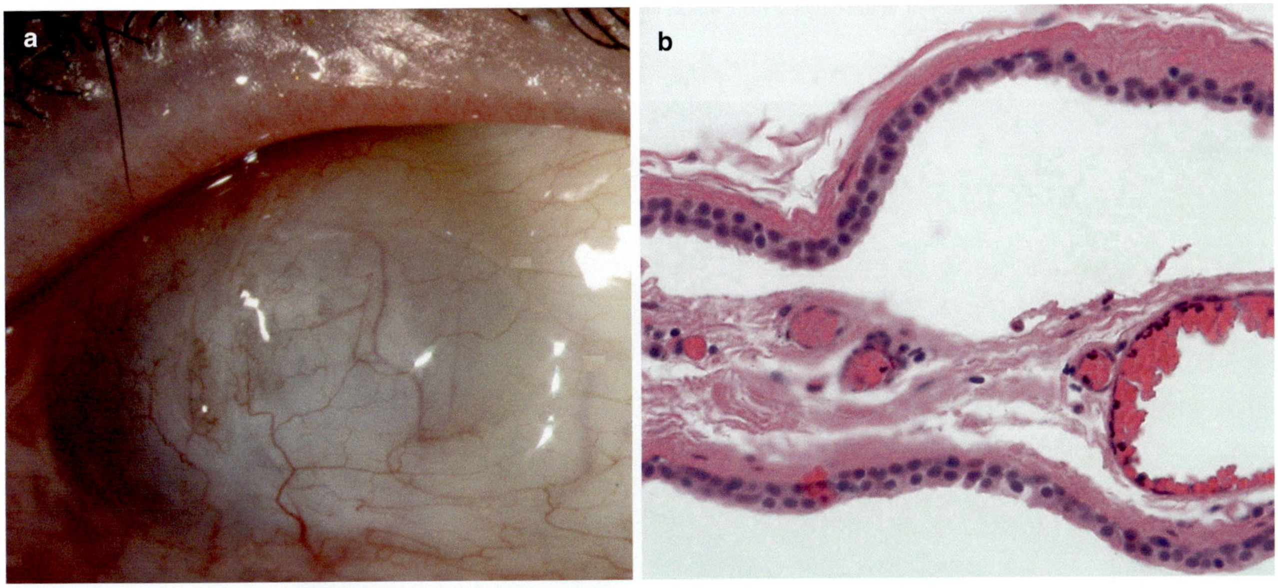

Fig. 3.5 Ductal cyst. (**a**) Bluish cyst in the temporal bulbar conjunctiva. The posterior margin of the cyst cannot be visualized. (**b**) The cyst is lined by two cell layers, with luminal cells showing apical snouts, consistent with apocrine differentiation. The double-cell lining is consistent with a ductal-type cyst, possibly from an accessory lacrimal gland. Apocrine differentiation may be metaplastic (hematoxylin and eosin stain, 40× magnification). (Reprinted with permission from Bryn Mawr Communications. Aponte EP, Schoenfield L, Stern RM, Singh AD. A ductal cyst of lacrimal origin. Adv Ocul Care. 2010:29–30)

3.1.9.1 Clinical Features

The conjunctival cyst is a smooth translucent lesion that contains clear fluid, although the fluid may be turbid (Fig. 3.6) or contain epithelial debris in the lumen that is layered like pseudohypopyon (Fig. 3.7). In dark-skinned patients, the cyst can be pigmented.

3.1.9.2 Histopathological Features

The epithelial inclusion cyst is lined by conjunctival epithelium. The lumen can be clear, or it can contain mucinous material, epithelial debris, and occasionally keratin. Ductal cysts are lined by two layers of epithelium, which is usually cuboidal in the inner layer and may contain PAS-positive material.

3.1.9.3 Treatment

The cyst can be stable and asymptomatic or can enlarge and become symptomatic, necessitating excision. In most cases, over a long-term follow-up, the cyst eventually undergoes spontaneous resolution. Successful removal of conjunctival cysts with high-frequency radio-wave electrosurgery was reported [50].

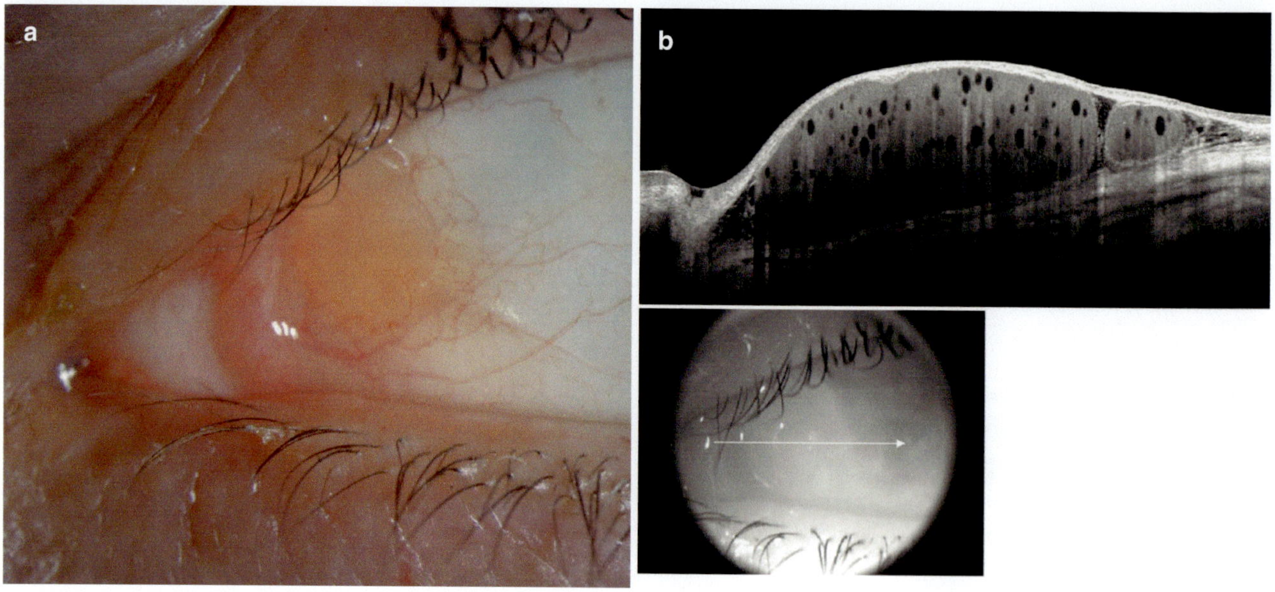

Fig. 3.6 Conjunctival epithelial cyst with lipid contents. (**a**) Clinical appearance. (**b**) Anterior-segment OCT reveals adipose connective tissue-filled content (droplets)

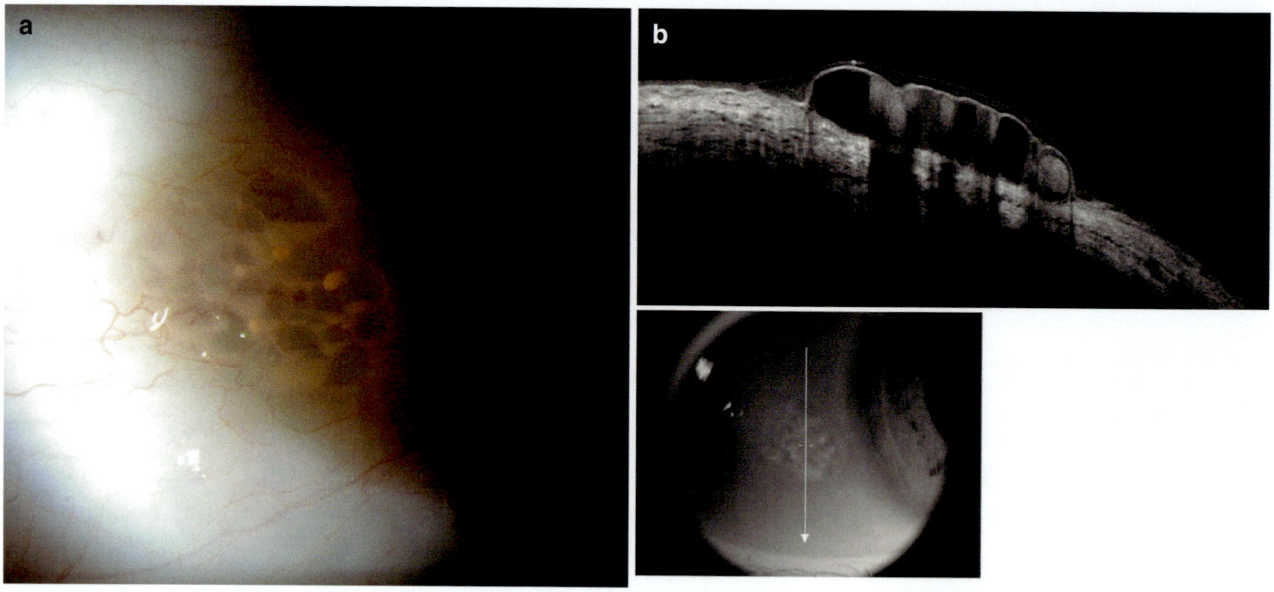

Fig. 3.7 Conjunctival epithelial cyst with layered contents. (**a**) Clinical appearance. (**b**) Anterior-segment OCT reveals multiple levels within cysts

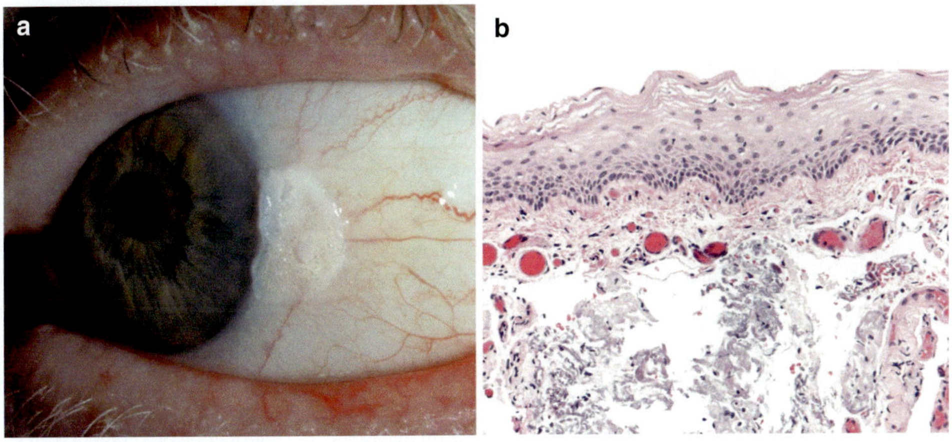

Fig. 3.8 Keratotic plaque. (**a**) Clinical appearance. (**b**) Histopathology: conjunctiva with loss of goblet cells, hyperkeratotic epithelium, and an underlying stroma with basophilic elastotic degeneration (hematoxylin & eosin x 20). (Courtesy of Gabreilla Yeaney, MD, Cleveland, Ohio)

3.1.10 Keratotic Plaque

This is a leukoplakic lesion that may develop in the limbal or bulbar conjunctiva, usually in the interpalpebral region (Fig. 3.8) [1, 2]. Histologically there is a focal thickening of keratin and epithelial layer, characterized mainly by acanthosis, hyperkeratosis, or parakeratosis. No dyskeratosis is seen. These lesions have little or no potential for carcinomatous changes.

3.1.11 Actinic Keratosis

Actinic keratosis of the conjunctiva is a rarely diagnosed focal leukoplakic lesion occurring at the intrapalpebral limbus, usually located over a chronically inflamed pinguecula or pterygium [2, 3, 51]. Rare cases of tarsal conjunctival involvement were reported [52, 53]. Actinic keratosis is classified among precancerous lesions, and it is also referred to as conjunctival dysplasia, actinic keratosis variety. Histologically the epithelium exhibits acanthosis, hyperkeratosis, and occasionally parakeratosis. The degree of dysplasia is minimal. Due to suspicion of a squamous cell carcinoma, these lesions are usually excised. Treatment by topical imiquimod was successful in one reported case [54] and by interferon α2b in another [53].

3.1.12 Sebaceous Adenoma

Sebaceous adenoma are rare, accounting for 1% of caruncular lesions and even fewer conjunctival lesions. Almost 50% of cases are associated with Muir–Torre syndrome [55], a rare autosomal-dominant condition defined by the association of cutaneous lesions (sebaceous neoplasms or keratoacanthoma) and Lynch syndrome-associated visceral malignancies. Those lesions should be tested for mismatch repair (MMR) proteins and the patients should undergo clinical investigation to rule out visceral neoplasms [55].

References

1. Spencer WH. Conjunctiva. In: Spencer WH, editor. Ophthalmic pathology, an atlas and textbook. 4th ed. Philadelphia: Saunders; 1996. p. 106–25.
2. Campbell RJ, Sobin LH. Tumors of the conjunctiva and caruncle. In: World Health Organization histological classification of tumours, editor. Histological typing of tumours of the eye and its adnexa. 2nd ed. Berlin: Springer; 1998. p. 9–15.
3. Shields CL, Shields JA. Tumors of the conjunctiva and cornea. Surv Ophthalmol. 2004;49:3–24.
4. Sjo N, Heegaard S, Prause JU. Conjunctival papilloma. A histopathologically based retrospective study. Acta Ophthalmol Scand. 2000;78:663–6.
5. Singh G. Conjunctival papilloma: a case report and a brief review of literature. Ann Transl Med. 2023;11(6):266.
6. Jian H, He W. Clinical features and factors affecting prognosis and partial deterioration of ocular papilloma: a retrospective study of 298 cases. Graefes Arch Clin Exp Ophthalmol. 2023;261(8):2395–402.
7. Yazu H, Dogru M, Miyauchi J, et al. Association of epithelial atypia with recurrence after surgical excision in conjunctival papilloma. Eye Contact Lens. 2018;44(Suppl 1):S77–81.
8. Shields CL, Shields JA. Tumors of the conjunctiva and cornea. Indian J Ophthalmol. 2019;67(12):1930–48.
9. Theotoka D, Morkin MI, Galor A, Karp CL. Update on diagnosis and management of conjunctival papilloma. Eye Vis (Lond). 2019;18(6):18.
10. Sripawadkul W, Khzam RA, Tang V, et al. Anterior segment optical coherence tomography characteristics of conjunctival papilloma as compared to papilliform ocular surface squamous neoplasia. Eye (Lond). 2023;37(5):995–1001.
11. Lass JH, Jenson AB, Papale JJ, et al. Papillomavirus in human conjunctival papillomas. Am J Ophthalmol. 1983;95:364–8.
12. Sjo NC, von Buchwald D, Cassonnet P, et al. Human papillomavirus in normal conjunctival tissue and in conjunctival papilloma: types and frequencies in a large series. Br J Ophthalmol. 2007;91:1014–5.

13. Mlakar J, Kocjan BJ, Hošnjak L, et al. Morphological characteristics of conjunctival squamous papillomas in relation to human papillomavirus infection. Br J Ophthalmol. 2015;99:431–6.
14. Peterson C, Parikh RN, Ahmad MT, et al. Detection of human papillomavirus in squamous lesions of the conjunctiva using RNA and DNA in-situ hybridization. Int J Mol Sci. 2022;23(13):7249.
15. Schechter BA, Rand WJ, Velazquez GE, et al. Treatment of conjunctival papillomata with topical interferon alfa-2b. Am J Ophthalmol. 2002;134:268–70.
16. Lass JH, Foster CS, Grove AS, et al. Interferon-alpha therapy of recurrent conjunctival papillomas. Am J Ophthalmol. 1987;103:294–301.
17. Rodríguez-Cabrera L, García-Regil P, Velasco-Levy A, Serna-Ojeda JC. Conjunctival papillomatosis in children treated with co-adjuvant topical interferon alpha-2b. Arch Soc Esp Oftalmol. 2019;94(7):352–4.
18. Hawkins AS, Yu J, Hamming NA, et al. Treatment of recurrent conjunctival papillomatosis with mitomycin C. Am J Ophthalmol. 1999;128:638–40.
19. Sripawadkul W, Theotoka D, Zein M, et al. Conjunctival papilloma treatment outcomes: a 12-year-retrospective study. Eye (Lond). 2023;37(5):977–82.
20. Bosniak SL, Novick NL, Sachs ME. Treatment of recurrent squamous papillomata of the conjunctiva by carbon dioxide laser vaporization. Ophthalmology. 1986;93:1078–82.
21. Kaliki S, Arepalli S, Shields CL, et al. Conjunctival papilloma: features and outcomes based on age at initial examination. JAMA Ophthalmol. 2013;131:585–93.
22. Belfort Neto R, Isenberg J, Castillejos AG, et al. Novel treatment of papillomatous conjunctival lesions using pattern scanning laser photocoagulation: 1-year results. Ocul Surf. 2018;16:337–40.
23. Shields CL, Lally MR, Singh AD, et al. Oral cimetidine (Tagamet) for recalcitrant, diffuse conjunctival papillomatosis. Am J Ophthalmol. 1999;128:362–4.
24. Lee CY, Chen HC, Meir YJ, et al. Subconjunctival injection of bevacizumab for recurrent conjunctival papilloma: a case report. Can J Ophthalmol. 2017;52(5):e156–9.
25. Sripawadkul W, AlBayyat G, Galor A, et al. Resolution of a presumed conjunctival papilloma after therapeutic treatment with the human papillomavirus vaccine. JAMA Ophthalmol. 2022;140(4):434–5.
26. Seth I, Roberts P, Cadieux D. Gardasil-9 vaccine as a possible treatment option for human papillomavirus Conjunctival papilloma. Ophthalmology. 2023;130(5):532.
27. Streeten BW, Carrillo R, Jamison R, et al. Inverted papilloma of the conjunctiva. Am J Ophthalmol. 1979;88:1062–6.
28. Stagner AM, Jakobiec FA, Chi A, et al. Conjunctival inverted squamous papilloma: a case report with immunohistochemical analysis and review of the literature. Surv Ophthalmol. 2015;60:263–8.
29. Singh V, Parwaiz A, Radotra BD, Singh M. Inverted mucoepidermoid papilloma of conjunctiva: a rare histological entity. Indian J Pathol Microbiol. 2019;62:481–2.
30. Jakobiec FA, Harrison W, Aronian D. Inverted mucoepidermoid papillomas of the epibulbar conjunctiva. Ophthalmology. 1987;94:283–7.
31. Ramberg I, Sjö NC, Bonde JH, Heegaard S. Inverted papilloma of the conjunctiva. BMJ Open Ophthalmol. 2019;4(1):e000193.
32. Lassalle S, Maschi C, Caujolle JP, et al. Inverted conjunctival papilloma: a certainly underestimated high-risk lesion for carcinomatous transformation-a case report. Can J Ophthalmol. 2017;52(1):e30–1.
33. Tseng SH, Chen YT, Huang FC, et al. Seborrheic keratosis of conjunctiva simulating a malignant melanoma: an immunocytochemical study with impression cytology. Ophthalmology. 1999;106:1516–20.
34. Kim JH, Bae HW, Lee KK, et al. Seborrheic keratosis of the conjunctiva: a case report. Korean J Ophthalmol. 2009;23(4):306–8.
35. Charles NC, Belinsky I. Pigmented inflamed seborrheic keratosis of the bulbar conjunctiva. Ophthalmic. Plast Reconstr Surg. 2023;39(3):e89–91.
36. Gündüz AK, Mirzayev I, Okcu Heper A, et. Al. Anterior segment optical coherence tomography in ocular surface tumours and simulating lesions. Eye (Lond). 2023;37(5):925–37.
37. Munro S, Brownstein S, Liddy B. Conjunctival keratoacanthoma. Am J Ophthalmol. 1993;116:654–5.
38. AlBayyat GJ, Venkateswaran N, Arreaza D, et al. Spontaneous regression of conjunctival keratoacanthoma. BMJ Case Rep. 2019;12(7):e228833.s.
39. Oellers P, Karp CL, Shah RR, et. al. Conjunctival keratoacanthoma. Br J Ophthalmol. 2014;98:275–6.
40. Díaz Díaz AL, Tello A, Chaparro Tapias TA, et al. Malignant transformation of a conjunctival keratoacanthoma requiring enucleation. Clin Ter. 2019;170(2):e81–3.
41. Allingham RR, Seo B, Rampersaud E, et al. A duplication in chromosome 4q35 is associated with hereditary benign intraepithelial dyskeratosis. Am J Hum Genet. 2001;68:491–4.
42. Seely M, Jackson K, Meeker A, Daluvoy M. Case series of patients with hereditary benign intraepithelial Dyskeratosis. Cornea. 2022;41(11):1451–4.
43. Dandar R, Silverberg M, Cheung AY. Surgical management of a recurrent hereditary benign intraepithelial dyskeratosis lesion involving a Boston keratoprosthesis. Can J Ophthalmol. 2023;58:e46–8.
44. Milman T, Jakobiec FA, Lally SE, et al. Lacrimal gland hamartoma (formerly termed Dacryoadenoma). Am J Ophthalmol. 2020;217:189–97.
45. Jakobiec FA, Perry HD, Harrison W, et al. Dacryoadenoma. A unique tumor of the conjunctival epithelium. Ophthalmology. 1989;96:1014–20.
46. Say EA, Shields CL, Bianciotto C, et al. Oncocytic lesions (oncocytoma) of the ocular adnexa: report of 15 cases and review of literature. Ophthalmic Plast Reconstr Surg. 2012;28:14–21.
47. Østergaard J, Prause JU, Heegaard S. Oncocytic lesions of the ophthalmic region: a clinicopathological study with emphasis on cytokeratin expression. Acta Ophthalmol. 2011;89:263–7.
48. Kapil JP, Proia AD, Puri PK. Lesions of the lacrimal caruncle with an emphasis on oncocytoma. Am J Dermatopathol. 2011;33:227–35.
49. Kalantzis GK, Verity DH, Rose GE. Periocular implantation cysts: a late complication of ophthalmic surgery. Eye (Lond). 2014;28:1004–7.
50. Park J, Lee S, Suh E. Removal of conjunctival cyst with high-frequency radio-wave electrosurgery. Can J Ophthalmol. 2015;50:378–83.
51. Mauriello JA Jr, Napolitano J, McLean I. Actinic keratosis and dysplasia of the conjunctiva: a clinicopathological study of 45 cases. Can J Ophthalmol. 1995;30:312–6.
52. Khan S, Chak M. A rare presentation of actinic keratosis affecting the tarsal conjunctiva and review of the literature. Case Rep Ophthalmol Med. 2018;12:4375354.
53. Gimeno-Carrero M, Suárez-Fernández MJ, Alonso-Martín B, et al. Conjunctival tarsal actinic keratosis treated with interferon alfa-2b: a rare case report and literature review. Case Rep Ophthalmol Med. 2021;2021(22):6616021.
54. Rowlands MA, Giacometti JN, Servat J, et al. Topical Imiquimod in the treatment of Conjunctival actinic keratosis. Ophthalmic Plast Reconstr Surg. 2017;33:e21–3.
55. Dias MBB, Morales MC, Fernandes AG, et al. Sebaceous adenoma of the conjunctiva and caruncle: a clinicopathological report of three cases and literature review. Arq Bras Oftalmol. 2021;85(2):174–7.

4 Conjunctival Tumors: Benign Melanocytic Tumors

Maya Eiger-Moscovich, Shahar Frenkel, and Jacob Pe'er

4.1 Benign Melanocytic Tumors

Conjunctival nevi are the most common conjunctival lesions. The various types of nevi are discussed herein, together with other benign melanocytic lesions of the conjunctiva, the episclera and sclera, such as complexion-associated melanosis, ocular melanocytosis, and primary acquired melanosis (PAM) without atypia and melanocytoma. There are many other pigmented conjunctival lesions that are not of melanocytic origin and should always be included in the differential diagnosis of melanocytic conjunctival lesions (see Chap. 5).

4.1.1 Conjunctival Nevus

4.1.1.1 Introduction

The circumscribed nevus is the most common melanocytic conjunctival tumor [1, 2]. It appears in all races, although it is more common in Caucasians. Many ophthalmic oncologists and pathologists will consider nevi that appear at birth or within the first 6 months of life as congenital nevi and those that appear more than 6 months after birth to be acquired. Most acquired conjunctival nevi will appear during the first two decades of life. Melanocytic conjunctival lesions that appear later in life should be suspicious for PAM or melanoma (Box 4.1).

Box 4.1 Clinical Features of Conjunctival Nevus that Are Suspicious for Melanoma

- Onset in adulthood
- Recent growth of the nevus
- Recent color change of the nevus
- Location in the tarsal conjunctiva
- Prominent feeder vessels
- Recurrence of an excised lesion

4.1.1.2 Clinical Features

Conjunctival nevi are typically located in the interpalpebral bulbar conjunctiva, commonly near the limbus, and rarely involve the cornea [2, 3]. The finding of melanocytic tumors in the tarsal conjunctiva is rare and should raise suspicion for PAM or malignant melanoma. Clinically, conjunctival nevus is a discrete, variably pigmented, slightly elevated sessile lesion, which in most cases contains cystic structures that can be seen by the naked eye, slit-lamp biomicroscopy (Fig. 4.1), anterior-segment OCT (Fig. 4.2), or ultrasound biomicroscopy [4]. OCT angiography [5], in vivo confocal microscopy [6], and dermoscopy [7] may also aid the diagnosis. Conjunctival nevi may vary in size from tiny lesions to ones that occupy large parts of the bulbar conjunctiva (Fig. 4.3) [8]. Nevi may become darker or lighter but usually will not change in size and color after adolescence. Changes in adulthood should raise suspicion for malignant transformation, although rapidly growing nevi in adults are rarely described [9]. The overall risk of malignant transformation is about 1% [2]. The presence of cystic structures can help differentiate nevi from other possible amelanotic conjunctival lesions. In childhood and adolescence, conjunctival nevi may become pinker and more congested due to inflammatory infiltration. These inflamed nevi will be discussed separately.

4.1.1.3 Histopathological Features

Conjunctival nevi range from junctional through compound to subepithelial nevi and reflect stages in the evolution of the nevus. Most excised nevi that are examined in the ophthalmic pathology laboratories are compound nevi. Spindle-shaped melanocytes are typically oriented parallel to the surface. In addition to the spindle cells, distinctive types of

M. Eiger-Moscovich · S. Frenkel · J. Pe'er (✉)
Ocular Oncology Service and Ophthalmic Pathology Laboratory, Department of Ophthalmology, Hadassah—Hebrew University Medical Center, Jerusalem, Israel
e-mail: peer@hadassah.org.il

© The Author(s), under exclusive license to Springer Nature Switzerland AG 2024
J. Pe'er et al. (eds.), *Clinical Ophthalmic Oncology*, https://doi.org/10.1007/978-3-031-72443-5_4

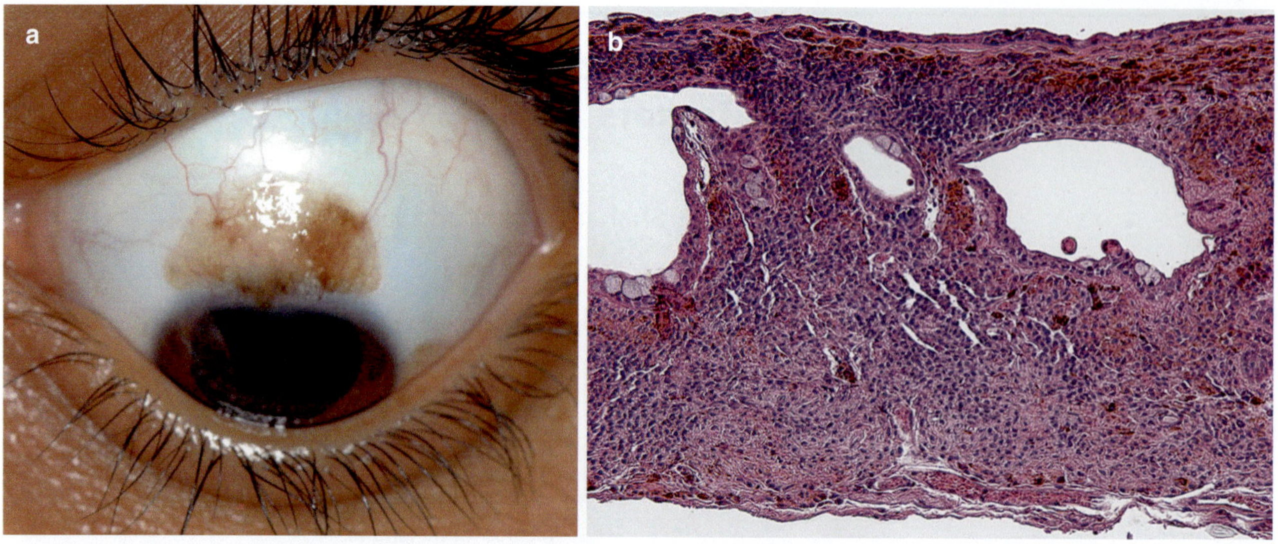

Fig. 4.1 (**a**) A typical partially pigmented compound conjunctival nevus with cystic elements, in an atypical location in the upper bulbar conjunctiva at the limbus. (**b**) Histopathology of a compound nevus of the conjunctiva with cystic structures lined by conjunctival epithelium (hematoxylin and eosin, original magnification ×10)

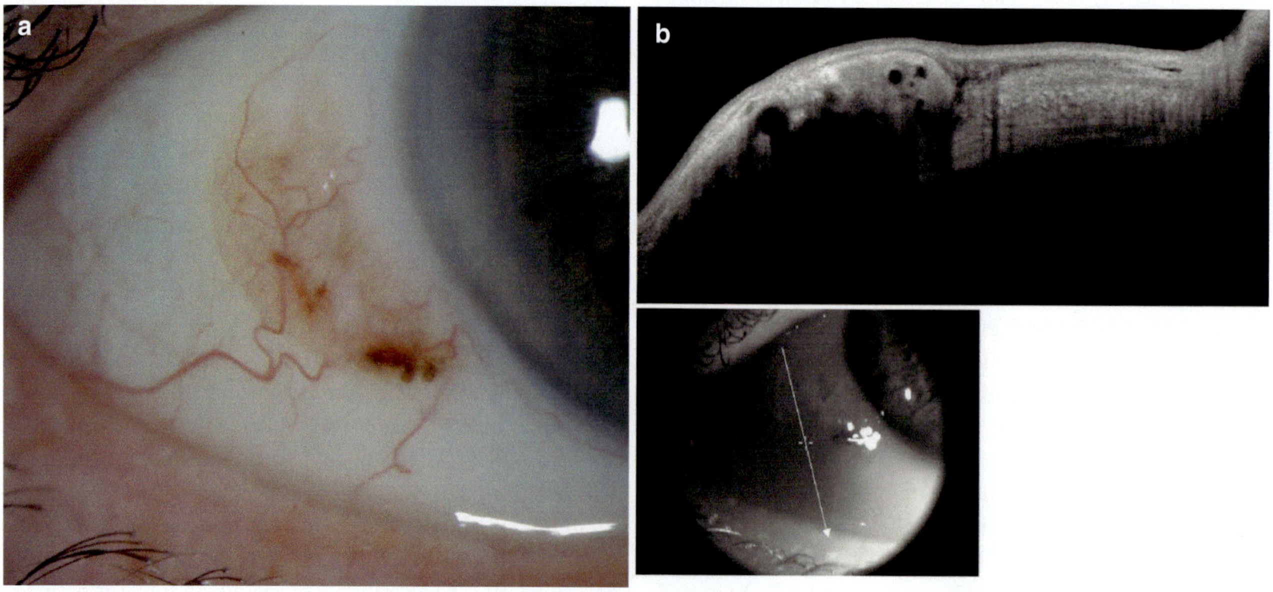

Fig. 4.2 A partially pigmented conjunctival nevus. (**a**) Intrinsic cysts are not readily identified. (**b**) Anterior-segment OCT reveals multiple cysts within the nevus

nevus cells were described in the conjunctiva as balloon cells, granular cell change, and deep penetrating nevus [10–14]. These cells usually appear in otherwise typical conjunctival nevi. About half of the conjunctival nevi express either BRAF or NRAS mutations, suggesting the driver mutations of conjunctival nevi are similar to those of skin nevi [15]..

Junctional Nevus

The junctional nevi usually appear as focal, flat, well-circumscribed lesions with various amounts of pigmentation. They are found only early in life and show nests of nevus cells along the interface of the epithelium and the substantia propria. The cells in junctional nevus can be round to oval, plump, epithelioid, cuboidal, or lymphocyte-like cells. They can form single, confluent, or irregular nests anterior to the epithelial basement membrane, which is, in general, intact. The epithelium overlying the nests is commonly reduced to a thin rim. These lesions may be confused with primary acquired melanosis; the latter usually appears in adults.

Compound Nevus

Compound conjunctival nevi represent an intermediate stage between the early junctional and late subepithelial nevus stage.

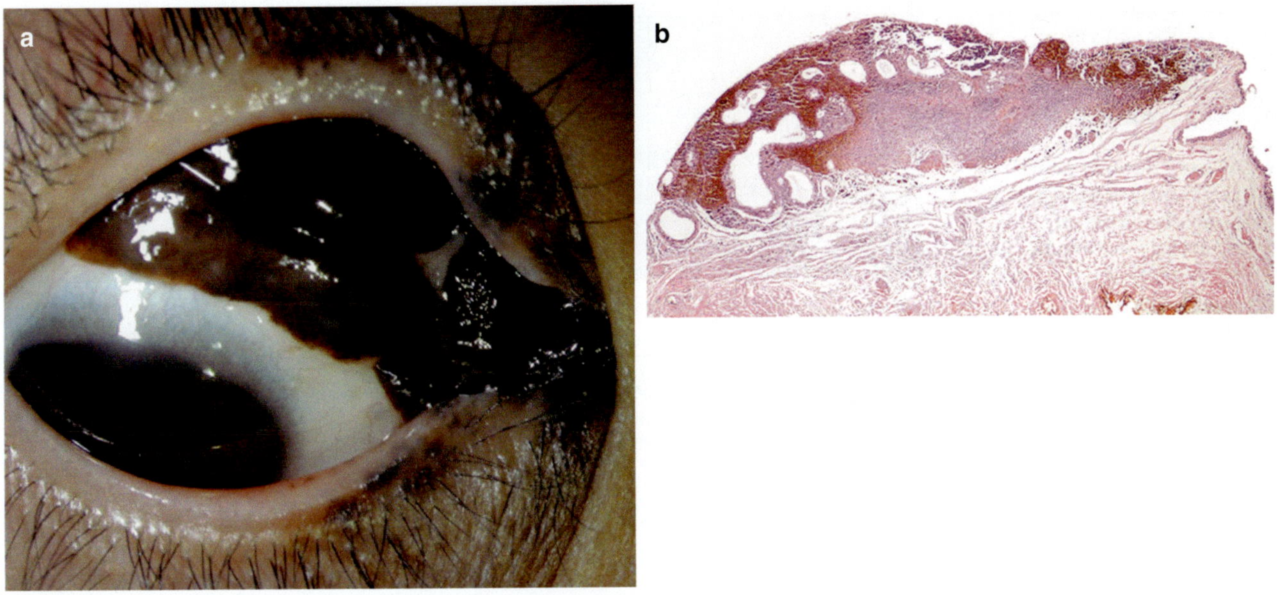

Fig. 4.3 (**a**) Clinical appearance. Large conjunctival nevus. (**b**) Histopathology revealed a compound nevus with cystic structures lined by conjunctival epithelium (hematoxylin and eosin, original magnification ×10)

They usually appear as elevated, well-circumscribed pigmented lesions. Nests of nevus cells are found in the substantia propria in addition to the junctional area and have less cytoplasm, which may reflect maturation. Solid nests of epithelium and epithelial cysts are very common within a compound nevus and may confuse the pathologist who is unfamiliar with conjunctival nevi (Fig. 4.3). Nevi in patients under 30 years old more frequently contain lymphocytic and eosinophilic infiltrates and have a smaller stromal component [16].

Subepithelial Nevus

Subepithelial nevi are believed to represent the last stage of conjunctival nevus, characterized by the migration of intraepithelial nevus cells into the substantia propria, followed by the disappearance of the junctional component. They appear as elevated, well-circumscribed pigmented lesions. Microscopically, these nevi typically appear as a symmetrically arranged intrastromal proliferation of predominantly small lymphocytoid melanocytes, often organized in large nests. Cystic and solid nests of conjunctival epithelium entrapped in melanocytic proliferation are seen in about half of the lesions [1].

4.1.1.4 Clinicopathological Variants

Spitz Nevus

A more distinctive type of conjunctival nevus is the Spitz nevus, which has been reported only in childhood and adolescence [17, 18]. Clinically, these lesions are rapidly growing nonpigmented lesions that should be differentiated from granulation tissue ("pyogenic granuloma") and, more importantly, from melanoma, which is extremely uncommon in children. Histologically, conjunctival Spitz nevi feature fascicles of spindle nevus cells that are usually oriented perpendicular to the epithelial surface and are uniformly and symmetrically arranged, unlike spindle cells in typical conjunctival nevi that are oriented parallel to the surface. Mitotic figures reflect the rapid clinical growth and do not indicate malignancy [1].

Blue Nevus

Blue and cellular blue nevi are rare conjunctival lesions that arise from neural crest cells like other melanocytic lesions, are situated in the deep conjunctival substantia propria, and do not reach the surface epithelium (Fig. 4.4). Clinically, they appear brown or black and have a benign clinical course [1, 19, 20]. Similar to other conjunctival nevi, they are commonly located in the bulbar conjunctiva, and they can be located in any part of the conjunctiva, including the palpebral conjunctiva [20, 21]. Histologically, the blue nevus comprises spindle-shaped cells with uniform melanin pigmentation. Elements of a blue nevus may be present in a typical conjunctival nevus. Such lesions have been termed "combined nevus." In cellular blue nevi, the fascicles of spindle-shaped cells are admixed with fibrillar collagen. There has been only one report of conjunctival melanoma arising from a blue nevus [22].

Deep Penetrating Nevus and Nevus with Granular Cell Change

Deep penetrating nevus and nevus with granular cell change were previously classified as "indeterminate" lesions but demonstrated benign behavior [23]. Deep penetrating nevus is clinically darkly pigmented and frequently shows growth, prompting excision. Nevertheless, it usually does not recur or undergo malignant transformation [14]. Histologically, the deep penetrating component is composed of larger mela-

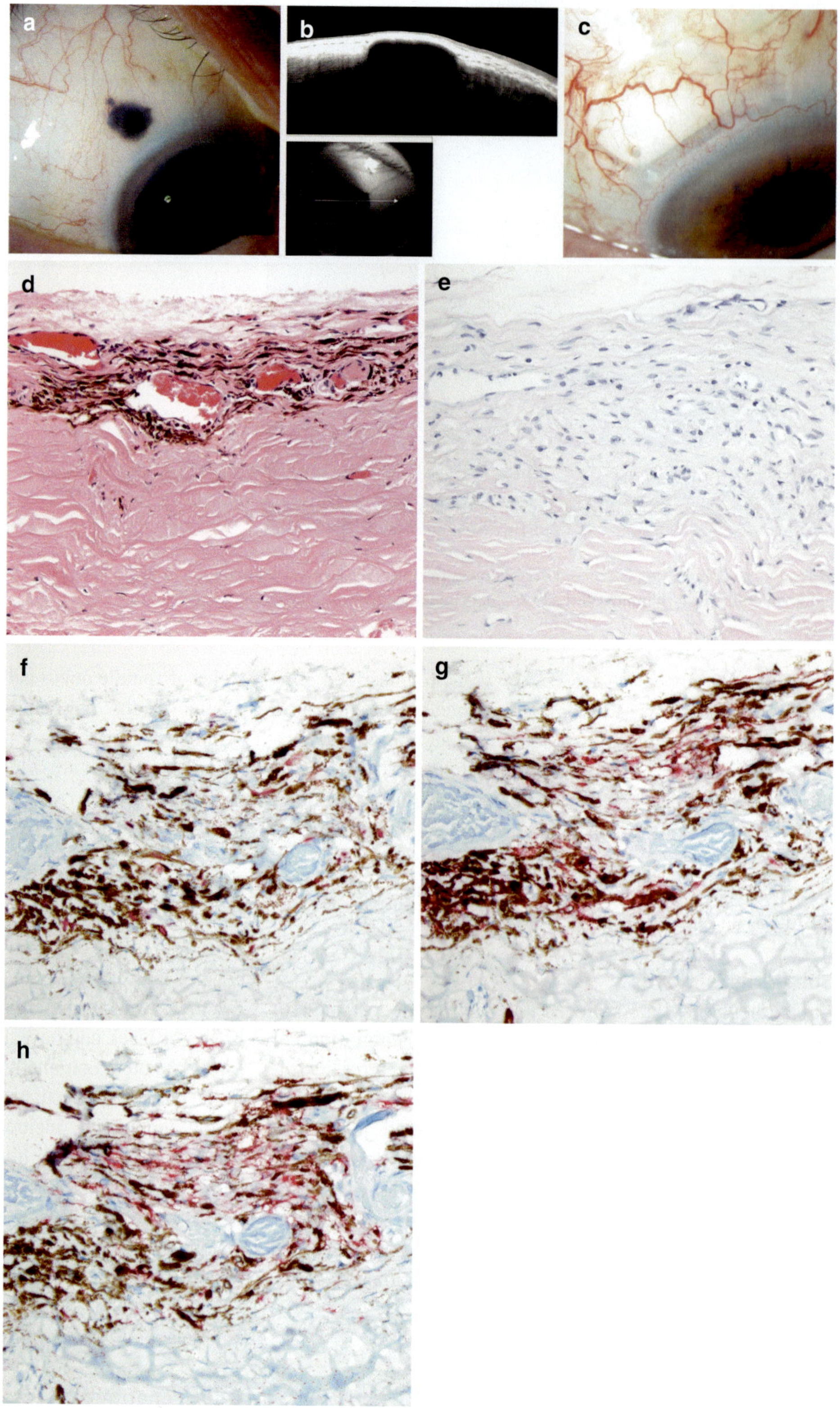

Fig. 4.4 Conjunctival blue nevus. (**a**) The nevus is located under the conjunctival stroma confirmed by anterior-segment OCT (**b**). (**c**) Appearance following excision that involved partial thickness scleral dissection, requiring scleral graft. (**d**) Histopathology showing flat collection of densely pigmented spindle melanocytes and melanophages on scleral surface (hematoxylin and eosin x 20). (**e**) Bleached stain reveals abundant cytoplasm, bland nuclei and inconspicuous nucleoli (×40). Immunohistochemistry for SOX10 (**f**) highlights the melanocytic nuclei (×40 red chromogen) HMB45, (**g**) the melanocytic cytoplasm (×40 red chromogen), and CD163 (**h**) highlights admixed macrophages (×40 red chromogen). (Courtesy of Gabreilla Yeaney, MD, Cleveland, Ohio)

nocytes with abundant lightly pigmented cytoplasm, with intensely pigmented melanophages in the background [23]. Nevi with the deep penetrating component are characterized by BRAF mutation and activation of the beta-catenin pathway [14]. Nevus with granular cell change may be a variant of deep penetrating nevus [24].

Inflamed Juvenile Conjunctival Nevus

Inflamed juvenile conjunctival nevus (IJCN) is a benign, juxta-limbal nevus that appears in children and adolescents, can grow rapidly, shows lesional redness, often shows cystic structures, and can be surrounded by vascular congestion [24]. Therefore, these lesions are frequently approached with

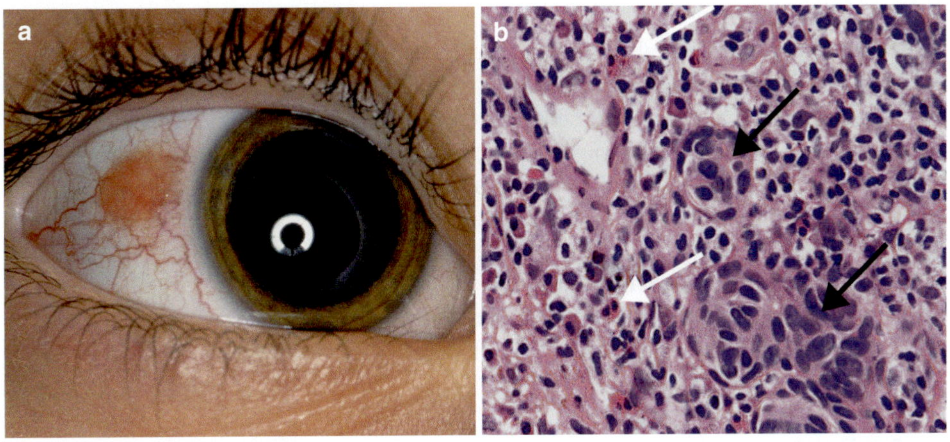

Fig. 4.5 Inflamed juvenile conjunctival nevus (IJCN). (**a**) Clinical pictures of an amelanotic inflamed juvenile conjunctival nevus in the temporal conjunctiva with cystic elements and dilated vessels around it. (**b**) Histopathology shows nevus nests (black arrows) with marked chronic inflammation around them and a remarkable number of eosinophils (white arrows) (hematoxylin and eosin, original magnification ×40)

undue concern by patients and clinicians, usually suspecting malignancy. More than half of these nevi are amelanotic, and changes in the pigmentation of amelanotic lesions have been documented (Fig. 4.5a).

Histologically, these rapidly growing lesions do not differ from simple compound conjunctival nevi in their benign histopathological features [24]. Cystic and solid epithelial elements are found in most of these nevi. In all lesions, there is significant polyclonal lymphocytic infiltration in and around the nevus, and significant infiltration of eosinophils is found in areas in most of these nevi (Fig. 4.5b) [24, 25]. Periods of rapid growth of inflamed nevi represent inflammatory infiltration and cystic enlargement, rather than malignant proliferation.

IJCNs are almost always associated with symptomatic allergic conjunctivitis or asymptomatic conjunctival papillary reaction. Increased expression of nerve growth factor (NGF), eosinophils, and mast cells in IJCN and modulation of eosinophil properties by lesion fibroblasts partly through NGF suggest a possible association between IJCN and allergic inflammation [26].

Typical cases of IJCN can be differentiated on clinical grounds from conjunctival melanoma. IJCN should also be differentiated from "salmon patch" lesions of conjunctival lymphoma, which is exceedingly rare in childhood, and the polyclonality of the lymphoid infiltrate that rule out the diagnosis of lymphoma [25]. The patient's young age and the cystic nature of typical lesions are indicators of a benign lesion.

4.1.1.5 Treatment

Most conjunctival nevi do not require excision since most patients relate that the lesion has been present and stable for many years, often since childhood or adolescence. In rare cases, spontaneous regression is observed [27]. The best management is usually periodic observation with a photographic comparison, although prolonged follow-up may not be necessary as most lesions do not change [28]. If growth is documented, local excision of the lesion should be considered [25]. In general, incisional biopsy is contraindicated in lesions that can be resected entirely. Some of the indications for excisional biopsy of conjunctival nevi include recent growth of the nevus, recent color change of the nevus, cosmetic concerns, recurrence of an excised lesion, and clinical suspicion of malignant melanoma. Parts of the lesion can be amelanotic, which may lead to an incomplete surgical resection. At the time of excision, the entire mass is removed, and if adherent to the globe, a thin lamella of the underlying sclera can also be removed with the lesion. Excision of wide margins and cryotherapy to the tumor bed and the resection margins are employed by some surgeons to prevent recurrence, as most cases that are excised are due to suspicion of malignant transformation. Others prefer to avoid cutting into the sclera and the application of cryotherapy and administer adjuvant local treatment only if histopathology indicates a diagnosis of PAM with atypia (for a discussion on adjuvant local treatment options for PAM with atypia, see Volume 4 Chap. 6). Laser photoablation of conjunctival nevi has been shown to be a safe and effective treatment [29, 30], and so has atmospheric low-temperature plasma-assisted noninvasive surgery [31].

In cases of typical IJCN, observation alone may suffice, and topical antiallergic agents may reduce tumor size [32]. Excisional biopsy is recommended in atypical lesions or whenever the clinician cannot make a definite diagnosis of IJCN. Similarly, lesions causing functional problems, such as dellen, interference with contact lens wear, or a significant cosmetic blemish, should be excised.

4.1.2 Complexion-Associated Conjunctival Pigmentation (Racial Melanosis)

Complexion-associated conjunctival pigmentation, also known as racial melanosis, is a common, bilateral condition of flat conjunctival pigmentation found in individuals with a dark complexion [1, 33]. However, the distribution of pigmentation may be asymmetric.

4.1.2.1 Clinical Features

The pigmentation is commonly present at the limbus, sometimes only horizontally at the 3 and 9 o'clock meridians and often for 360°, and may involve the adjacent cornea and limbal conjunctiva. Uncommonly, pigmentation may involve the fornix and rarely the palpebral conjunctiva. The pigmentation can be mottled with a patchy appearance [34].

4.1.2.2 Histopathological Features

The basal layer of the conjunctival epithelium appears hyperpigmented due to benign melanocytes located in this layer.

4.1.2.3 Treatment

As malignant transformation is extremely rare in complexion-associated melanosis, apart from observation, there is no need for surgical treatment.

4.1.3 Congenital Melanosis Oculi (Congenital Ocular Melanocytosis)

Congenital melanosis oculi is a pigmentary condition of the sclera and uvea that can be associated with periocular skin, orbit, meninges, and soft palate pigmentation [1, 33]. In this condition, the conjunctiva is usually not pigmented; it is included here because it is often considered in the clinical differential diagnosis of a conjunctival pigmented lesion. Due to its diffuse pattern, congenital melanosis oculi is often confused with conjunctival primary acquired melanosis. When the periocular skin is involved, the condition is called "oculodermal melanocytosis" or "nevus of Ota"[35].

4.1.3.1 Clinical Features

The surface of the eye appears slate gray or blue and not brown or black as seen in conjunctival melanocytic lesions due to the Tyndall effect of the pigmented melanin that is seen through the layers of the episclera and sclera (Fig. 4.6). There can also be isolated choroidal melanocytosis [36].

4.1.3.2 Histopathological Features

Since the pigmentation is due to dendritic melanocytes that are present within the episcleral and scleral tissue, it does not move with the bulbar conjunctiva.

4.1.3.3 Treatment

Conjunctival melanoma has not been described in melanosis oculi. However, the risk of uveal melanoma is 1:400 in individuals with light complexion [37], with double the risk of metastases [38], and there may be multiple genetically distinct uveal melanomas [39].

Affected patients should be followed regularly for the development of uveal, orbital, or meningeal melanoma [34, 37, 40]. Optic nerve melanocytoma was also described in a patient with melanosis oculi in the same eye [41].

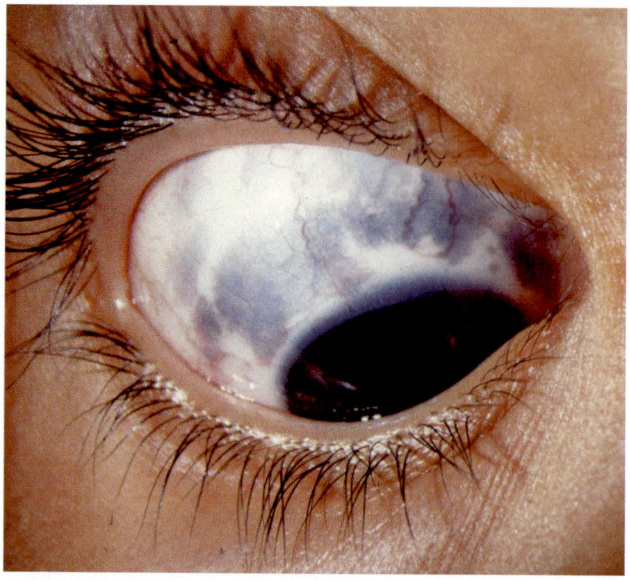

Fig. 4.6 Congenital melanosis oculi with gray-blue pigmentation of the sclera

4.1.4 Primary Acquired Melanosis (PAM) Without Atypia

Primary acquired melanosis is an important benign conjunctival pigmented lesion that, when with atypia, can give rise to conjunctival melanoma in individuals with light complexion. It is acquired in middle age and appears patchy, flat, noncystic, and variably brown, usually a unilateral lesion. The pigmentation can wax and wane over time [35].

Histologically, PAM lesions are flat, intraepithelial melanocytic lesions and divided into two major groups: PAM without atypia and PAM with atypia. Both types of PAM are discussed in Chap. 6.

4.1.5 Melanocytoma of the Conjunctiva

Melanocytoma (magnocellular nevus) is a rare, heavily pigmented benign lesion. Most melanocytomas occur in the optic nerve head, and conjunctival melanocytoma is extremely rare [42].

Histologically, it comprises polygonal tumor cells with small, inconspicuous nuclei and abundant cytoplasm filled with mature giant melanosomes that often can only be observed after bleaching due to abundant pigmentation. Mitotic figures are uncommon, and scattered melanophages have been described.

Routine follow-up is suggested since malignant transformation and infiltrative growth were described for melanocytomas of the optic disc and uvea [42].

4.1.6 Tumors of the Caruncle

The caruncle contains both conjunctival and cutaneous elements. Consequently, any tumor of the conjunctiva and skin may occur in the caruncle. In a large series of caruncular lesions [43–47], the vast majority were benign lesions, led by nevi and squamous papillomas. The caruncle is the most common site for oncocytoma [48, 49]. Only about 5% of the lesions in these series were premalignant and malignant tumors (for details, see Chap. 10).

References

1. Folberg R. Melanocytic lesions of the conjunctiva. In: Spencer WH, editor. Ophthalmic pathology, an atlas and textbook. 4th ed. Philadelphia: Saunders; 1996. p. 125–55.
2. Shields CL, Fasiudden AF, Mashayekhi A, et al. Conjunctival nevi: clinical features and natural course in 410 consecutive patients. Arch Ophthalmol. 2004;122:167–75.
3. Gupta A, Daigavane S. A rare case of conjunctival nevi involving the cornea. Pan Afr Med J. 2023;12(44):167.
4. Vizvári E, Skribek Á, Polgár N, et al. Conjunctival melanocytic naevus: diagnostic value of anterior segment optical coherence tomography and ultrasound biomicroscopy. PLoS One. 2018;14(13):e0192908.
5. Brouwer NJ, Marinkovic M, Bleeker JC, et al. Anterior segment OCTA of melanocytic lesions of the conjunctiva and iris. Am J Ophthalmol. 2021;222:137–47.
6. Cai J, Xu C, Ng TK, Li Z. Morphological characterization of nevi on the caruncle conjunctiva under *in vivo* confocal microscopy. Front Med (Lausanne). 2023;4(10):1166985.
7. Cinotti E, La Rocca A, Labeille B, et al. Dermoscopy for the diagnosis of conjunctival lesions. Dermatol Clin. 2018;36:439–49.
8. Shields CL, Regillo AC, Mellen PL, et al. Giant conjunctival nevus: clinical features and natural course in 32 cases. JAMA Ophthalmol. 2013;131:857–63.
9. Meyerov J, Levitz L, Haddad A. Pigmented nevus of the caruncle and plica Semilunaris: a case report. Case Rep Ophthalmol. 2023;14:83–6.
10. Thompson JM, Bermudez-Magner JA, Barker NH, et al. Balloon cell nevi of the conjunctiva: Clinicopathologic correlation and literature review. Surv Ophthalmol. 2015;60:481–5.
11. Seregard S. Pigmented spindle cell naevus of reed presenting in the conjunctiva. Acta Ophthalmol Scand. 2000;78:104–6.
12. Eiger-Moscovich M, Eagle RC Jr, Lally SE, et al. Conjunctival melanocytic nevi with granular cell change. Arch Pathol Lab Med. 2020;144:457–65.
13. Hohnen H, Singh S, Lam G, et al. Conjunctival combined deep penetrating naevus: a clinicopathological report. Pathology. 2023;55:721–3.
14. Šekoranja D, Vergot K, Hawlina G, Pižem J. Combined deep penetrating nevi of the conjunctiva are relatively common lesions characterised by BRAFV600E mutation and activation of the beta catenin pathway: a clinicopathological analysis of 34 lesions. Br J Ophthalmol. 2020;104:1016–21.
15. Francis JH, Grossniklaus HE, Habib LA, et al. BRAF, NRAS, and GNAQ mutations in conjunctival melanocytic nevi. Invest Ophthalmol Vis Sci. 2018;59:117–21.
16. Nebot L, Sáez A, Serret P, et al. Search for histopathological characteristics of inflammatory juvenile conjunctival nevus in conjunctival nevi related to age: analysis of 33 cases. Saudi J Ophthalmol. 2019;33:214–8.
17. Kantelip B, Boccard R, Nores JM, et al. A case of conjunctival Spitz nevus: review of literature and comparison with cutaneous locations. Ann Ophthalmol. 1989;21:176–9.
18. Vervaet N, Van Ginderdeuren R, Van Den Oord JJ, Foets B. A rare conjunctival Spitz nevus: a case report and literature review. Bull Soc Belge Ophtalmol. 2007;303:63–7.
19. Blicker JA, Rootman J, White VA. Cellular blue nevus of the conjunctiva. Ophthalmology. 1992;99:1714–7.
20. Sayed-Ahmed I, Murillo JC, Monsalve P, et al. Blue nevi of the ocular surface: clinical characteristics, pathologic features, and clinical course. Ophthalmology. 2018;125:1189–98.
21. Suller AL, Zhao J, Hodgson NM, et al. Blue nevi of the palpebral conjunctiva: report of 2 cases and review of literature. Orbit. 2022;41:527–34.
22. Demirci H, Shields CL, Shields JA, et al. Malignant melanoma arising from unusual conjunctival blue nevus. Arch Ophthalmol. 2000;118:1581–4.
23. Eder A, Milman T, Singh Mudhar H, et al. Unusual conjunctival melanocytic proliferations. Report of five cases and review of the literature. Surv Ophthalmol. 2023;27:S0039.
24. Zamir E, Mechoulam H, Micera A, et al. Inflamed juvenile conjunctival naevus: clinicopathological characterisation. Br J Ophthalmol. 2002;86:28–30.
25. Choi EK, Chévez-Barrios P. Inflamed conjunctival nevi: histopathological criteria. Arch Pathol Lab Med. 2014;138:1242–6.
26. Levi-Schaffer F, Micera A, Zamir E, et al. Nerve growth factor and eosinophils in inflamed juvenile conjunctival nevus. Invest Ophthalmol Vis Sci. 2002;43:1850–6.
27. Ho VW, Brunner M, Hussain RN, Heimann H. Regressing conjunctival nevus in a child. J Ophthalmic Vis Res. 2018;13:501–3.
28. Negretti GS, Roelofs KA, Damato B, et al. The natural history of conjunctival naevi in children and adolescents. Eye (Lond). 2021;35:2579–84.
29. Shin KH, Hwang JH, Kwon JW. Argon laser photoablation of superficial conjunctival nevus: results of a 3-year study. Am J Ophthalmol. 2013;15:823–8.
30. Park YM, Lee JE, Lee JS. Efficacy of pattern scan laser photocoagulation for superficial conjunctival nevi ablation. Lasers Med Sci. 20161;31:1037–9.
31. Nejat F, Jadidi K, Eghtedari S, Nabavi NS. Sublimation of benign conjunctival nevi using plasma-assisted noninvasive surgery: a clinical case series. Iran J Med Sci. 2023;48:85–90.
32. Kato K, Takeuchi M, Yonekawa Y, et al. Management of inflamed conjunctival nevus with topical antiallergic medications: case series. Clin Ophthalmol. 2021;12(15):559–64.
33. Shields CL, Shields JA. Tumors of the conjunctiva and cornea. Surv Ophthalmol. 2004;49:3–24.
34. Shields CL, Shields JA. Tumors of the conjunctiva and cornea. Indian J Ophthalmol. 2019;67:1930–48.
35. Plateroti AM, Scavella V, Abdolrahimzadeh B, et al. An update on oculodermal melanocytosis and rare associated conditions. Semin Ophthalmol. 2017;32:524–8.
36. Augsburger JJ, Brooks CC, Correa ZM. Isolated choroidal melanocytosis: clinical update on 37 cases. Graefes Arch Clin Exp Ophthalmol. 2020;258:2819–29.
37. Singh AD, De Potter P, Fijal BA, et al. Lifetime prevalence of uveal melanoma in white patients with ocula (dermal) melanocytosis. Ophthalmology. 1998;105:195–8.
38. Shields CL, Kaliki S, Livesey M, et al. Association of ocular and oculodermal melanocytosis with the rate of uveal melanoma metastasis: analysis of 7872 consecutive eyes. JAMA Ophthalmol. 2013;131:993–1003.

39. Wagley S, Belin PJ, Dollar JJ, et al. Multiple genetically distinct uveal melanomas Arise in the same eye of two patients with melanosis oculi. Am J Ophthalmol. 2022;234:1–5.
40. Doglietto F, Colosimo C, Lauriola L, et al. Intracranial melanocytic meningeal tumours and melanosis oculi: case report and literature review. BMC Cancer. 2012;6(12):220.
41. Maniar A, Jakati S, Kaliki S. Congenital choroidal melanocytoma in a child with ocular melanocytosis. BMJ Case Rep. 2019;30(12):e231376.
42. Herwig-Carl MC, Loeffler KU, Grossniklaus HE. Melanocytoma of the conjunctiva: Clinicopathologic features of three cases. Ocul Oncol Pathol. 2019;5:290–7.
43. Santos A, Gomez-Leal A. Lesions of the lacrimal caruncle. Clinicopathologic features. Ophthalmology. 1994;101:943–9.
44. Ostergaard J, Prause JU, Heegaard S. Caruncular lesions in Denmark 1978–2002: a histopathological study with correlation to clinical referral diagnosis. Acta Ophthalmol Scand. 2006;84:130–6.
45. Kaeser PF, Uffer S, Zografos L, et al. Tumors of the caruncle: a clinicopathologic correlation. Am J Ophthalmol. 2006;142:448–55.
46. Levy J, Ilsar M, Deckel Y, et al. Lesions of the caruncle: a description of 42 cases and a review of the literature. Eye (Lond). 2009;23:1004–18.
47. Yvon C, Balamurugan T, Bianchi E, et al. Caruncular lesions: a 16-year single Centre review in the United Kingdom. Eur J Ophthalmol. 2022;10:11206721221137938.
48. Say EA, Shields CL, Bianciotto C, et al. Oncocytic lesions (oncocytoma) of the ocular adnexa: report of 15 cases and review of literature. Ophthalmic Plast Reconstr Surg. 2012;28:14–21.
49. Østergaard J, Prause JU, Heegaard S. Oncocytic lesions of the ophthalmic region: a clinicopathological study with emphasis on cytokeratin expression. Acta Ophthalmol. 2011;89:263–7.

Ocular Surface Squamous Neoplasia

5

Jacob Pe'er, Shahar Frenkel, and Arun D. Singh

5.1 Introduction

Ocular surface squamous neoplasia (OSSN) is a term used for the precancerous and cancerous epithelial lesions of the conjunctiva and cornea [1, 2]. OSSN is a spectrum ranging from mild dysplasia, moderate dysplasia, severe dysplasia [also called carcinoma in situ (CIS)], and invasive squamous cell carcinoma (SCC). The most common previously used names for the intraepithelial lesions are "intraepithelial epithelioma," "Bowen's disease" of the conjunctiva, or "Bowenoid epithelioma." Because of differences in the histology of conjunctiva and skin, the term Bowen's disease should be reserved only for cutaneous lesions. Other terms for intraepithelial ocular surface neoplasia are conjunctival intraepithelial neoplasia (CIN) [3], corneal intraepithelial neoplasia, or both, corneal and conjunctival intraepithelial neoplasia (CCIN). Since the term OSSN does not distinguish between premalignant squamous epithelial dysplasia, including carcinoma in situ, and invasive SCC, it should not be used in surgical pathology reports to avoid mismanagement and can be used only clinically [4].

5.2 Epidemiological Aspects

OSSN is found in all races. It is uncommon in northern countries but common in countries that are closer to the equator and where exposure to sunlight is greater. The incidence of OSSN in the Northern hemisphere is highest at the latitude of 16° south and decreases by half for every 10° one travels north from there [5]. The incidence was 0.3 per million in the United States [6] but surprisingly higher in Canada with 0.45 per million per year [5]. In a study performed in Uganda, the incidence of OSSN was 1.3 per million, and in Australia, the incidence is reported to be as high as 19 per million population [1]. OSSN occurs predominantly in adults, although a few cases in children have been reported, especially in those with xeroderma pigmentosum [7]. In most series, OSSN is more common in men [5, 6], an occurrence that is explained by their greater exposure to sunlight. In one large series, men also showed higher-grade lesions [8]. According to some studies, patients with CIN are younger by 5–9 years than those with invasive SCC, a fact that implies the precancerous nature of the CIN [9].

5.3 Etiology and Associated Diseases

There are several possible factors and mechanisms that may explain or are associated with the development of OSSN. The most important ones are exposure to solar ultraviolet radiation, human papillomavirus, AIDS, and the stem cell theory.

5.3.1 Sunlight Exposure

Exposure to solar ultraviolet radiation has been identified in many studies as a major etiological factor in the development of OSSN [3, 9]. The rarity of OSSN in Europe and North America and its higher incidence in sub-Saharan African countries and in Australia [1], where people are more exposed to sunlight, suggests an important role of solar ultraviolet light in the development of OSSN. Lee and Hirst [1] observed a relationship between lifetime exposure to solar ultraviolet light and the risk of developing OSSN. Newton et al. [10] noted that the incidence of ocular SCC increases by 29% per unit increase in ambient solar ultraviolet light exposure, corresponding to a 49% increase in incidence with each 10° decline in latitude from north toward 16° south.

J. Pe'er (✉) · S. Frenkel
Ocular Oncology Service and Ophthalmic Pathology Laboratory, Department of Ophthalmology, Hadassah—Hebrew University Medical Center, Jerusalem, Israel
e-mail: Peer@hadassah.org.il

A. D. Singh
Department of Ophthalmic Oncology, Cole Eye Institute, Cleveland Clinic, Cleveland, OH, USA
e-mail: singha@ccf.org

© The Author(s), under exclusive license to Springer Nature Switzerland AG 2024
J. Pe'er et al. (eds.), *Clinical Ophthalmic Oncology*, https://doi.org/10.1007/978-3-031-72443-5_5

A history of actinic skin lesions such as solar keratoses and SCC is also strongly associated with the development of OSSN. It is well known that ultraviolet B rays cause damage to DNA in human epithelial cells. Failure of DNA repair, as occurs in xeroderma pigmentosum, leads to somatic mutations and the development of cancerous cells of OSSN. According to a study on the pathophysiology of OSSN [11], UV radiation damages DNA and produces pyrimidine dimers in the DNA chain. Specific CC — > TT base pair dimer transformations of the p53 tumor-suppressor gene occur in OSSN, allowing cells with damaged DNA past the G1-S cell cycle checkpoint. In recent years, several studies demonstrated that ultraviolet light signature—the telomerase reverse transcriptase (TERT) promoter mutations are common in OSSN lesions, supporting UV induction as the major source of mutagenesis in these lesions [12, 13].

5.3.2 Human Papillomavirus

In recent years, human papillomavirus (HPV), mainly type 16, has been demonstrated in tissues of OSSN [14]. DNA of HPV was found in fresh tissue of OSSN, using amplification with PCR and sequencing of the DNA, in ocular surface swabs of patients with OSSN, and in studies of formalin-fixed paraffin-embedded tissue, using immunostaining. However, HPV was also detected in uninvolved eyes with apparently healthy conjunctiva and in cases of persistence of infection many years after the successful eradication of OSSN lesions. In one study where evidence for HPV was analyzed by immunohistochemistry and multiplex polymerase chain reaction (PCR), no HPV was detected in OSSN lesions [15]. Another study showed no statistically significant association between anti-HPV antibody status and the risk of conjunctival neoplasia [16]. Recent studies from Denmark showed that HPV, mainly HPV16, increases the odds of conjunctival CIN and carcinoma by 8.4 folds, compared to healthy conjunctival mucosa [17], and that patients with HPV-positive tumors were significantly younger and had higher recurrence rates compared with HPV-negative tumors [18]. These findings and the geographical differences lead to the assumption that HPV alone may be incapable of causing OSSN [19] and that other factors in conjunction with HPV are involved in the causation of OSSN. According to a study from India, HPV was a predictor of better survival in OSSN patients [20].

5.3.3 Acquired Immunodeficiency Syndrome (AIDS)

The incidence of OSSN has increased significantly since the eruption of the AIDS epidemic, especially in sub-Saharan African countries [21]. In studies from Rwanda, Uganda, Congo, Kinshasa, and Zimbabwe, human immunodeficiency virus (HIV) infection was strongly associated with an apparent increase in the incidence of OSSN. In a study from Kenya, 74% of patients with OSSN were HIV-positive [22]. In recent studies, HIV infection has been attributed to 33% of SCC of the conjunctiva in sub-Saharan Africa [23]. In these countries, the OSSN occurs at a younger age than was previously reported, and the disease tends to be aggressive (Fig. 5.1). Although HIV infection seems to be an obvious

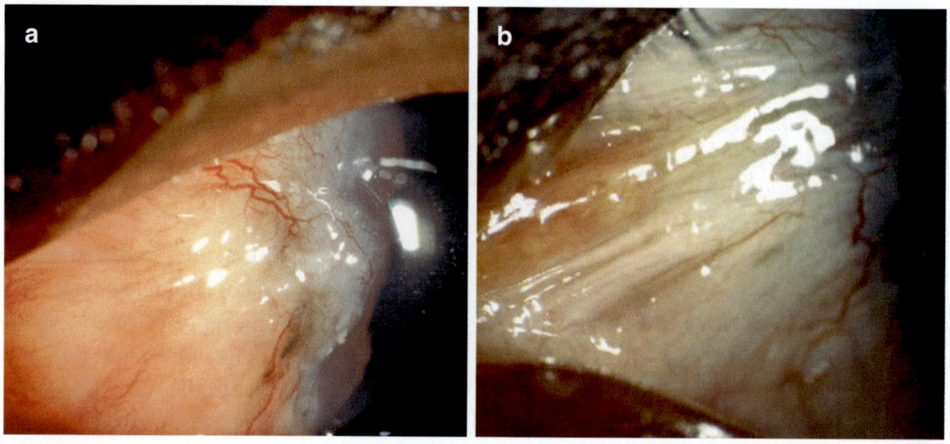

Fig. 5.1 A 52-year-old African woman was diagnosed with HIV, with a CD4 count of 56 × 10^6/mm^3 and viral load >100,000 copies/mL. At presentation, a fleshy conjunctival growth extending onto the cornea was initially diagnosed as a pterygium (**a**). The ocular symptoms worsened with enlargement of the mass, which on CT scan revealed extension into the medial rectus muscle insertion. Conjunctival biopsy confirmed diffusely infiltrating invasive, moderately differentiated squamous cell carcinoma. The patient declined lid-sparing exenteration. In the interim, she was started on antiretroviral therapy (zidovudine, lamivudine, and efavirenz). Over the next several months, her symptoms improved. At 12 months, the CD4 count was 221 × 10^6/mm^3, and the viral load was undetectable. The conjunctival mass had completely resolved (**b**). In the setting of HIV, even Kaposi's sarcoma and non-Hodgkin's lymphoma are recognized as responding to highly active antiretroviral therapy via immune restoration. (Reprinted from Holkar S, Mudhar HS, Jain A, Gupta M, Rogstad KE, Parsons MA, Singh AD, Rennie IG. Regression of invasive conjunctival squamous carcinoma in an HIV-positive patient on antiretroviral therapy. Int J STD AIDS. 2005;16(12):782–3. With permission from Sage Publications)

risk factor by itself, its interaction with ultraviolet light and HPV, which are also prevalent in African countries, can accelerate the development of OSSN.

5.3.4 Post-Transplantation and Immunosuppression

Solid organ transplantation and consequent immunosuppression are important risk factors for the development of squamous cell carcinoma, basal cell carcinoma, melanoma, and lymphoma [24–26]. The incidence of squamous cell carcinoma varies with the type, intensity, and duration of the immunosuppressive treatment [27]. OSSN has also been observed in the setting of immunosuppression [28]. Such tumors tend to be bilateral, aggressive, and nonresponsive to topical interferon therapy [29] (Fig. 5.2).

5.3.5 Xeroderma Pigmentosum and Other DNA Repair Disorders

Xeroderma pigmentosum is caused by autosomal-recessive inheritance of defective nucleotide excision repair genes related to Bloom syndrome, Nijmegen breakage, and other DNA repair disorders (Fig. 5.3). Patients with XP have severe sun sensitivity and are prone to develop skin cancers, including basal cell, skin SCC, and melanoma (Fig. 5.4) [30, 31]. Most patients with XP have parental consanguinity and require multidisciplinary care and monitoring for ocular manifestations [32]. The cornea undergoes progressive scarring, vascularization, pannus formation due to limbal stem cell deficiency, and even endothelial loss [30, 33, 34]. The conjunctival and corneal neoplasms tend to occur at an early age with bilateral, multiple, recurrent, aggressive, and invasive behavior, and are difficult to manage (Fig. 5.5) [30, 34, 35]. A wide-brimmed hat and sunglasses can reduce the exposure to UV irradiation.

5.3.6 Stem Cell Theory

Because of the tendency for OSSN to arise in the limbal area, where the stem cells for the corneal and conjunctival epithelium are located, Lee and Hirst [1] proposed the limbal transition zone/stem cell theory for the development of OSSN. Based on Tseng's concept of the long-living and high proliferation rate of stem cells in the limbal area, they postulated that alterations in this anatomical site influenced by other factors cause abnormal maturation of the conjunctival and corneal epithelium, resulting in the formation of OSSN. It has been postulated that limbal epithelial stem cells are the possible progenitor cells in OSSN [11].

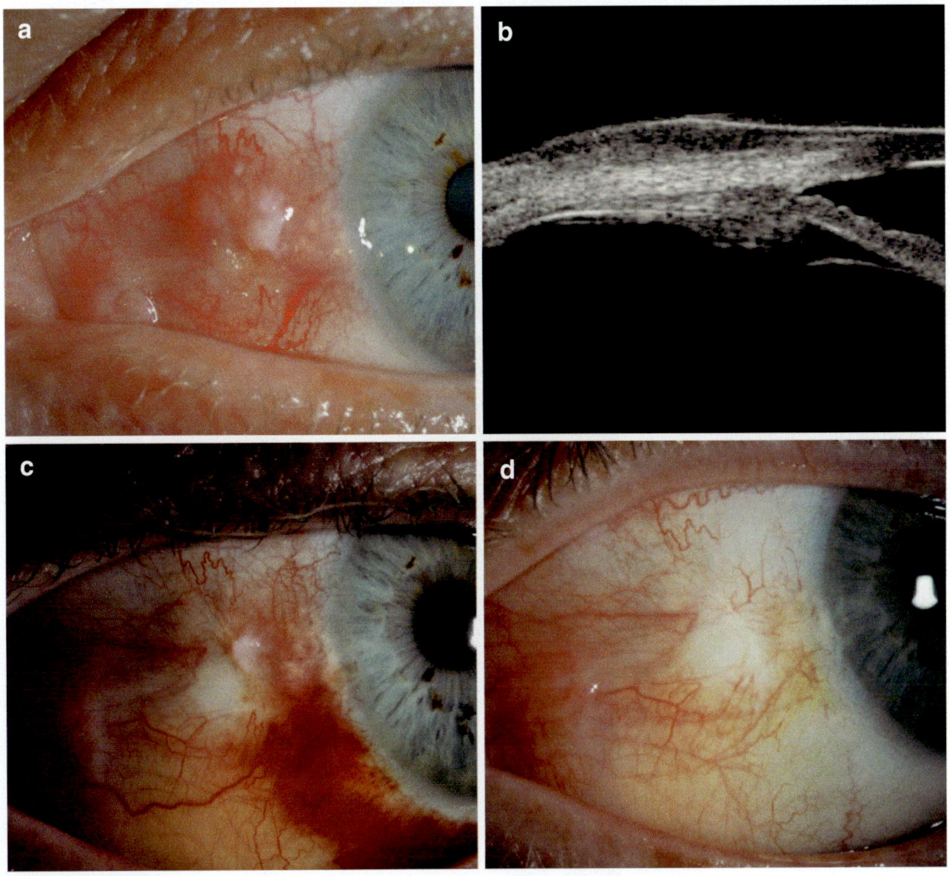

Fig. 5.2 A 55-year-old male s/p simultaneous liver-kidney transplant about 10 years prior with nodular thickening left lower eyelid (basal cell carcinoma) and biopsy-proven CIN right eye (**a**). The lesion was adherent to the underlying sclera. UBM excluded deep scleral extension (**b**). He was treated with six subconjunctival injections of interferon alpha 2b (IFN α-2b, three million units/0.5 mL) given at 1–2 weeks intervals. (**c**) The response is evident after second injection. Note subconjunctival hemorrhage. (**d**) There was total resolution after the sixth injection. The patient has remained recurrence-free at 6 months after the last injection

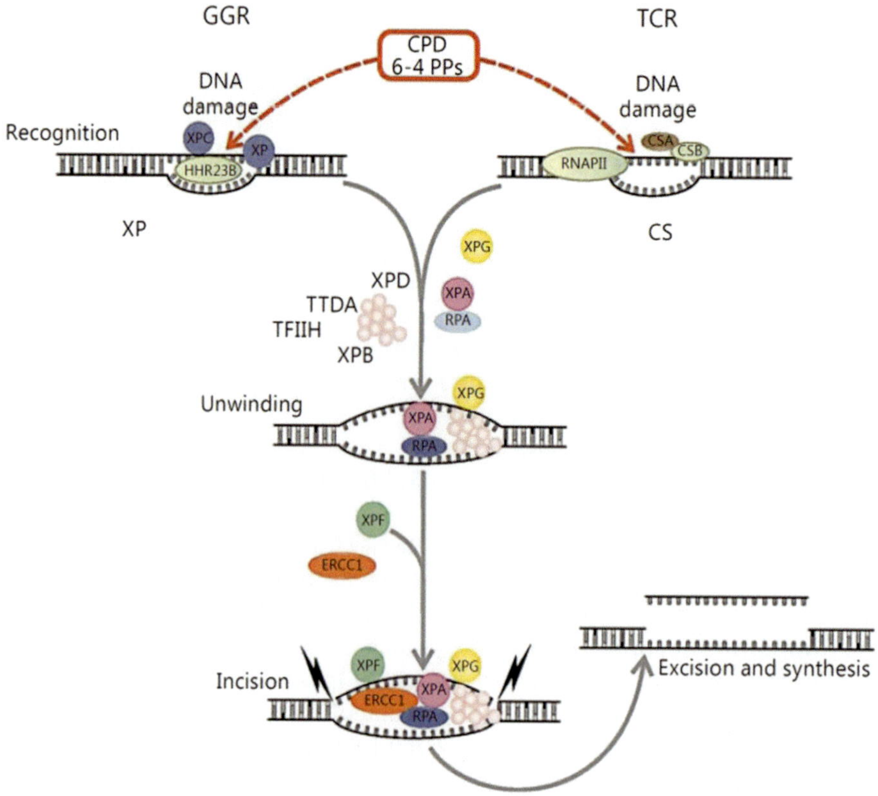

Fig. 5.3 Overview of the nucleotide excision repair (NER) system as the genetic basis for XP and related disorders. Transcription-coupled repair (TCR) removes damaged DNA from genes that are actively transcribed, while the slower global genome repair (GGR) system works in the remaining genome. In GGR, the DNA damage by UV radiation leads to the formation of cyclobutane pyrimidine dimers (CPDs) or 6–4 photoproducts (PPs), which are recognized by XPC proteins. Meanwhile, in TCR, DNA damage blocks RNA polymerase II function. Pathways overlap after initial damage recognition in a process involving XPB, XPG, XPA, and replication protein A (RPA). Finally, XPF and XPG remove the damaged regions by making incisions of ~ 30 nucleotides, followed by DNA synthesis to fill the gaps. (Reprinted from Suarez MJ, Rivera-Michlig R, Dubovy S, Rodriguez FJ. Clinicopathological Features of Ophthalmic Neoplasms Arising in the Setting of Xeroderma Pigmentosum. Ocul Oncol Pathol. 2015 Dec;2(2):112–21. With permission from S. Karger AG, Basel © 2016) [36]

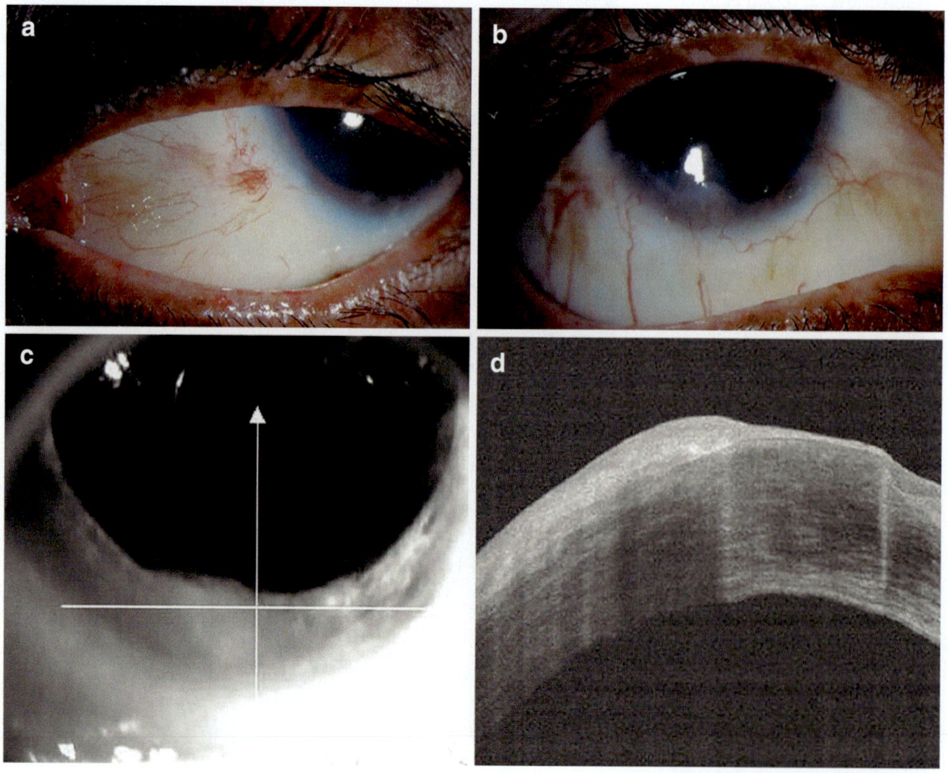

Fig. 5.4 A 33-year-old Asian woman with xeroderma pigmentosum. Note (**a**) pterygium-like changes in the left eye and peripheral corneal opacification and (**b**) vascularization of the right cornea attributed to limbal stem cell deficiency. OCT at 6 clock position (**c**) shows thickened corneal epithelium indicating CIN within the corneal pannus (**d**)

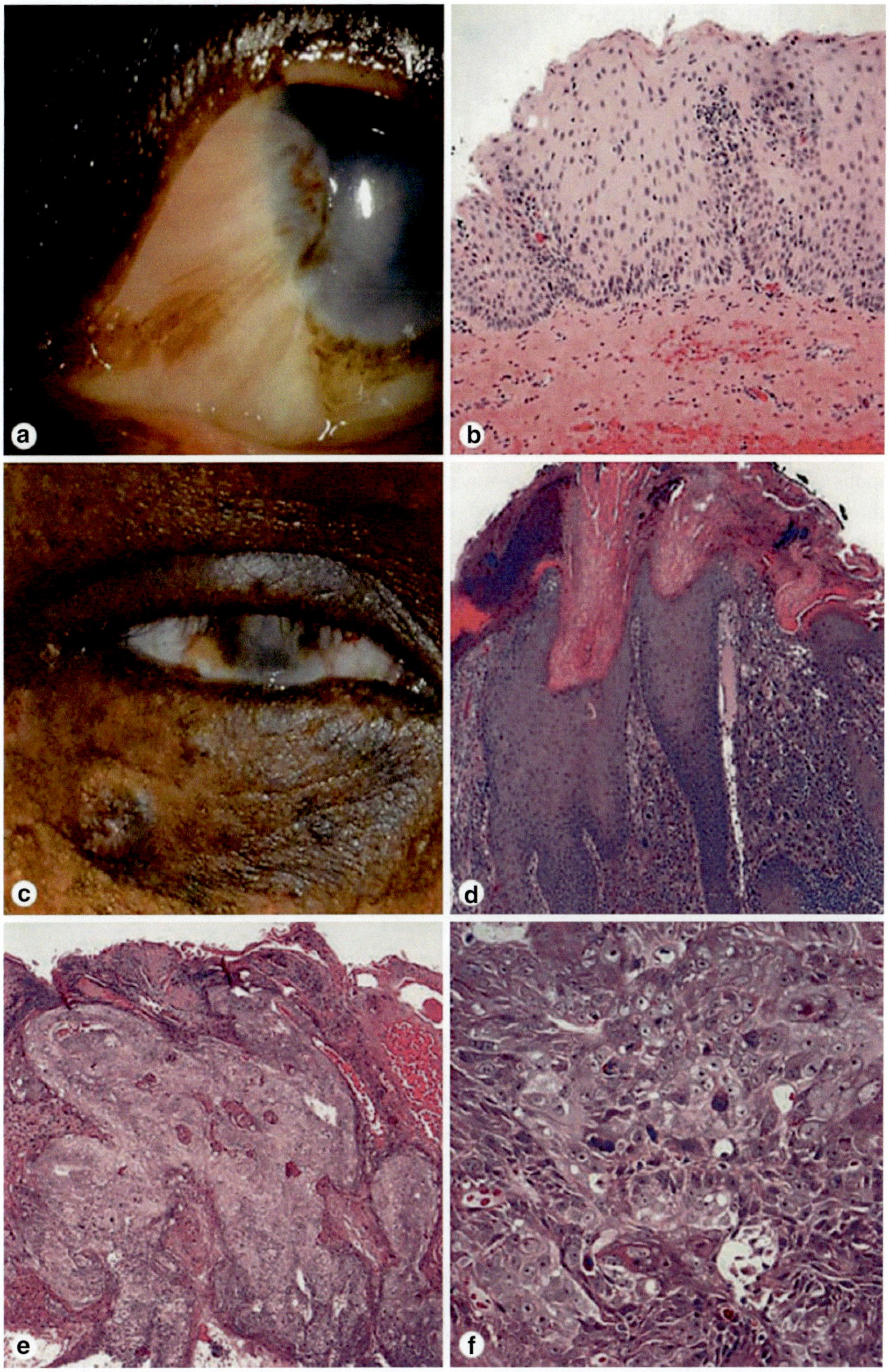

Fig. 5.5 Spectrum of differentiation of squamous neoplasia in XP. XP patients develop a variety of squamous lesions, including CIN with variable dysplasia (**a**, **b**) and well-differentiated, highly keratinized eyelid SCCs (patient 3; **c**, **d**). A subset of tumors may be less differentiated and demonstrate increased pleomorphism (**e**, **f**). (Reprinted from Suarez MJ, Rivera-Michlig R, Dubovy S, Rodriguez FJ. Clinicopathological Features of Ophthalmic Neoplasms Arising in the Setting of Xeroderma Pigmentosum. Ocul Oncol Pathol. 2015 Dec;2(2):112–21. With permission from S. Karger AG, Basel © 2016)

5.4 Clinical Features

5.4.1 Symptoms

In addition to the presence of the lesion on the ocular surface, other symptoms include ocular redness and irritation. Visual acuity is usually not reduced unless the center of the cornea is affected [37]. OSSN may grow within weeks to years; in most cases, the history is of several months.

5.4.2 Signs

Clinically, it may be difficult to distinguish between conjunctival epithelial dysplasia, carcinoma in situ, and invasive squamous cell carcinoma, although suspicion toward one of these three lesions may exist. These lesions arise commonly within the interpalpebral fissure, mostly at the limbus (Figs. 5.6 and 5.7). OSSN may appear gelatinous with superficial vessels, papilliform when it has a papillary appearance (Fig. 5.8), or leukoplakic, with a white keratin plaque covering the lesion [3] (Fig. 5.9). It may also appear as a nodular lesion (Fig. 5.10), especially when it is an invasive SCC or as a diffuse lesion masquerading as chronic conjunctivitis. OSSN may rarely occur in the tarsal or forniceal conjunctiva (Fig. 5.11). The limbal component may be inconspicuous with predominant corneal extension (Fig. 5.12). Usually, OSSN appears as a nonpigmented lesion, although pigmented conjunctival SCC has been reported, mostly in more pigmented individuals [38] (Fig. 5.13). According to one study, clinical characteristics that may predict high-grade lesions are temporal and superior location, papillomatous and nodular-appearing lesions, and size of the lesional area [7]. Bilateral disease and intraocular tumor extension are more common in patients with XP and HIV infection [39, 40]. An unexpected incidence of OSSN,

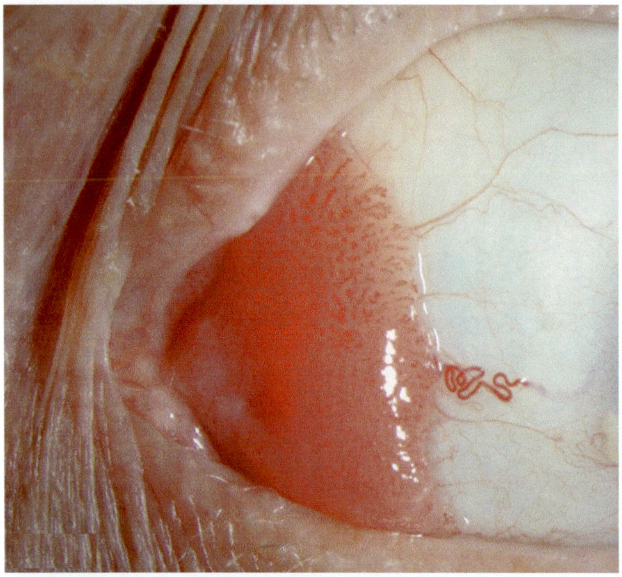

Fig. 5.6 Papillomatous ocular surface squamous neoplasia

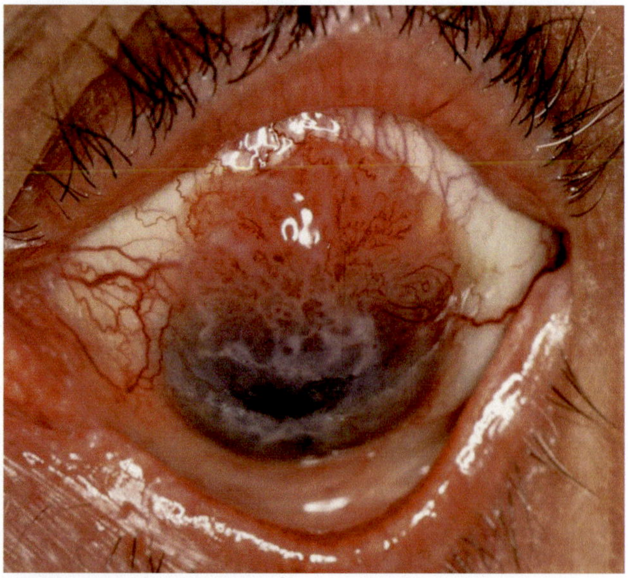

Fig. 5.7 Papillary conjunctival SCC invading into the upper half of the cornea

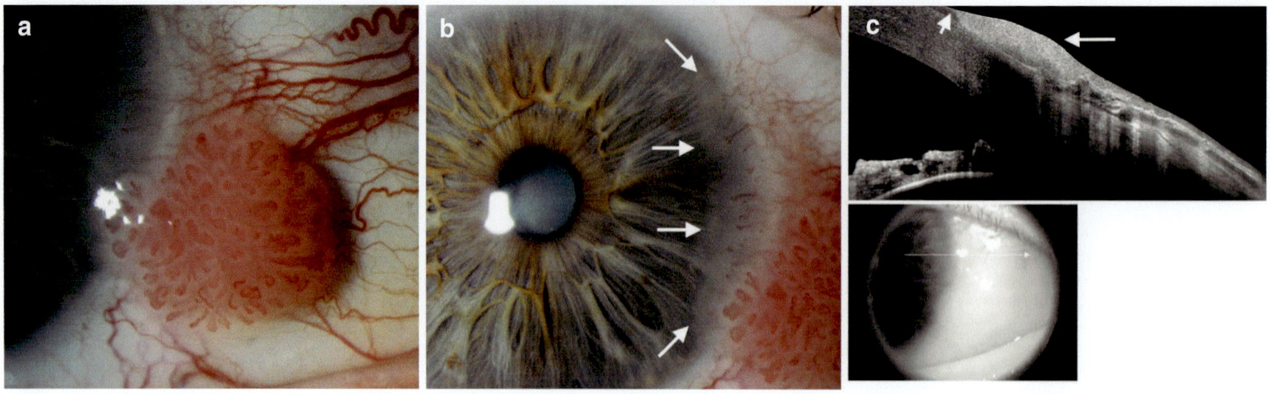

Fig. 5.8 (**a**) Papillomatous limbal CIN with prominent intrinsic and feeder vessels. (**b**) Note subtle corneal extension (arrows) visualized by OCT (**c**) as abruptly (small arrow) thickened hyper-reflective epithelium (large arrow)

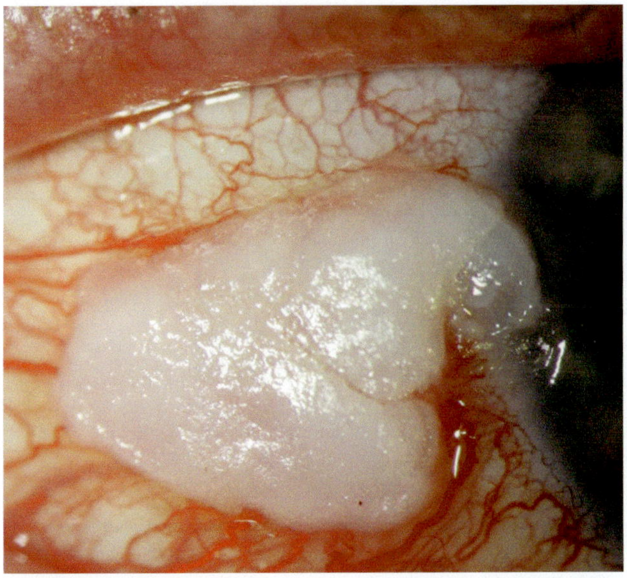

Fig. 5.9 Leucoplakic CIN

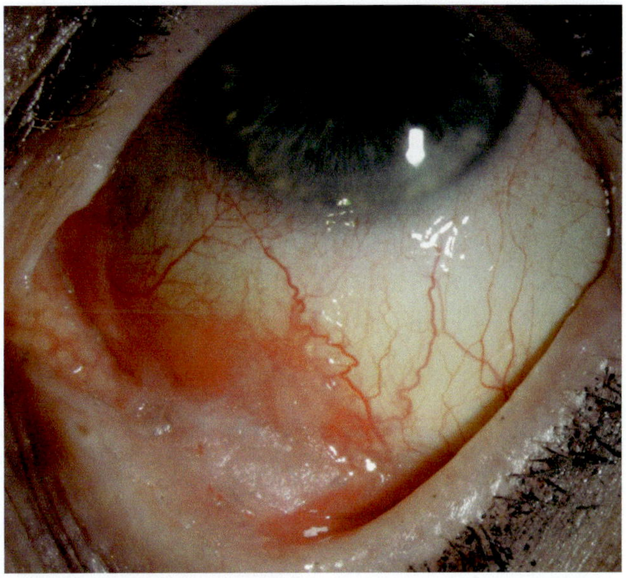

Fig. 5.11 CIN originating in the inferior fornix

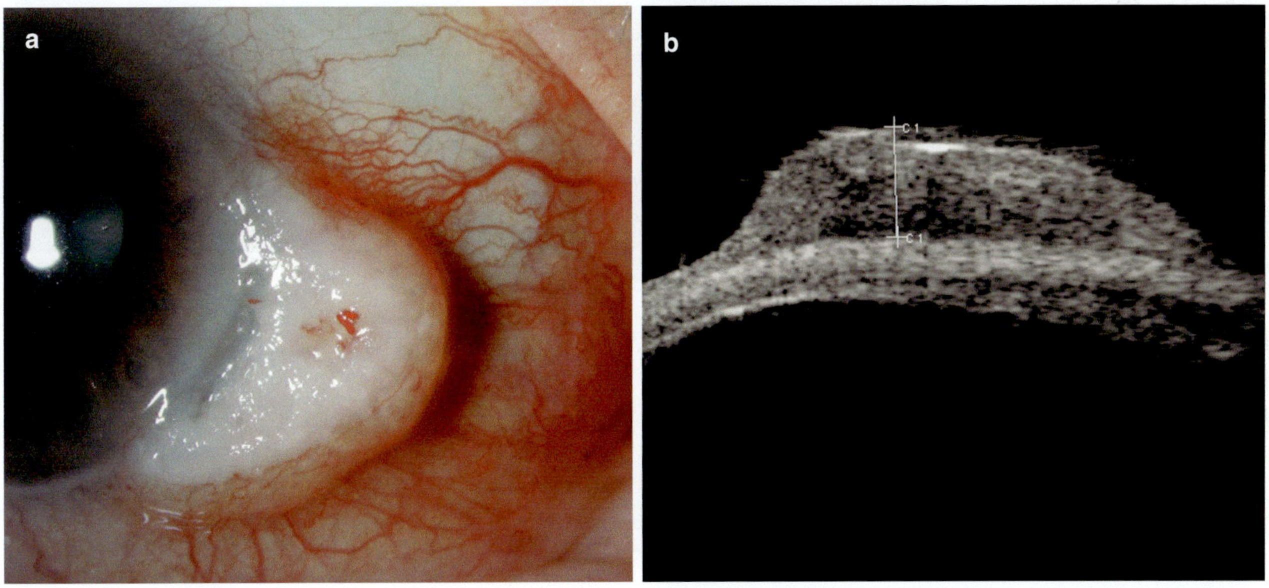

Fig. 5.10 (**a**) Nodular CIN. (**b**) UBM excluded deep scleral or intraocular extension

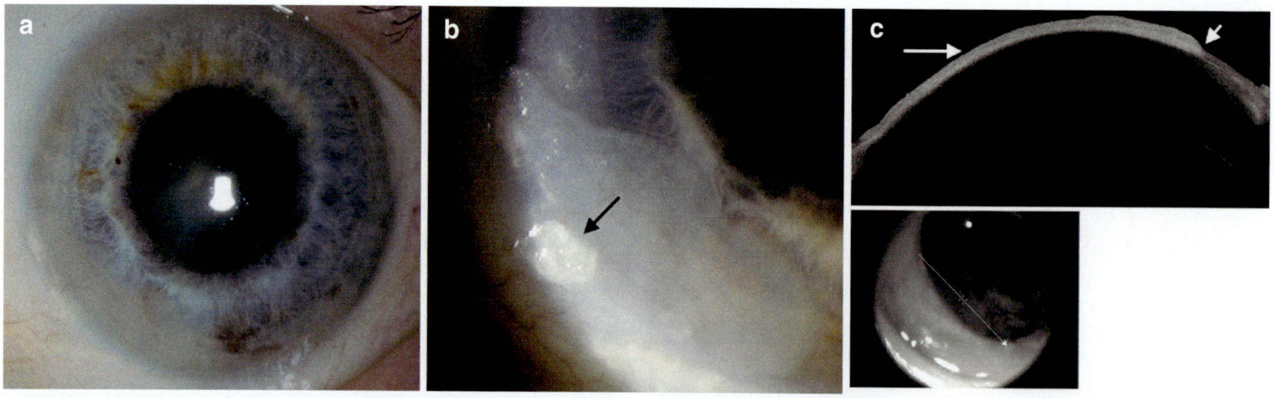

Fig. 5.12 (**a**) CIN presenting as limbal/ peripheral corneal opacity. (**b**) A small area of leukoplakia (arrow) offers the diagnostic clue. (**c**) OCT reveals abruptly (small arrow) thickened and hyper-reflective epithelium (large arrow)

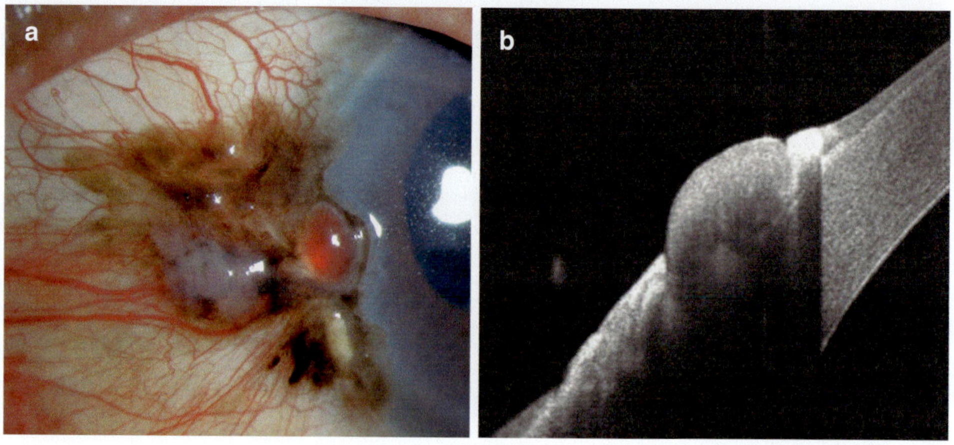

Fig. 5.13 Invasive conjunctival squamous carcinoma in an Indian man. (**a**) The lesion is pigmented, resembling conjunctival melanoma. (**b**) Anterior-segment OCT indicates superficial epithelial involvement with shadowing due to pigmentation

between 3.6% and 15%, was found in pterygium specimens [41, 42]. Thus, histopathological evaluation of all pterygium removed is indicated.

5.5 Differential Diagnosis

The main lesions in the differential diagnosis of OSSN are pinguecula (Fig. 5.14), pterygium (Fig. 5.15), and squamous papilloma (Fig. 5.16) [3].

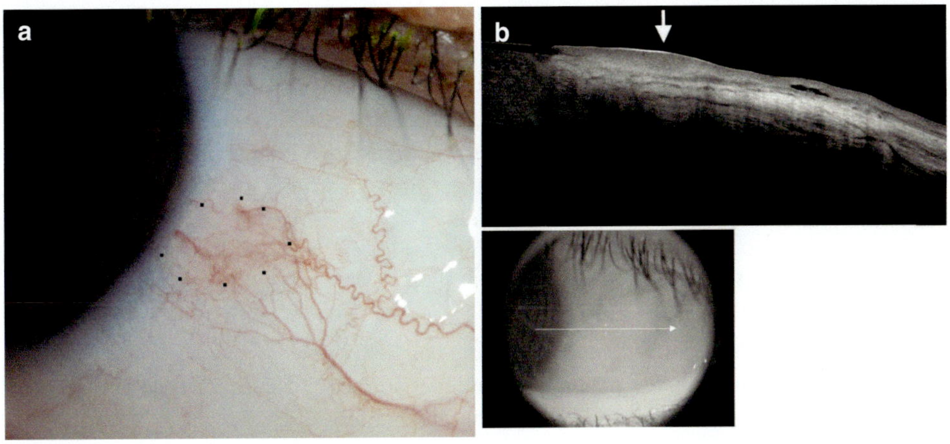

Fig. 5.14 (**a**) A faint yellow-white lesion of conjunctiva resembling pinguecula (encircled by dots). (**b**) OCT reveals an abrupt transition into a thickened and hyper-reflective epithelium (arrow)

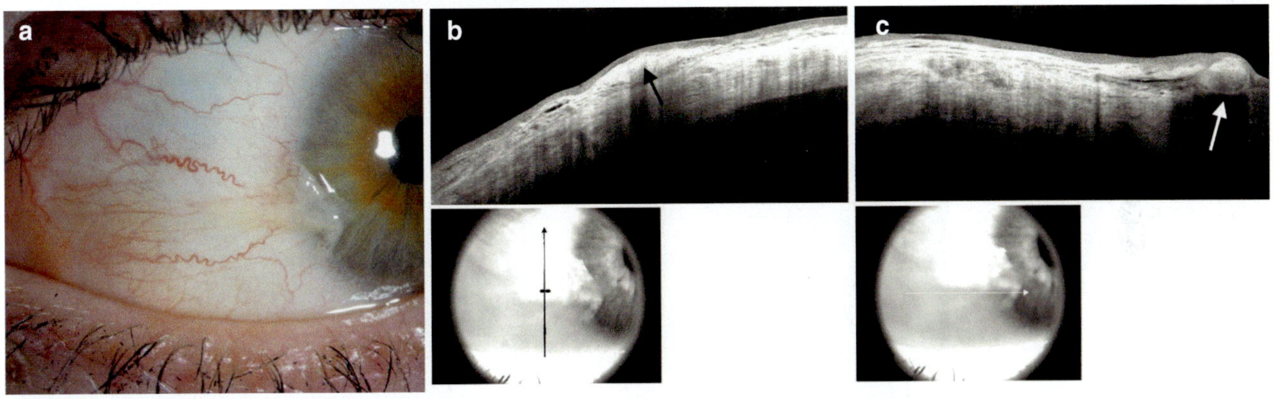

Fig. 5.15 (**a**) Pterygium with nodular thickening mimicking CIN. OCT reveals normal corneal epithelium over a stromal nodular change both in the transverse (**b**, arrow) and longitudinal scan (C, arrow)

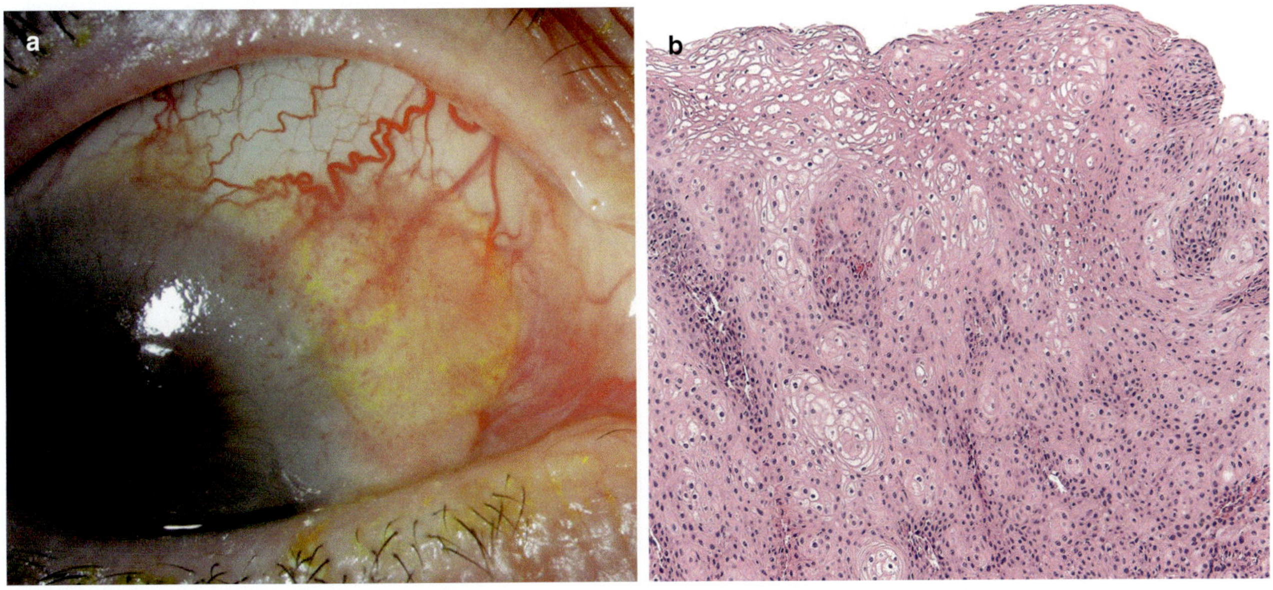

Fig. 5.16 Squamous papilloma. (**a**) A lesion with limbal involvement from 11 to 4 o'clock, with corneal and conjunctival extension. (**b**) Histopathology demonstrated a papillary squamo-proliferative lesion characterized by acanthotic squamous epithelium and fibrovascular cores. No goblet cells were present within the lesion. Features of high-grade dysplasia, such as full-thickness basaloid population lacking orderly maturation, were not identified (hematoxylin and eosin, 100x). (Reprinted from Ganapathy PS, Plesec T, Singh AD. Conjunctival squamous papilloma refractory to interferon α-2b in a patient on systemic immunosuppression (tacrolimus). Am J Ophthalmol Case Rep. 2017 Feb 3;6:1–3. With permission from Elsevier)

5.6 Diagnostic Evaluation

It may be clinically difficult to distinguish between intraepithelial and invasive squamous neoplasia and between these and other lesions such as pinguecula and pterygium, especially with leukoplakia and squamous papilloma.

5.6.1 Staining Patterns

In our experience, the use of fluorescein staining can help in the diagnosis, emphasizing the papillary or granular surface of part of the OSSN lesion and delineating its borders (Fig. 5.17) [37, 43]. Others have used rose bengal, lissamine green [44, 45], or 1% toluidine blue eye drops [46] (Fig. 5.18).

5.6.2 Imaging Techniques

Recent publications have described the use of high-frequency ultrasound in the diagnosis of OSSN and particularly in estimating the depth of invasion [47]. Others have used confocal microscopy [48] or ultra-high-resolution optical coherence tomography [49], even with coexisting ocular surface diseases (Figs. 5.12, 5.13, 5.14, 5.15 and 5.16) [50] (Chap. 1). However, the definitive diagnosis must be a histological one.

5.6.3 Diagnostic Cytology

Preoperative cytological diagnosis may be of value in planning surgery in order to prevent unnecessary removal of

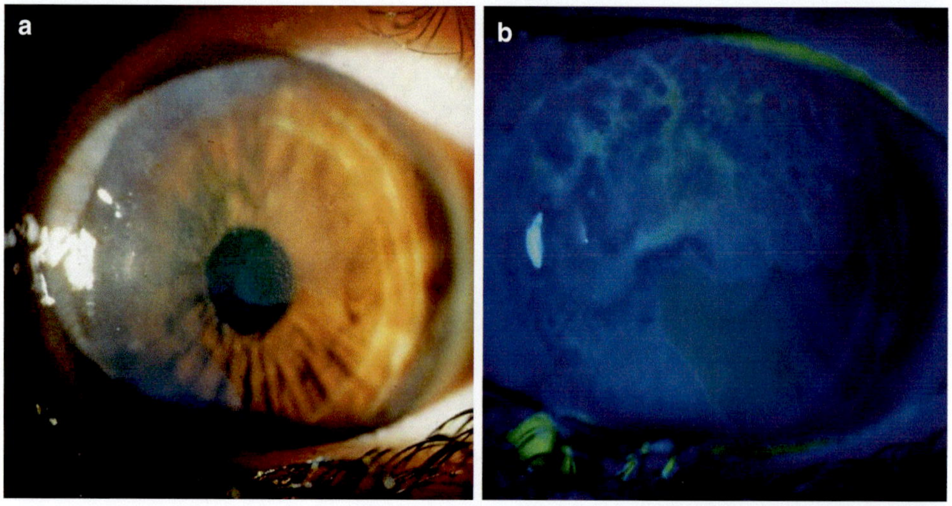

Fig. 5.17 (**a**) A diffuse corneal involvement by CIN showing hazy and irregular corneal surface. (**b**) Staining with fluorescein shows the granular surface of the involved cornea and clearly delineates the border between the affected and nonaffected areas

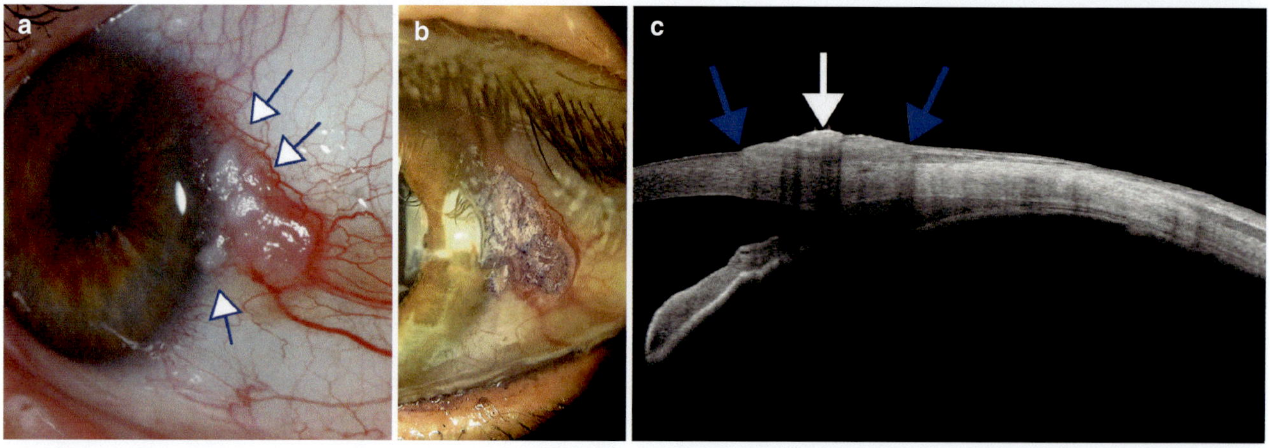

Fig. 5.18 A limbal OSSN. (**a**) A clinical picture of a limbal OSSN. Note the three white areas of hyperkeratosis (arrows). (**b**) A toluidine blue staining highlights the irregular epithelium with a specific speckled staining pattern. Staining with fluorescein before toluidine blue helps reduce nonspecific staining in an unknown mechanism. (**c**) An anterior-segment OCT (Cassia) image shows the lesion between the blue arrows and an area of hypoerkeratosis (white arrow)

large areas of normal conjunctiva in the case of a benign lesion and to prevent partial excision of malignant lesions.

5.6.3.1 Exfoliative Cytology

Cells from the conjunctival surface are obtained with a platinum spatula, brush, or cotton wool tip. The cells are then smeared onto slides and fixed in 90% alcohol. Papanicolaou and Giemsa stains are used to examine the specimen [51, 52]. The advantages of this technique are the ability to obtain prospective cytological information on the nature of the lesion, mainly in differentiating between benign and malignant lesions, and in the ability to sample multiple sites, also simplifying follow-up evaluation after treatment. The major disadvantage is that only superficial cells are obtained with this technique. Sometimes, only keratinized cells are obtained. Exfoliative cytology does not provide information on the degree of the tumor invasion, which may be crucial in the overall management.

5.6.3.2 Impression Cytology

Another method of obtaining cells from the surface of the conjunctival lesion is by impression cytology [53]. With this technique, several types of filter paper, such as cellulose acetate filter paper, millipore filter paper, or biopore membrane device, are gently placed in contact with the ocular surface, sampling the most superficial cells. These are fixed and stained with Papanicolaou stain. The advantages and disadvantages of exfoliation cytology also apply to impression cytology.

5.7 Histopathological Features

Only histological evaluation of excised lesions, either from incisional or excisional biopsy, can differentiate between the three lesions in the spectrum of OSSN [1, 2, 54].

5.7.1 Dysplasia

Dysplastic lesions exhibit mild, moderate, or severe degrees of cellular atypia that may involve various thicknesses of the epithelium, starting from the basal layer outward (Fig. 5.19). These lesions show a modification of epithelial cell organization with various degrees of loss of the normal cellular polarity. Usually, the most superficial layers are uninvolved. In cases with severe dysplastic changes, it may be difficult to distinguish the lesion from carcinoma in situ.

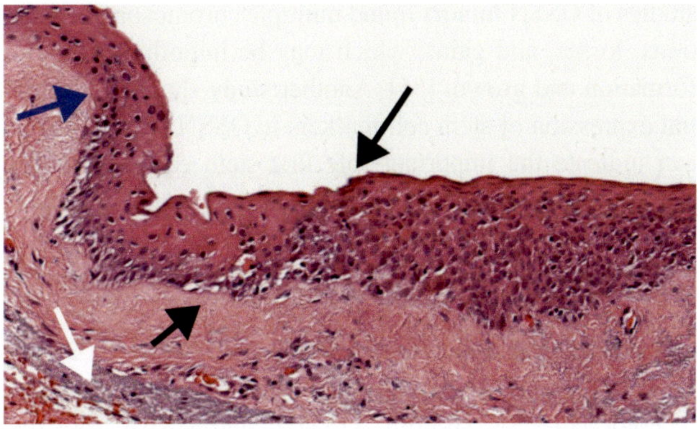

Fig. 5.19 A histological picture of conjunctival intraepithelial dysplasia (CIN) overlying pterygium. The epithelium lost its normal cellular polarity. The normal conjunctival epithelium is seen on the left side of the blue arrow, with mild dysplasia between the blue and black arrows and marked acanthosis (thickening) with dysplasia of almost the entire epithelial thickness (severe dysplasia, carcinoma in situ) to the right of the line connecting the two black arrows (hematoxylin and eosin, original magnification × ~ 20). Note the underlying blueish solar elastosis of the substantia propria, making the diagnosis of pterygium (white arrow)

5.7.2 Carcinoma in Situ

Carcinoma in situ may show all the histological features of SCC; however, it is usually confined to the epithelium, respecting the basement membrane. Carcinoma in situ usually shows a total loss of normal cellular maturation and affects the full thickness of the epithelium. The cells are large and usually elongated. Keratinized cells may be identified, and mitotic figures can be present in all layers.

5.7.3 Invasive Squamous Cell Carcinoma

Invasive squamous cell carcinoma shows features similar to carcinoma in situ, but the basement membrane of the epithelium is breached, and the subepithelial tissue of the conjunctiva is invaded. Most conjunctival SCCs are well differentiated, and they often show surface keratinization. The tumor may show various degrees of cellular pleomorphism. In examining such lesions, hyperplastic and hyperchromatic cells, individually keratinized cells (dyskeratosis), concentric collections of keratinized cells (horn pearls), loss of cellular cohesiveness, and atypical mitotic figures may be observed. The subepithelial tissue in invasive SCC is usually inflamed and contains islands of atypical epithelial cells. In pigmented individuals, OSSN can be pigmented due to abnormal proliferation of melanocytes in the lesions. Genetic studies of OSSN tumors found multiple chromosomal alterations, losses, and gains, which may be important in tumor formation and growth [55]. Another study showed differential expression of stem cell markers in OSSN tumors, which can indicate the important role that stem cells, especially limbal epithelium stem cells, play in the genesis of OSSN [56]. Recent studies found increased expression of biomarkers, which have implications for the prognosis and treatment of conjunctival SCC. These include expression of programmed cell death ligands 1 and 2 (PD-L1, PD-L2) and programmed cell death 1 (PD1), epidermal growth factor receptor (EGFR), stratifin, FOXP3, and CXCR4-positive regulatory T cells [57–61].

5.7.4 Staging

In the recent edition of the American Joint Committee on Cancer (AJCC) staging system, the primary OSSN tumors are classified according to the degree of depth of invasion, as found in histopathological evaluation; the size of the lesions; and the involvement of neighboring structures (Table 5.1) [62]. The OSSN lesions are divided into carcinoma in situ–Tis, and four stages of invasive SCC: T1 for tumors <5 mm in greatest dimension; T2 for tumors >5 mm in the greatest dimension; T3 for tumors invading adjacent structures (excluding the orbit); and T4 for tumors invading the orbit with or without further extension, divided into four substaging, T4a, b, c, d. While some studies found that the AJCC category of OSSN is a reliable predictor of clinical outcome [63], others did not find this staging a useful guide for initial management, and these authors suggest a partial reclassification [64]. The intraepithelial neoplasia, which is not subdivided in the AJCC staging, has been categorized by others as mild dysplasia (grade 1/3), moderate dysplasia (grade 2/3), and severe dysplasia (grade 3/3 or carcinoma in situ) [64, 65]. Most cases are classified by the AJCC as grade T3, which includes a spectrum of tumors ranging from small tumors with minimal corneal involvement on one end to tumors with an intraocular extension on the other end [65]. Therefore, the suggestion is to reclassify this group.

Table 5.1 AJCC (eighth ed.) definition of primary tumor (T) [45, 46]

T category	T criteria
TX	The primary tumor cannot be assessed
T0	No evidence of a primary tumor
Tis	Carcinoma in situ
T1	Tumor (< 5 mm in greatest dimension) invades through the conjunctival basement membrane without invasion of adjacent structures
T2	Tumor (> 5 mm in greatest dimension) invades through the conjunctival basement membrane without invasion of adjacent structures
T3	Tumor invades adjacent structures (excluding the orbit)
T4	Tumor invades the orbit with or without further extension
T4a	Tumor invades orbital soft tissue without bone invasion
T4b	Tumor invades bone
T4c	Tumor invades adjacent paranasal sinuses
T4d	Tumor invades brain

Used with permission of the American Joint Committee on Cancer (AJCC), Chicago, Illinois. The original and primary source for this information is the AJCC Cancer Staging Manual, Seventh Edition (2010) published by Springer Science+Business Media

Used with permission of the American College of Surgeons, Chicago, Illinois. The original and primary source for this information is the AJCC Cancer Staging Manual, Eighth Edition (2017) published by Springer International Publishing

5.7.5 Histopathological and Clinical Variants

Several types of invasive conjunctival SCC with rather aggressive behavior have been reported [2]. Because of the aggressiveness of these variants, which often invade the eyeball and the orbital tissue and even metastasize to lymphatics and distant sites, they should be histopathologically differentiated from less aggressive, conventional SCC.

5.7.5.1 Spindle Cell Squamous Carcinoma

The spindle cell variant of SCC exhibits spindle-shaped cells, which may be difficult to distinguish from fibroblasts.

5.7.5.2 Mucoepidermoid Carcinoma

Mucoepidermoid carcinoma is a variant of conjunctival SCC that shows, besides the squamous cells, mucus-secreting cells that are positively stained for mucopolysaccharides. In a recent evaluation, Mudhar et al. found that these tumors are not real mucoepidermoid carcinoma but represent predominantly SCC with mucinous differentiation and adenosquamous carcinoma [66].

5.7.5.3 Adenoid Squamous Cell Carcinoma

Another aggressive variant of conjunctival SCC is the adenoid squamous carcinoma, which histologically shows extracellular hyaluronic acid but no intracellular mucin.

5.7.5.4 Squamous Cell Carcinoma of Cornea

OSSN arising in the corneal epithelium is rare [9, 67]. There is controversy about its origin. Some authors support the possible potential of the corneal epithelium to undergo dysplastic and cancerous changes, while others believe that the origin of corneal OSSN is at the limbus (Fig. 5.20). Histologically, the corneal intraepithelial neoplasia is similar to that in the limbal region and conjunctiva. Usually, the Bowman's layer is intact. Corneal intraepithelial neoplasia

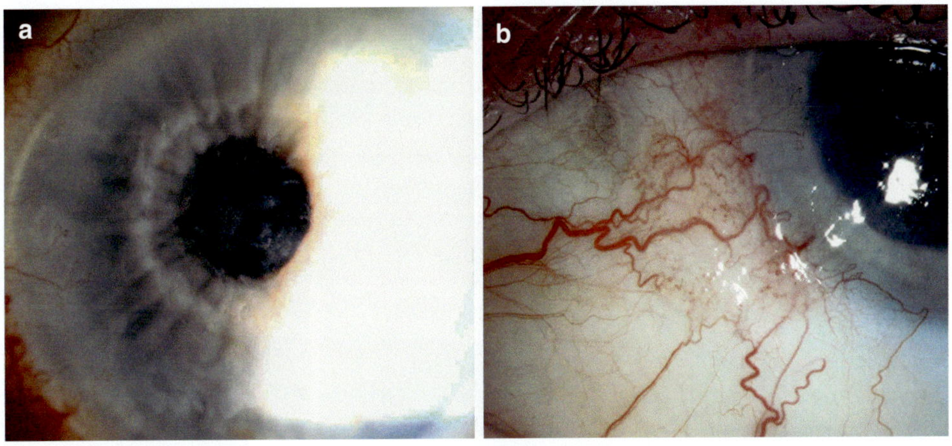

Fig. 5.20 (**a**) Squamous cell carcinoma of cornea resembling filamentary keratitis. (**b**) Examination of the limbus reveals a small area of conjunctival thickening with fine intrinsic vascularity

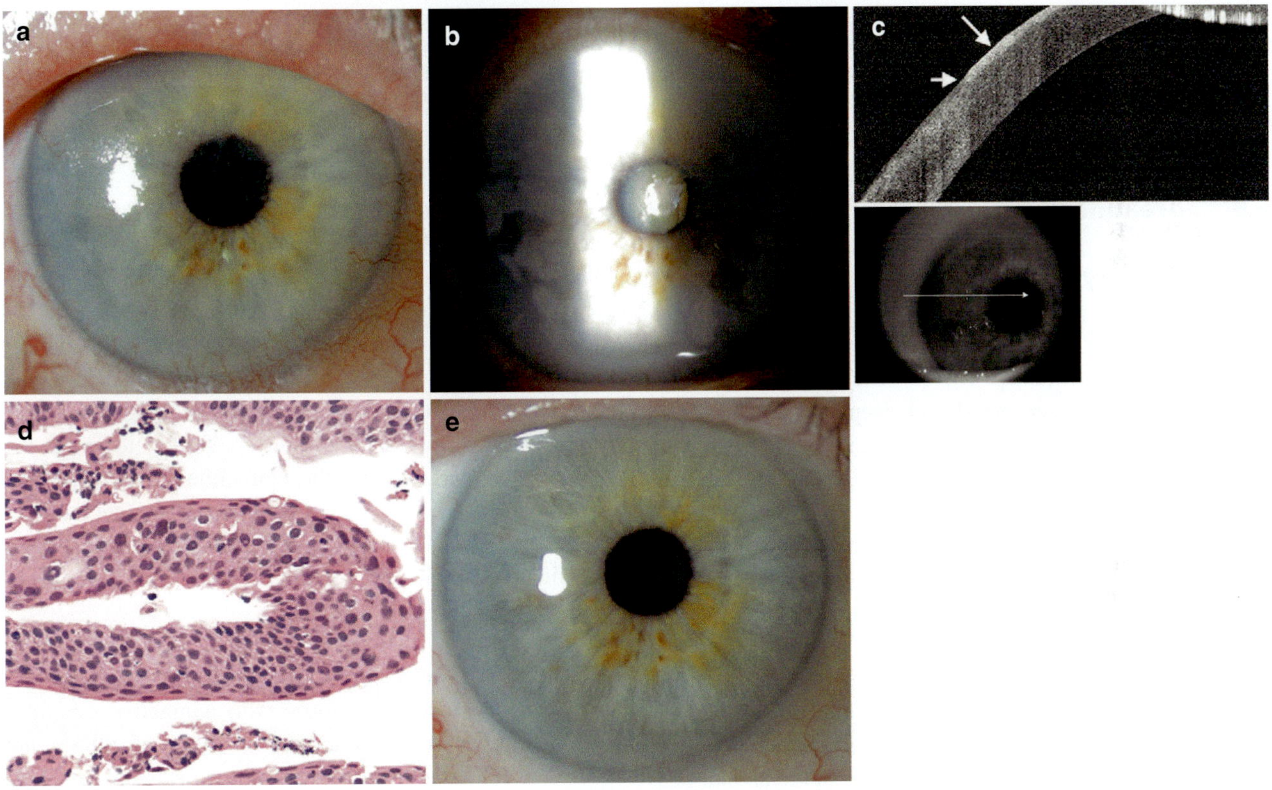

Fig. 5.21 Corneal CIN. (**a**) A patient was treated for nonspecific keratitis with topical steroids for several months. (**b**) Note superficial corneal opacity on transillumination. (**c**) OCT reveals an abruptly thickened (small arrow) and hyper-reflective epithelium (large arrow). (**d**) A diagnostic biopsy shows strips of thickened epithelium with nuclei that are large, hyperchromatic, and haphazardly arranged, suggestive of CIN. (**e**) Topical treatment with interferon alpha-2b (one million units/mL) led to total resolution within 3 months

has a tendency to recur because of inadequate scraping, but with current methods of treatment (topical therapy), this rarely occurs (Fig. 5.21) [37, 43].

5.7.5.5 Squamous Cell Carcinoma in Anophthalmic Socket

A review of nine published cases indicates a long interval between enucleation and the diagnosis of SCC (mean, 45 years), predominant diffuse involvement of the upper eyelid, advanced stage at diagnosis, and tendency for metastases (Fig. 5.22). It is speculated that the presence of prosthesis-induced chronic inflammation may be a factor in initiating and masking the signs and symptoms of OSSN [68].

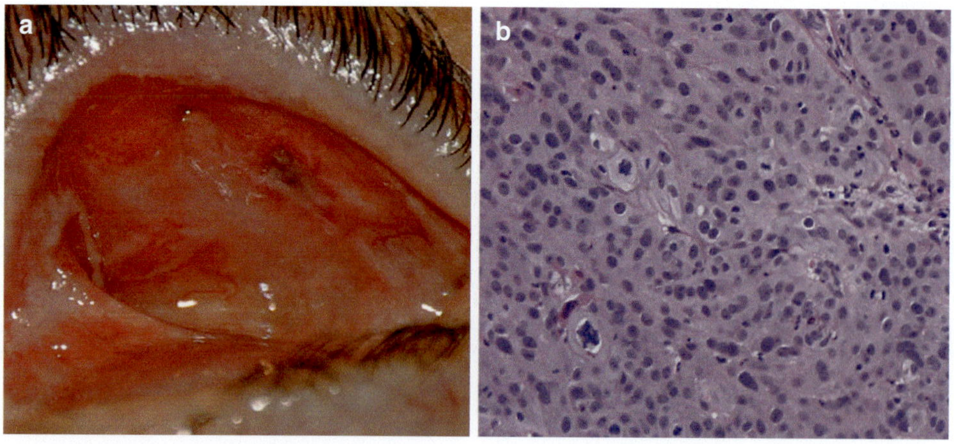

Fig. 5.22 (**a**) A recurrent squamous cell carcinoma in the superior nasal aspect of the tarsal conjunctiva of the upper lid in an anophthalmic socket. (**b**) Poorly differentiated invasive carcinoma without keratinization was associated with an overlying squamous carcinoma in situ. Although some areas were suggestive of sebaceous differentiation, *oil red* O and immunostaining for androgen receptor were both negative (40× magnification, hematoxylin and eosin). (Reprinted from Espana EM, Levine M, Schoenfield L, Singh AD. Ocular surface squamous neoplasia in an anophthalmic socket 60 years after enucleation. Surv Ophthalmol. 2011;56(6):539–43. With permission from Elsevier)

5.8 Treatment

5.8.1 Surgery

Surgical excision of the OSSN lesion is the traditional method of treatment (Chap. 13). Its success depends on the involvement of the peripheral and deep surgical margins. One approach to avoid recurrence is to excise the tumor tissue with wide surgical margins of 2–3 mm [3, 69, 70] (Fig. 5.23a, b). When the deep cornea or sclera are involved, deep lamellar keratectomy or sclerectomy is performed. Recurrence rates following excision of OSSN alone range from 15 to 52%, with an average of 30% [1]. Erie et al. [9] found 5% recurrence when the surgical margins were free and 53% recurrence when they were involved. Similarly, Pizzarello and Jakobiec found 69% recurrence when dysplastic tissues were left at the surgical margins [3].

Therefore, techniques to ensure clear surgical margins have been applied. Frozen sections were used by Char et al. to assess the surgical margins [71]. However, there was a disparity between the apparently free surgical margins and the recurrence of the OSSN. Buus et al. have used a modified Mohs' micrographic technique that was developed for cutaneous tumors to ensure clear surgical margins [72]. No recurrences were documented in their series of 19 patients. Excision with large margins, especially when cryotherapy is applied to the tumor bed and the margins, may necessitate the use of an amniotic membrane graft to close the surgical wound.

An alternative approach requires minimal margins no larger than 0.5 mm around the lesion, and pending the histopathological report, administering adjuvant topical treatment [chemotherapy with 0.02% mitomycin C (MMC) or 1% 5-fluorouracil (5FU), or immunotherapy with interferon alpha 2 (IFN α2)]—see below (5.8.4). Of note, one should take care to scrape off the involved corneal epithelium without cutting into Bowman's layer, which serves as a barrier from invasions into the stroma. This can be achieved with a blunt instrument such as a hockey blade or with the application of alcohol over the involved epithelium to break the hemi-desmosomes binding the epithelium to its basement membrane (Fig. 5.23c, d). Deep lamellar keratectomy or sclerectomy should be avoided, and a histopathological diagnosis of invasive SCC mandates adjuvant brachytherapy—see below (5.8.3).

Two cases of OSSN with intraocular involvement were managed by local excision. Char et al. [71] reported a successful iridocyclochoroidectomy with adjunctive cryotherapy. Most eyes with intraocular invasion of OSSN are enucleated [73], and in cases with orbital invasion, exenteration is required.

5.8.2 Cryotherapy

Because of the high recurrence rate of OSSN after surgical excision alone, Fraunfelder et al. advocated the use of cryosurgery in the treatment of eyelid and ocular surface tumors [74]. Later on, he and others reported the use of combined excision and cryotherapy treatment for OSSN with a recurrence rate as low as 0–12%. Cryotherapy acts both by destroying the tumor cells and obliterating its microcirculation, resulting in ischemic infarction of both normal and tumor tissue. Side effects include iritis, alterations in intra-

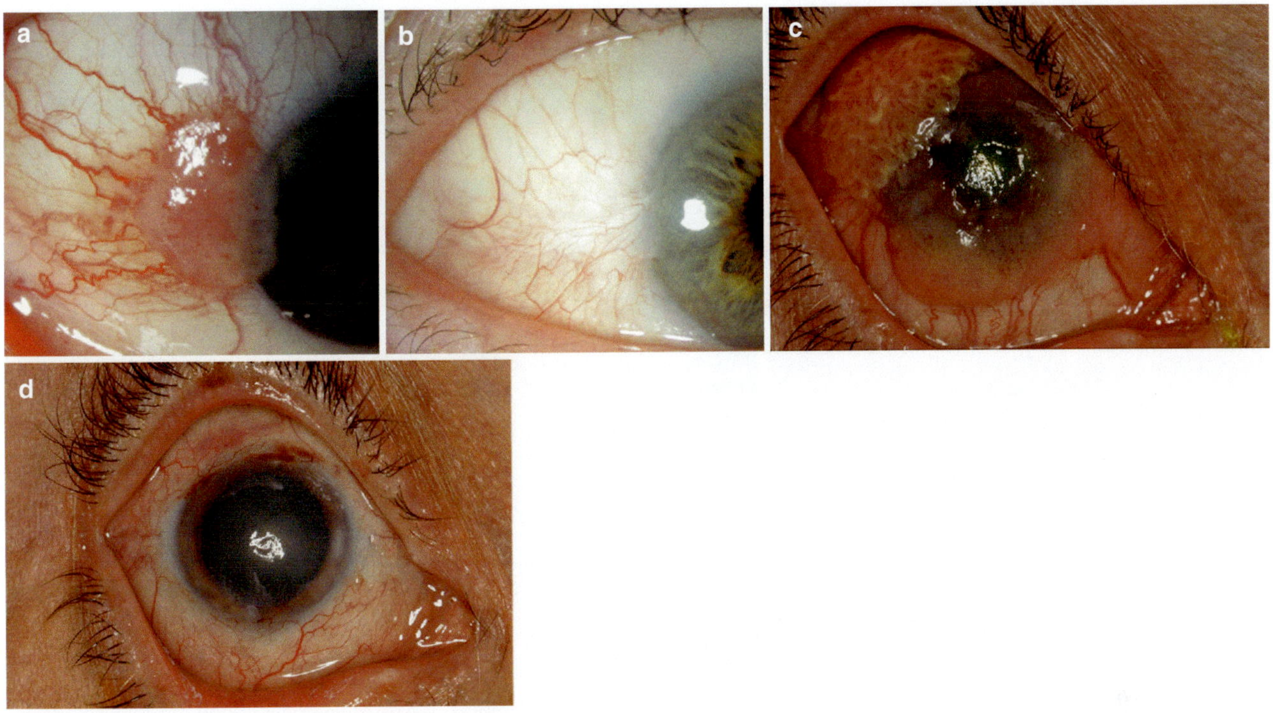

Fig. 5.23 CIN Local excision. (**a**) Pretreatment appearance. (**b**) Following excision with 2 mm clear margins, alcohol epitheliectomy, double freeze–thaw cryotherapy applications and primary closure. A 360-degree conjunctival SCC before (**c**) and after (**d**) surgical excision with minimal (~0.5 mm) margins, a blunt hockey-blade removal of the involved cornea epithelium (without alcohol), and no cryotherapy or amniotic membrane

ocular pressure, inflammation, corneal edema, scarring, and superficial corneal vascularization, sector iris atrophy, ablation of the peripheral retina, and ectropion.

5.8.3 Brachytherapy

Brachytherapy has been used for many years in the treatment of OSSN. A radioactive plaque is placed over the tumor bed (and over the now-closed surgical wound), and the radiation dose is calculated to a depth of 1 mm if the sclera was not involved or 2 mm if the tumor invaded the sclera. The most commonly used radioactive material in the past was strontium 90, with a recommended dose of 20–180 Gy to the tumor surface [75]. The current more popular geta source is ruthenium-106, with a recommended dose of 50–320 Gy to the tumor bed with complete tumor regression (Fig. 5.24) [76–78]. Sources for gamma radiation include phosphorus 32 [79] and iodine 125 applicators [80] (Fig. 5.25). Reported complications include post-irradiation conjunctivitis, dry eye, conjunctival telangiectasis and scarring, symblepharon, scleral ulceration, corneal perforation, and cataract. However, with lower doses, the side effects are minor. Brachytherapy is recommended only after a histopathological diagnosis and is usually used as adjuvant therapy following the tumor resection. In cases of intraocular invasion, brachytherapy can effectively treat the invasion and preserve the eye. Treatment of cases of invasive SCC with proton beam therapy was also reported [81, 82].

5.8.4 Topical Chemotherapy and Immunotherapy

Because of the possible complications of surgical excision, cryotherapy, and brachytherapy, topical medical therapy has become an expanding field. Topical drops of mitomycin C (MMC), 5-fluorouracil (5FU), and interferon alpha-2b (INF-α2b) (which can also be administered as intralesional injections) have shown promising and comparable results as primary therapy for OSSN, suggesting similar long-term clinical benefits. They have also been used as an adjuvant to surgical excision. Recently, newer and less studied agents, such as immune checkpoint inhibitors, retinoic acid, aloe vera, and antivascular endothelial growth factor, have been shown to have antineoplastic properties and potential for the treatment of OSSN [83] (Chap. 12).

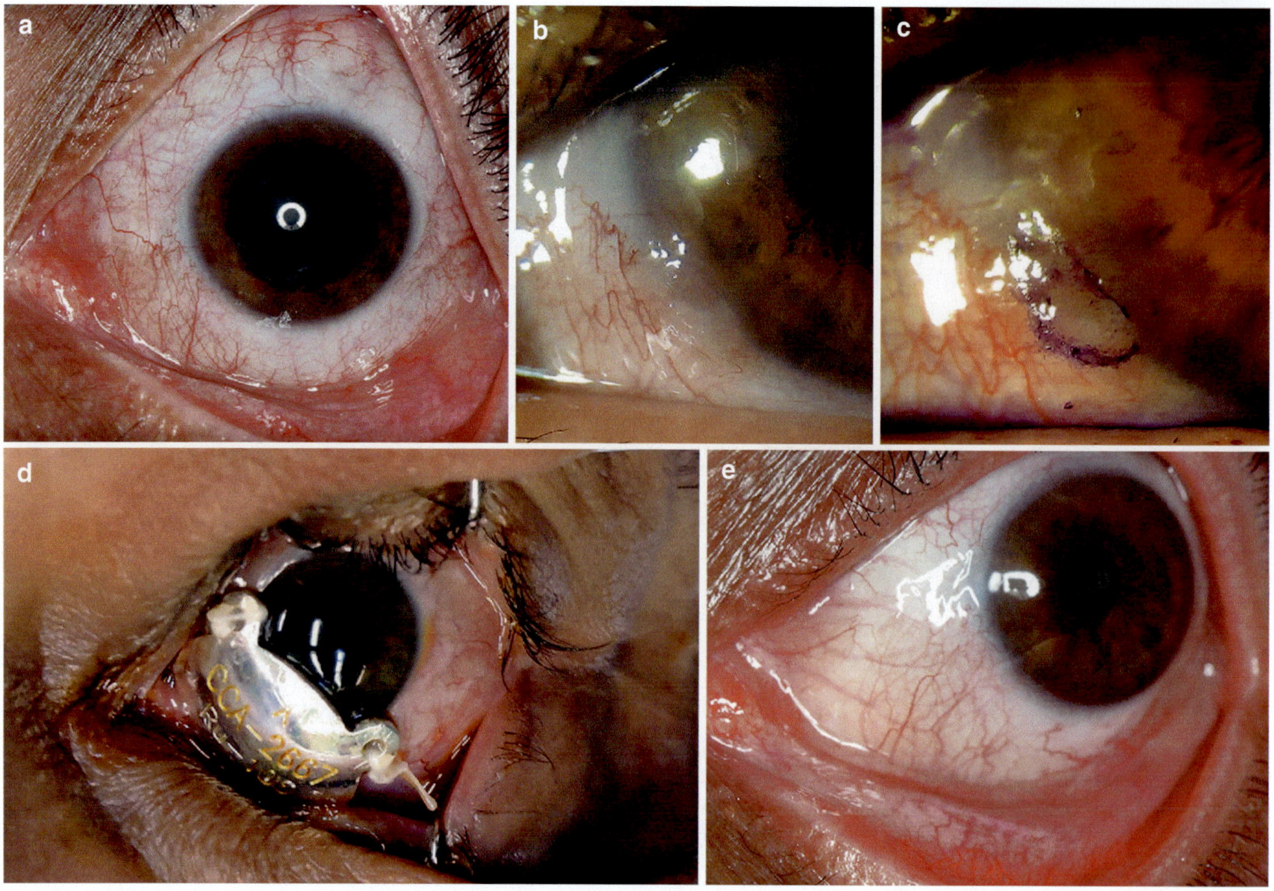

Fig. 5.24 Recurrent CIN treated with Ru-106 plaque brachytherapy. (**a**) A limbal lesion was excised and pathologically diagnosed as CIN grade I–II. Adjuvant treatment with three cycles of 0.02% mitomycin C (MMC) resulted in no evidence of disease at the end of the 12 weeks of treatment. However, 14 weeks later, there was a local recurrence: (**b**) a gelatinous lesion re-appeared on the 8 o'clock limbus. (**c**) The lesion strained in a fine granular pattern with toluidine blue, indicating a 90% risk for malignancy. The patient elected treatment over continued follow-up. (**d**) A small 15 mm in diameter, round-shaped (CCA) ruthenium (Ru-106) plaque was sutured to the sclera over the conjunctiva and limbus (14 h—5000 cGy to a depth of 1 mm). There is no need to use temporary donor tissue to cover the plaque and the eyelids close comfortably over the plaque with no need for tarsorrhaphy. (**e**) At 8 months of follow-up, there is no sign of a local recurrence or melting of the sclera

5.8.4.1 Mitomycin C Drops

Mitomycin C is an antineoplastic/antibiotic drug that acts as an alkylating agent. Our group introduced and promoted the use of topical MMC since the early 1990s [37]. Our protocol since then includes the use of 0.02% (0.2 mg/mL) MMC drops four times daily for 2 weeks of treatment and then 2 weeks without it [2, 37, 43], with repetitions as needed, with a response rate of 95%. Throughout an entire cycle of 4 weeks, we give topical steroids four times daily to ameliorate the side effects. Other groups have used 0.04% MMC in various lengths of cycles and periods between cycles with a good response (Fig. 5.26) [84–86]. The use of a low dose of 0.002% has also been reported [87].

The main adverse reactions to MMC are conjunctival hyperemia, superficial punctate epithelial erosions, allergic conjunctivitis, pain, photophobia, and blepharospasm. In using the higher concentration of 0.04% MMC, there was one case of punctal stenosis [84], and repeating this concentration in multiple courses, limbal cell deficiency was reported [84, 86, 88]. In treating OSSN, there is no reason to use 0.04% MMC. In using 0.02% MMC, the side effects disappear within 2 weeks of stopping the treatment with or without the addition of lubricants and topical steroids. Even in the treatment of pigmented conjunctival lesions, we now limit the concentration to 0.03% to avoid limbal stem cell deficiency.

MMC is the most potent topical drug for treating OSSN, showing a fast response. It is cheap and stable. Because of its superficial effect, it should not be used for invasive SCC as a primary treatment. However, it has been used successfully in treating patients with partially excised invasive conjunctival SCC without evidence of recurrence [89]. It has also been used intraoperatively [90, 91].

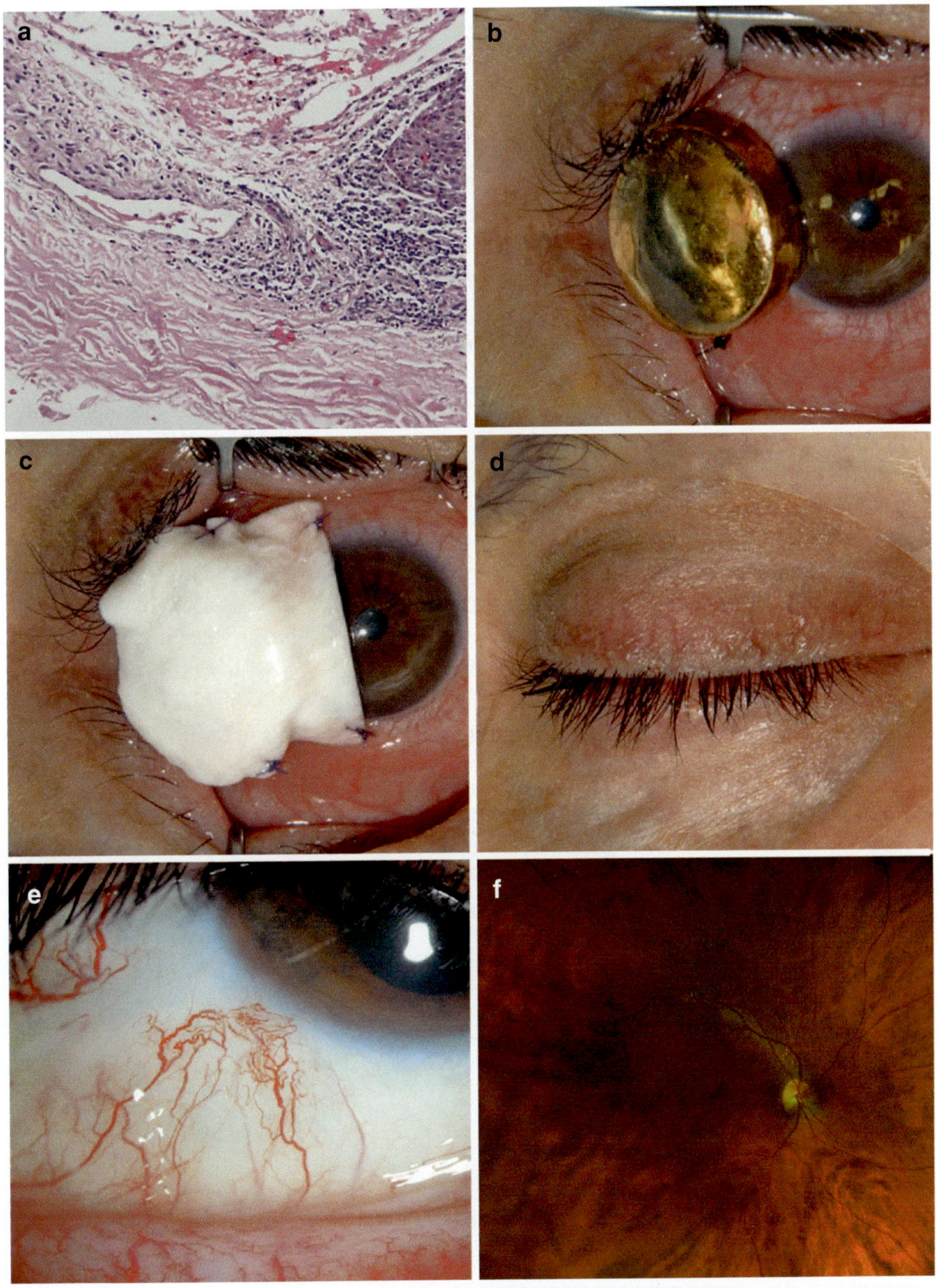

Fig. 5.25 Invasive conjunctival SCC with extension into sclera (**a**) treated with iodine 125 brachytherapy (45 Gy to the depth of 3 mm) (**b**). The plaque was covered with donor pericardium (**c**) followed by temporary trans-marginal tarsorrhaphy (**d**) to minimize postoperative discomfort for the duration of the implant placement (48 h). The patient is recurrence-free at 5 years with visual acuity of 20/25 due to minimal cataract (**e**) and without radiation retinopathy (**f**)

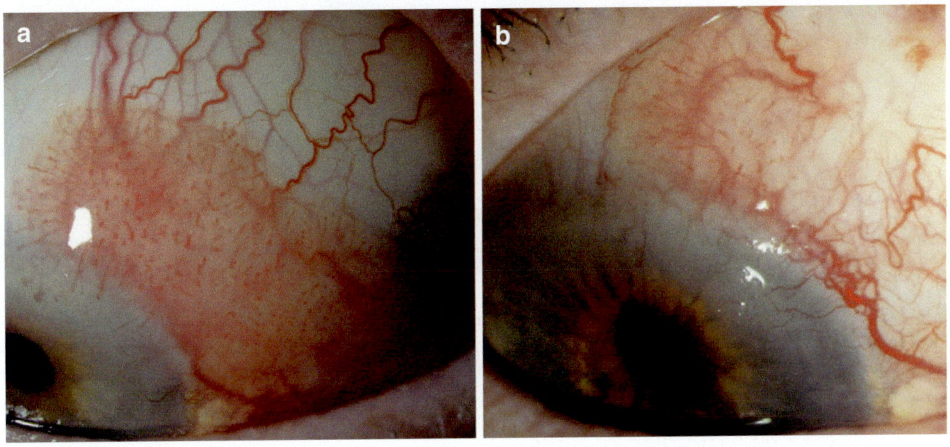

Fig. 5.26 Diffuse CIN treated with MMC. (**a**) Pretreatment appearance. (**b**) Post-treatment appearance: note the partial resolution after 1 week of topical MMC (0.04% qid)

5.8.4.2 5-Fluorouracil (5FU) Drops

5FU has been used for OSSN as a sole treatment or as an adjuvant treatment to surgical excision, with a good response and a low recurrence rate [90–93]. 5FU 1% has been administered in different protocols, such as four times daily for 1 week followed by 3 weeks off with repetitions up to four cycles [92]. Others used it four times daily for 4 weeks [93]. In these recent reports, complete tumor regression was achieved in 82–83%, and in a more recent study, the recurrence rate was 19% in 2 years [94].

With 5FU, patients experience toxic keratoconjunctivitis, including conjunctival hyperemia, superficial keratitis, filamentary keratitis, and sometimes pain, tearing, and photophobia, but usually, no long-term side effects are found [91–93]. 5FU is a potent, relatively cheap, and stable drug.

5.8.4.3 Interferon Alpha-2b

The use of recombinant interferon alpha-2b (IFN-α2b), initially by intralesional injections and later by topical applications, was pioneered and promoted by Karp and colleagues for the treatment of CIN [95]. In using interferon alpha-2b four times daily with a dose of one million IU/ml, the response rate was 81%; and in using three million IU/ml, the response rate was 92% (Figs. 5.21 and 5.27). There was no response of invasive SCC to topical interferon alpha-2b [96]. Shields and colleagues used interferon alpha-2b as an adjuvant treatment to surgical excision with complete control in 95% [97]. Krilis et al. [98] showed a higher response to treatment by interferon alpha-2b when combining it with topical retinoic acid every other day, achieving a 97.75% response rate.

Topical INF-α2b eye drops are well tolerated with minimal side effects such as conjunctival hyperemia and occasional follicular conjunctivitis [96]. When injecting subconjunctivally, the patients also experience systemic side effects such as a "flu-like" syndrome (Figs. 5.2 and 5.28) [99].

Using INF-α2b, tumor resolution takes longer than with MMC and 5FU, on average 4 months, with a high response rate of 92.5% and recurrence of 0–17% [97–101]. The downsides of topical INF-α2b are its high cost and that it must be refrigerated. Unfortunately, following its market withdrawal, there is a worldwide supply shortage of interferon alpha-2b [102]. Recently, pegylated interferon alpha-2a was used successfully [103].

Table 5.2 compares the main features of MMC, 5FU, and INF-α2b. (For more details, see Chap. 12.)

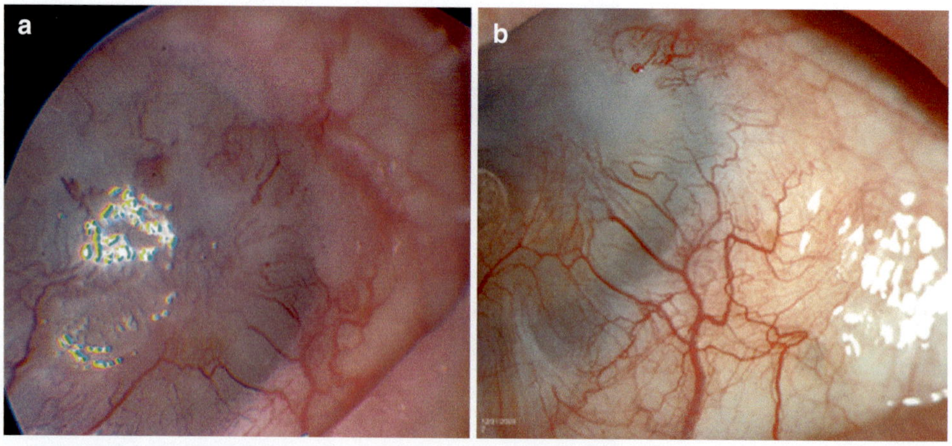

Fig. 5.27 Multiple recurrent CIN associated with limbal stem cell deficiency due to multiple previous excisions. (**a**) Pretreatment clinical picture. (**b**) Following treatment with topical interferon alpha-2b one million units/ml for 3 months, there was complete regression of the focal CIN

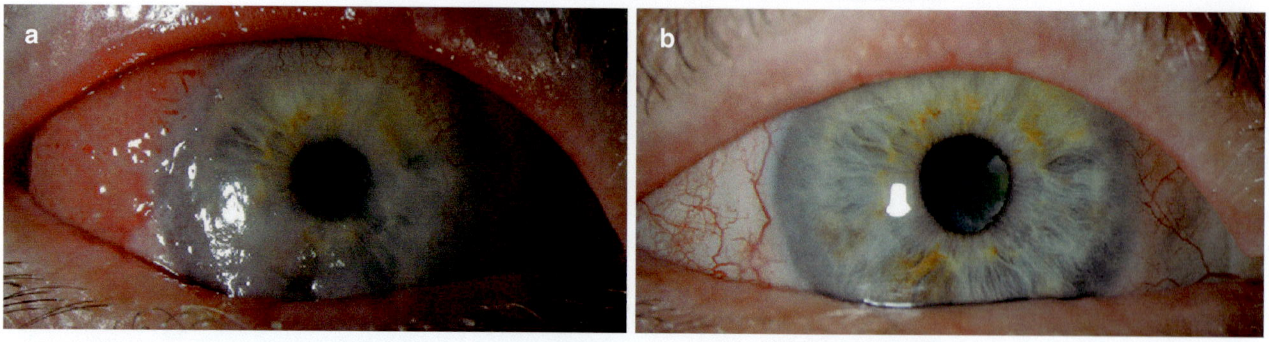

Fig. 5.28 Diffuse conjunctival and corneal CIN right eye. (**a**) A pretreatment clinical picture. He was treated with four subconjunctival injections of interferon alpha 2b (three million units/0.5 mL) given at 1–2 weeks intervals combined with topical interferon alpha 2b (one million units/mL). (**b**) There was total resolution after 6 months of topical therapy. The patient has remained recurrence-free for 24 months

Table 5.2 Local chemotherapy for OSSN

	MMC	5FU	INF-α2b
Response rate	82–100%	80–93%	80–100%
Time to resolution	Fast	Medium	Slow
Side effects	+++ (0.04%) ++ (0.02%)	++	+
Systemic side effects	–	–	–
Availability	+++	+++	+/–
Cost	Low	Low	High
Stability at room temperature	High	High	Low

5.8.5 The Combined Approach

The fact that tumors recur after the most meticulous surgery, even with the addition of cryotherapy, hints that not all the tumor cells have been destroyed. Thus, our group and others combined a surgical approach without wide surgical margins or cryotherapy, but adding local chemotherapy using mitomycin C, 5FU, or interferon alpha-2b or 2a for intraepithelial diseases and adding, irrespective of histological clearance, and brachytherapy for invasive disease. This combinatorial approach was successful in preserving the ocular surface and effective in treating the OSSN.

5.8.6 Reconstruction

Reconstruction of the ocular surface may be needed after a large excision of ocular surface tumors, and the use of autologous conjunctival transplantation and autologous limbal transplants to restore corneal and limbal areas after treating OSSN by surgery and cryotherapy have been described (Chap. 22). Amniotic membrane transplantation has been used for reconstruction after excision of large ocular surface neoplasia [104–106].

5.9 Prognosis

5.9.1 Local Recurrence

OSSN is considered to be of low-grade malignancy [3, 9]. Conjunctival intraepithelial neoplasias (CIN), including dysplasia and carcinoma in situ, are regarded as precancerous lesions that rarely progress to invasive SCC. However, recurrences of these lesions are common after surgical excision, depending on the involvement of the surgical margins [3, 9]. Erie et al. [9] reported 24% recurrence after the excision of CIN and 41% after the excision of SCC. Lee and Hirst [1] found a recurrence rate of 17% for conjunctival dysplasia, 40% for carcinoma in situ, and 30% for SCC. In this series, 31% had a second recurrence and 8% had more than two recurrences. Galor et al. [107] found that higher-grade lesions, tarsal involvement, and positive margins in the histopathological evaluation are predictors of recurrence. Superior tumor location and leukoplakia also decrease the chance of tumor resolution [94]. Most recurrences develop within 2 years, but later recurrences have been reported. New methods of adjuvant treatment reduce the recurrence rate significantly, as was discussed in the treatment section.

5.9.2 Intraocular Invasion

Intraocular invasion, although rare, may occur in OSSN [70, 108]. It occurs in older patients who had SCC located near the corneoscleral limbus with one or more recurrences after surgical excision [40] (Fig. 5.29a). Ultrasound biomicroscopy is a useful tool to detect intraocular extension of OSSN and reveals uveal thickening and blunting of the anterior chamber's angle. Histopathological examination may show growth of the SCC through the limbus with involvement of the Schlemm's canal, trabecular meshwork, anterior chamber, iris, ciliary body, suprachoroidal space, and choroid, sometimes extending even behind the equator. In very advanced cases, the tumor may involve the entire orbit (Fig. 5.29b).

Brachytherapy is an effective treatment when the tumor is located intraocularly, but in very advanced cases with extraocular extension, extended enucleation or orbital exenteration is required for tumor control [40]. Orbital exenteration has failed to demonstrate overall survival benefits, but it allows local control of the disease [109].

5.9.3 Metastasis

Metastasis of conjunctival SCC is very rare [9, 40, 69, 110]. The main sites of metastasis include preauricular, submandibular, and cervical lymph nodes, parotid gland, lungs, and bones (Fig. 5.30). The main cause of metastasis is a delay in the diagnosis and treatment. Regional lymph node involvement preceded the development of distant metastases; there-

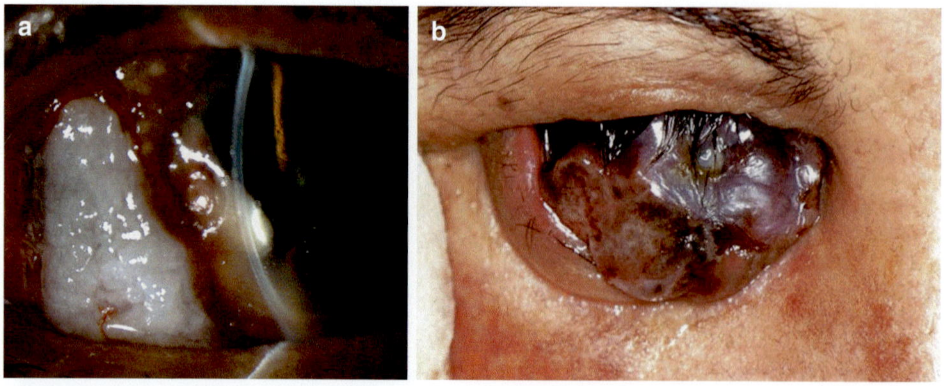

Fig. 5.29 Intraocular invasion of conjunctival SCC. (**a**) The peri-limbal tumor invaded into the anterior chamber and can be seen as a white mass near the anterior chamber's angle and over the iris. (**b**) Advanced conjunctival SCC protruding through the eyelid aperture. The tumor invaded the eyeball and the orbit

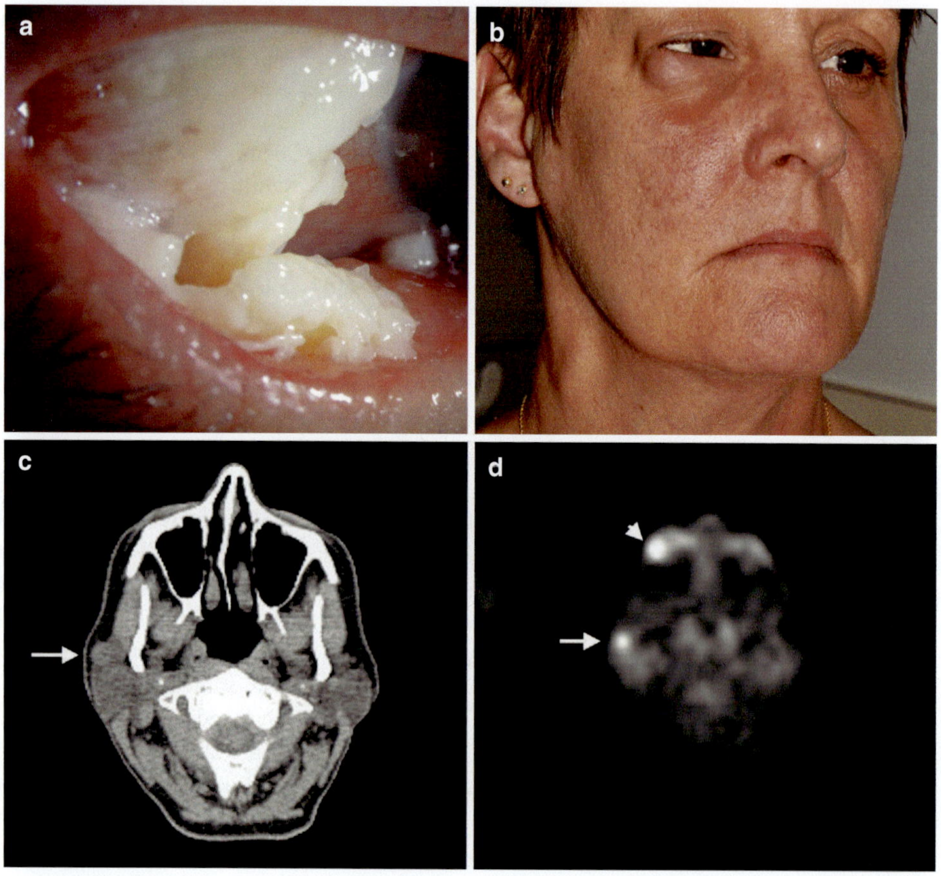

Fig. 5.30 Conjunctival SCC with orbital extension. (**a**) A white mass over the bulbar and tarsal conjunctiva. (**b**) A frontal picture of the head and neck shows the mass under the lower eyelid and the enlargement of the parotid and cervical lymph nodes. (**c**) CT shows an enlarged parotid lymph node (arrow). (**d**) The same lymph node is hypermetabolic on PET scan (large arrow). The conjunctival/orbital tumor is also hypermetabolic on the PET scan (small arrow)

fore, regular examination of these lymph nodes should be performed in suspicious lesions to enable lymph node and radical neck dissection in cases of nodal involvement. Sentinel lymph node biopsy (SLNB) has been used in suspicious cases, but at present, insufficient evidence exists to show that SLNB improves patients' outcomes and survival [111]. When distant metastasis occurs, it leads to the patients' death in most cases [40, 69, 110, 112].

References

1. Lee GA, Hirst LW. Ocular surface squamous neoplasia. Surv Ophthalmol. 1995;39(6):429–50.
2. Pe'er J. Ocular surface squamous neoplasia. Ophthalmol Clin N Am. 2005;18(1):1–13.
3. Pizzarello LD, Jakobiec FA. Bowen's disease of the conjunctiva: a misnomer. In: Jakobiec FA, editor. Ocular and adnexal tumors. Birmingham: Aesculapius; 1978. p. 553–71.

4. Margo CE, White AA. Ocular surface squamous neoplasia: terminology that is conceptually friendly but clinically perilous. Eye. 2014;28:507–9.
5. Sun EC, Fears TR, Goedert JJ. Epidemiology of squamous cell conjunctival cancer. Cancer Epidemiol Biomarkers Prev. 1997;6(2):73–7.
6. Darwhich R, Ghazawi FM, Le M, et al. Epidemiology of invasive ocular surface squamous neoplasia in Canada during 1992-2010. Br J Ophthalmol. 2020;104:1368–72.
7. Gupta N, Sachdev R, Tandon R. Ocular surface squamous neoplasia in xeroderma pigmentosum: clinical spectrum and outcome. Graefes Arch Clin Exp Ophthalmol. 2011;249(8):1217–21.
8. Kao AA, Galor A, Karp CL, et al. Clinicopathologic correlation of ocular surface squamous neoplasms at Bascom Balmer eye institute: 2001 to 2010. Ophthalmology. 2012;119:1773–6.
9. Erie JC, Campbell RJ, Liesegang J. Conjunctival and corneal intraepithelial and invasive neoplasia. Ophthalmology. 1986;93(2):176–83.
10. Newton R, Ferlay J, Reeves G, et al. Effect of ambient solar ultraviolet radiation on incidence of squamous cell carcinoma of the eye. Lancet. 1996;347(9013):1450–1.
11. Gichuhi S, Ohnuma S, Sagoo MS, Burton MJ. Pathophysiology of ocular surface squamous neoplasia. Exp Eye Res. 2014;129:172–82.
12. Scholz SL, Thomasen H, Reis H, et al. Frequent TERT promoter mutations in ocular surface squamous neoplasia. Invest Ophthalmol Vis Sci. 2015;56:5854–61.
13. Lin SY, Liao SL, Hong JB, et al. TERT promoter mutations in periocular carcinomas: implications of ultraviolet light in pathogenesis. Br J Ophthalmol. 2016;100:274–7.
14. McDonnell JM, Mayr AJ, Martin WJ. DNA of human papillomavirus type 16 in dysplastic and malignant lesions of the conjunctiva and cornea. N Engl J Med. 1989;320(22):1442–6.
15. Guthoff R, Marx A, Stroebel P. No evidence for a pathogenic role of human papillomavirus infection in ocular surface squamous neoplasia in Germany. Curr Eye Res. 2009;34(8):666–71.
16. Waddell K, Magyezr J, Boursaghin L, et al. Antibodies against human papillomavirus type 16 (HPV-16) and conjunctival squamous cell neoplasia in Uganda. Br J Cancer. 2003;88(12):2002–3.
17. Ramberg I, Moller-Hansen M, Toft PB, et al. Human papillomavirus infection plays a role in conjunctival squamous cell carcinoma: a systematic review and meta-analysis of observational studies. Acta Ophthalmol. 2021;99:478–88.
18. Ramberg I, Toft PB, Georgsen JB, et al. Conjunctival intraepithelial neoplasia and carcinoma: distinct clinical and histological features in relation to human papilloma virus status. Br J Ophthalmol. 2021;105:878–83.
19. Hanbazazh M, Gyure KA. Ocular human papillomavirus infections. Arch Pathol Lab Med. 2018;142:706–10.
20. Chauhan S, Sen S, Sharma A, et al. Human papillomavirus: a predictor of better survival in ocular surface squamous neoplasia patients. Br J Ophthalmol. 2012;96(12):1517–21.
21. Goedert JJ, Cote TR. Conjunctival malignant disease with AIDS in USA. Lancet. 1995;346(8969):257–8.
22. Gichuhi S, Macharia E, Kabiru J, et al. Clinical presentation of ocular surface squamous neoplasia in Kenya. JAMA Ophthalmol. 2015;133:1305–13.
23. Muchengeti M, Bohlius J, Dhokotera TG. Conjunctival cancer in people living with HIV. Curr Opin Infect Dis. 2021;34:1–7.
24. Perry JD, Polito SC, Chundury RV, Singh AD, Fritz MA, Vidimos AT, Gastman BR, Koyfman SA. Periocular skin cancer in solid organ transplant recipients. Ophthalmology. 2016;123(1):203–8.
25. Dahlke E, Murray CA, Kitchen J, Chan AW. Systematic review of melanoma incidence and prognosis in solid organ transplant recipients. Transplant Res. 2014;6(3):10.
26. Clarke CA, Morton LM, Lynch C, et al. Risk of lymphoma subtypes after solid organ transplantation in the United States. Br J Cancer. 2013;9:109.
27. Kim C, Cheng J, Colegio OR. Cutaneous squamous cell carcinomas in solid organ transplant recipients: emerging strategies for surveillance, staging,and treatment. Semin Oncol. 2016;43:390–4.
28. Shields CL, Ramasubramanian A, Mellen PL, Shields JA. Conjunctival squamous cell carcinoma arising in immunosuppressed patients (organ transplant, human immunodeficiency virus infection). Ophthalmology. 2011;118:2133–7.
29. Ashkenazy N, Karp CL, Wang G, et al. Immunosuppression as a possible risk factor for interferon nonresponse in ocular surface squamous neoplasia. Cornea. 2017;36:506–10.
30. Nandyala S, Mohamed A, Chaurasia S, et al. Ocular features in a large cohort of Indians eith xeroderma pigmentosum. Cornea. 2021;40:571–7.
31. Lehmann J, Seebode C, Martens MC, Emmert S. Xeroderma Pigmentosum—facts and perspectives. Anticancer Res. 2018;38:1159–64.
32. Lim R, Sethi M, Morley AMS. Ophthalmic manifestations of Xeroderma Pigmentosum: a perspective from the United Kingdom. Ophthalmology. 2017;124:1652–61.
33. Chaurasia S, Mulay K, Ramappa M, et al. Corneal changes in xeroderma pigmentosum: a clinicopathologic report. Am J Ophthalmol. 2014;157:495–500.
34. Brooks BP, Thompson AH, Bishop RJ, et al. Ocular manifestations of xeroderma pigmentosum: long-term follow-up highlights the role of DNA repair in protection from sun damage. Ophthalmology. 2013;120:1324–36.
35. Kaliki S, Jajapuram SD, Maniar A, Mishra DK. Ocular and periocular tumors in xeroderma pigmentosum: a study of 120 Asian Indian patients. Am J Ophthalmol. 2019;198:146–53.
36. Suarez MJ, Rivera-Michlig R, Dubovy S, Rodriguez FJ. Clinicopathological features of ophthalmic neoplasms arising in the setting of Xeroderma Pigmentosum. Ocul Oncol Pathol. 2015;2:112–21.
37. Frucht-Pery J, Rozenman Y. Mitomycin C therapy for corneal intraepithelial neoplasia. Am J Ophthalmol. 1994;117:164–8.
38. Kaliki S, Vempuluru VS, Ghose N, et al. Ocular surface squamous neoplasia in India: a study of 438 patients. Int Ophthalmol. 2022;42:1915–26.
39. Vempuluru VS, Pattnaik M, Ghose n, Kaliki S. Bilateral ocular surface squamous neoplasia: a study of 25 patients and review of literature. Eur J Ophthalmol. 2022;32:620–7.
40. Kaliki S, Jajapuram SV, Maniar A, et al. Ocular surface squamous neoplasia with intraocular tumour extension: a study of 23 patients. Eye. 2020;34:319–26.
41. Zhu C, Weiss M, Scribbick FW, et al. Occurrence of occult neoplasia in pterygium specimens among Hispanic and non-Hispanic patients. Curr Eye Res. 2022;47:978–81.
42. Mejia LF, Zapata M, Gil JC. An unexpected incidence of ocular surface neoplasia on pterygium surgery: a retrospective clinical and histopathological report. Cornea. 2021;40:1002–6.
43. Frucht-Pery J, Sugar J, Baum J, et al. Mitomycin C treatment for conjunctival-corneal intraepithelial neoplasia: a multicenter experience. Ophthalmology. 1997;104(12):2085–93.
44. Wilson FM 2nd. Rose bengal staining of epibulbar squamous neoplasms. Ophthalmic Surg. 1976;7(2):21–3.
45. Machado LM, Castro RS, Fontes BM. Staining patterns in dry eye syndrome: rose bengal versus lissamine green. Cornea. 2009;28:732–4.
46. Romero IL, Barros JD, Martins MC, et al. The use of 1% toluidine blue eye drops in the diagnosis of ocular surface squamous neoplasia. Cornea. 2012;32(1):36–9.

47. Finger PT, Tran HV, Turbin RE, et al. High-frequency ultrasonographic evaluation of conjunctival intraepithelial neoplasia and squamous cell carcinoma. Arch Ophthalmol. 2003;121(2):168–72.
48. Xu Y, Zhou Z, Xu Y, et al. The clinical value of in vivo confocal microscopy for diagnosis of ocular surface squamous neoplasia. Eye (Lond). 2012;26(6):781–7.
49. Kieval JZ, Carp CL, Abou Shousha M, et al. Ultra-high resolution optical coherence tomography for differentiation of ocular surface squamous neoplasia and pterygia. Ophthalmology. 2012;119(3):481–6.
50. Atallah M, Joag M, Galor A, et al. Role of high resolution optical coherence tomography in diagnosing ocular surface squamous neoplasia with coexisting ocular surface diseases. Ocul Surf. 2017;15:688–95.
51. Spinak M, Friedman AH. Squamous cell carcinoma of the conjunctiva. Value of exfoliative cytology in diagnosis. Surv Ophthalmol. 1977;21(4):351–5.
52. Semenova EA, Milman T, Finger PT, et al. The diagnostic value of exfoliative cytology vs. histopathology for ocular surface squamous neoplasia. Am J Ophthalmol. 2009;148(5):772–8.
53. Nolan GR, Hirst LW, Bancroft BJ. The cytomorphology of ocular surface squamous neoplasia by using impression cytology. Cancer. 2001;93(1):60–7.
54. Mishra DK, Taneja S, Singh V, et al. Histopathological spectrum of ocular surface squamous neoplasia: a retrospective study of 776 lesions. Indian J Pathol Microbiol. 2022;65:3–7.
55. Asnaghi L, Alkatan H, Mahale A, et al. Identification of multiple DNA copy number alterations including frequent 8p11.22 amplification in conjunctival squamous cell carcinoma. Invest Ophthalmol Vis Sci. 2014;9(55):8604–13.
56. Mishra DK, Veena U, Kaliki S, et al. Differential expression of stem cell markers in ocular surface squamous neoplasia. PLoS One. 2016;11:e0161800.
57. Wolkow N, Jakobiec FA, Afroghen AH, et al. Programmed cell death 1 ligand 1 and programmed cell death 1 ligand 2 are expressed in conjunctival invasive squamous cell carcinoma: therapeutic implications. Am J Ophthalmol. 2019;200:226–41.
58. Nagarajan P, El-Hadad C, Gruschkus SK, et al. PD-L1/PD1 expression, composition of tumor-associated immune infiltrate, and HPV status in conjunctival squamous cell carcinoma. Invest Ophthalmol Vis Sci. 2019;60:2388–98.
59. Sakai A, Tagami M, Kakehashi A, et al. Expression, intracellular localization, and mutation of EGFR in conjunctival squamous cell carcinoma and the association with prognosis and treatment. PLoS One. 2020;15:e0238120.
60. Chauhan S, Sen S, Chauhan SS, et al. Stratifin in ocular surface squamous neoplasia and its association with p53. Acta Ophthalmol. 2021;99:e1483–91.
61. Tagami M, Kakehashi A, Katsuyama-Yoshikawa A, et al. FOXP3 and CXCR$-positive regulatory cells in the tumor stroma as indicators of tumor immunity in the conjunctival squamous cell carcinoma microenvironment. PLoS One. 2022;17:e0263895.
62. Conway RM, Graue GF, Pelaye DE, et al. Conjunctiva carcinoma. American Joint Committee on Cancer (AJCC) Cancer staging manual, vol. Chapter 65. 8th ed. New York: Springer; 2017. p. 787–93.
63. Chauhan S, Sen S, Sharma A, et al. American joint committee on cancer staging and clinicopathological high-risk predictors of ocular surface squamous neoplasia: a study from a tertiary eye center in India. Arch Pathol Lab Med. 2014;138:1488–94.
64. Bellerive C, Berry JL, Polski A, Singh AD. Conjunctival squamous neoplasia: staging and initial treatment. Cornea. 2018;37:1287–91.
65. Meel R, Dhiman R. Proposal for a new classification for ocular surface squamous neoplasia. Eye. 2018;32:1284–5.
66. Mudhar HS, Milman T, Zhang PJL, et al. Conjunctival 'mucoepidermoid carcinoma' revisited: a revision of terminology, based on morphologic, immunohistochemical and molecular findings of 14 cases, and the 2018 WHO classification of tumours of the eye. Mod Pathol. 2020;33:1242–55.
67. Waring GO III, Roth AM, Ekins MB. Clinical and pathologic description of 17 cases of corneal intraepithelial neoplasia. Am J Ophthalmol. 1984;97(5):547–59.
68. Espana EM, Levine M, Schoenfield L, Singh AD. Ocular surface squamous neoplasia in an anophthalmic socket 60 years after enucleation. Surv Ophthalmol. 2011;56(6):539–43.
69. Iliff WJ, Marback R, Green WR. Invasive squamous cell carcinoma of the conjunctiva. Arch Ophthalmol. 1975;93(2):119–22.
70. Bowen RC, Soto H, Raval V, Bellerive C, Yeaney G, Singh AD. Ocular surface squamous neoplasia: outcomes following primary excision with 2 mm margin and cryotherapy. Eye (Lond). 2021;35(11):3102–9.
71. Char DH, Crawford JB, Howers EL, et al. Resection of intraocular squamous cell carcinoma. Br J Ophthalmol. 1992;76(2):123–5.
72. Buus DR, Tse DT, Folberg R. Microscopically controlled excision of conjunctival squamous cell carcinoma. Am J Ophthalmol. 1994;117(1):97–102.
73. Shields JA, Shields CL, Gunduz K, et al. The 1998 pan American lecture. Intraocular invasion of conjunctival squamous cell carcinoma in five patients. Ophthalmic Plast Reconstr Surg. 1999;15(3):153–60.
74. Fraunfelder FT, Wallace TR, Farris HE, et al. The role of cryosurgery in external ocular and periocular disease. Trans Sect Ophthalmol Am Acad Ophthalmol Otolaryngol. 1977;83(4 Pt. 1):713–24.
75. Lommatzsch P. Beta-ray treatment of malignant epithelial tumors of the conjunctiva. Am J Ophthalmol. 1976;81(2):198–206.
76. Zehetmayer M, Menapace R, Kulnig W. Combined local excision and brachytherapy with ruthenium-106 in the treatment of epibulbar malignancies. Ophthalmologica. 1993;207(3):133–9.
77. Rao R, Honavar SG, Lahane S, et al. Histopathology-guided management of ocular surface squamous neoplasia with corneal stromal or scleral invasion using ruthenium-106 plaque brachytherapy. Br J Ophthalmol. 2023;107:621–6.
78. Rahal A, Meller D, Manthey A, et al. Brachytherapy as a curative option for ocular surface squamous neoplasia. Int Ophthalmol. 2023;43:1861–5.
79. Marr BP, Abramson DH, Cohen GN, Williamson MJ, McCormick B, Barker CA. Intraoperative high-dose rate of radioactive phosphorus 32 brachytherapy for diffuse recalcitrant conjunctival neoplasms: a retrospective case series and report of toxicity. JAMA Ophthalmol. 2015;133:283–9.
80. Arepalli S, Kaliki S, Shields CL, et al. Plaque radiotherapy in the management of scleral-invasive conjunctival squamous cell carcinoma: an analysis of 15 eyes. JAMA Ophthalmol. 2014;132:691–6.
81. El-Assal KS, Salvi SM, Rundle PA, et al. Treatment of invasive ocular surface squamous neoplasia with proton beam therapy. Eye (Lond). 2013;27:1223–4.
82. Santoni A, Thariat J, Maschi C, et al. Management of invasive squamous cell carcinoma of the conjunctiva. Am J Ophthalmol. 2019;200:1–9.
83. Monroy D, Serrano A, Galor A, Karp CL. Medical treatment for ocular surface squamous neoplasia. Eye. 2023;37:885–93.
84. Khong JJ, Muecke J. Complications of mitomycin C therapy in 100 eyes with ocular surface neoplasia. Br J Ophthalmol. 2006;90(7):819–22.
85. Hirst LW. Randomized controlled trial of topical mitomycin C for ocular surface squamous neoplasia: early resolution. Ophthalmology. 2007;114(5):976–82.
86. Russell HC, Chadha V, Lockington D, et al. Topical mitomycin C chemotherapy in the management of ocular surface neoplasia:

a 10-year review of treatment outcomes and complications. Br J Ophthalmol. 2012;94(10):1316–21.
87. Prabhasawat P, Tarinvorakup P, Tesavibul N, et al. Topical 0.002% mitomycin C for the treatment of conjunctival-corneal intraepithelial neoplasia and squamous cell carcinoma. Cornea. 2005;24:443–8.
88. Lichtinger A, Pe'er J, Frucht-Pery J, Solomon A. Limbal stem cell deficiency after topical mitomycin C therapy for primary acquired melanosis with atypia. Ophthalmology. 2010;117:431–7.
89. Frucht-Pery J, Rozenman Y, Pe'er J. Topical mitomycin-C for partially excised conjunctival squamous cell carcinoma. Ophthalmology. 2002;109(3):548–52.
90. Siganos CS, Kozobolis VP, Christodoulakis EV. The intraoperative use of mitomycin-C in excision of ocular surface neoplasia with or without limbal autograft transplantation. Cornea. 2002;21:12–6.
91. Sarici AM, Arvas S, Pazarli H. Combined excision, cryotherapy, and intraoperative mitomycin C (EXCRIM) for localized intraepithelial and squamous cell carcinoma of the conjunctiva. Graefes Arch Clin Exp Ophthalmol. 2013;251:2201–4.
92. Joag MG, Sise A, Murillo JC, et al. Topical 5-fluorouracil 1% as primary treatment for ocular surface squamous neoplasia. Ophthalmology. 2016;123:1442–8.
93. Parrozzani R, Frizziero L, Trainiti S, et al. Topical 1% 5-fluoruracil as a sole treatment of corneoconjunctival ocular surface squamous neoplasia: long-term study. Br J Ophthalmol. 2017;101:1094–9.
94. Wylegala A, Sripawadkul W, Zein M, et al. Topical 1% 5-fluorouracil eye drops as primary treatment for ocular surface squamous neoplasia: long-term follow-up study. Ocul Surf. 2023;27:67–74.
95. Karp CL, Moore JK, Rosa RH Jr. Treatment of conjunctival and corneal intraepithelial neoplasia with topical interferon alpha-2b. Ophthalmology. 2001;108(6):1093–8.
96. Galor A, Karp CL, Chhabra S, et al. Topical interferon alpha 2b eye-drops for treatment of ocular surface squamous neoplasia; a dose comparison study. Br J Ophthalmol. 2010;94(5):551–4.
97. Shields CL, Kaliki S, Kim HJ, et al. Interferon for ocular surface squamous neoplasia in 81 cases: outcomes based on the American joint committee on cancer classification. Cornea. 2013;32(3):248–56.
98. Krilis M, Tsang H, Coroneo M. Treatment of conjunctival and corneal epithelial neoplasia with retinoic acid and topical interferon alfa-2b: long-term follow-up. Ophthalmology. 2012;119:1969–73.
99. Karp CL, Galor A, Chhabra S, et al. Subconjunctival/perilesional recombinant interferon α2b for ocular surface squamous neoplasia: a 10-year review. Ophthalmology. 2010;117:2241–6.
100. Nanji AA, Moon CS, Galor A, et al. Surgical versus medical treatment of ocular surface squamous neoplasia: a comparison of recurrences and complications. Ophthalmology. 2014;121:994–1000.
101. Sripawadkul W, Reyes-Capo D, Zein M, et al. Long-term study of topical interferon alpha-2b eye drops as primary treatment of ocular surface squamous neoplasia. Ocul Surf. 2022;30:108–14.
102. Jiang J, Bohringer D, Auw-Hadrich C, et al. Current practice in the treatment of epithelial and melanocytic tumours with interferone-alpha-2b: a survey of tertiary eye centers in Germany. Klin Monatsbl Augenheilkd. 2023;240:891–6.
103. Park J, Han J, Chung TY, et al. Pegylated interferone alpha-2a for the treatment of ocular surface squamous neoplasia. Cornea. 2022;41:1271–5.
104. Espana EM, Prabhasawat P, Grueterich M, et al. Amniotic membrane transplantation for reconstruction after excision of large ocular surface neoplasias. Br J Ophthalmol. 2002;86(6):640–5.
105. Palamar M, Kaya E, Egrilmez S, et al. Amniotic membrane transplantation in surgical management of ocular surface squamous neoplasia: long-term results. Eye. 2014;28:1131–5.
106. Furdova A, Czanner G, Koller J, et al. Amniotic membrane application in surgical treatment of conjunctival tumors. Sci Rep. 2023;13:2835.
107. Galor A, Karp CL, Oellers P, et al. Predictors of ocular surface squamous neoplasia recurrence after excisional surgery. Ophthalmology. 2012;119(10):1974–81.
108. Murillo JC, Galor A, Wu MC, et al. Intracorneal and intraocular invasion of ocular surface squamous neoplasia after intraocular surgery: report of two cases and review of the literature. Ocul Oncol Pathol. 2017;3:66–72.
109. Martel A, Hamedani M, Lagier J, et al. Does orbital exenteration still has a place in 2019? J Fr Ophthalmol. 2020;43:152–74.
110. El-Hadad C, Rubin ML, Nagarajan P, et al. Prognostic factors for orbital exenteration, local recurrence, metastasis, and death from disease in conjunctival squamous cell carcinoma. Ophthalmic Plast Reconstr Surg. 2021;37:262–8.
111. Freitag SK, Aakalau VK, Tao JP, et al. Sentinel lymph node biopsy for eyelid and conjunctival malignancy: a report by the American Academy of ophthalmology. Ophthalmology. 2020;127:1757–65.
112. Vempuluru VS, Indusekhar H, Mohamed A, Kaliki S. Metastatic conjunctival squamous cell carcinoma: a study of 5 cases. Int Ophthalmol. 2022;42:3097–108.

Primary Acquired Melanosis

6

Jacob Pe'er and Robert Folberg

6.1 Introduction

The name applied to the condition described in this chapter has evolved over many years. Each name carried with it implications for diagnosis and therapy. Hutchinson, who was the first to describe these lesions clinically in 1892, called them "senile freckle" or "lentigo melanosis" [1], while Dubreuilh, who was the first to describe these lesions histologically in 1912, used the term "melanose circonscrite pre-cancereuse" [1]. In 1936, Miescher used the term "melanotische precancerose" [1]; and in 1966, Reese used the term "precancerous melanosis" [2]. The name itself—"precancerous"—prompted surgeons at that time to perform radical surgery, including orbital exenteration, to treat a condition that is confined to the epithelium and that poses no risk of metastasis. In reaction to the overtreatment of these lesions, Zimmerman proposed the name "benign acquired melanosis" in 1966 [3, 4], but the inclusion of the word "benign" led ophthalmologists to treat these lesions conservatively, and patients managed by observation often developed malignant melanoma. In 1978, Silvers used the terms "intraepithelial melanocytic hyperplasia" and "atypical melanocytic hyperplasia" [5] to describe the histology of lesions that were predisposed to evolve into melanoma if not treated appropriately. The histological name, however, could not be applied in a clinical setting by ophthalmologists.

The term "primary acquired melanosis" (PAM) was adopted by the World Health Organization in 1980, representing flat, brown, intraepithelial conjunctival lesions in its International Histological Classification of Tumors [6]. "Primary" denotes that the lesion is not the result of generalized (racial) dark pigmentation, systemic disease (e.g., Addison's disease), or local factors (foreign body, injury, inflammation, medication, etc.). "Acquired" distinguishes these lesions from those that are congenital, and "melanosis" indicates that the pigment in the lesion is explicitly derived from the production of melanin rather than another pigment or a drug deposit (Table 6.1) [7].

Table 6.1 Types of conjunctival melanosis

Category	Subtype	Etiology		
Congenital	Ocular melanosis	Developmental episcleral hyperpigmentation		
	Oculodermal melanosis			
Acquired	Complexion associated	Normal pigmentation in darker races		
	Primary	Idiopathic		
	Secondary	Localized	Post-inflammatory	Post-traumatic
			Foreign body	Drug deposition
		Systemic	Addison's disease	Ochronosis
		Syndromic	Carney complex	Peutz–Jeghers syndrome

J. Pe'er (✉)
Ocular Oncology Service and Ophthalmic Pathology Laboratory, Department of Ophthalmology, Hadassah—Hebrew University Medical Center, Jerusalem, Israel
e-mail: peer@hadassah.org.il

R. Folberg
Ophthalmology and Pathology, Oakland University William Beaumont School of Medicine, Rochester, MI, USA

© The Author(s), under exclusive license to Springer Nature Switzerland AG 2024
J. Pe'er et al. (eds.), *Clinical Ophthalmic Oncology*, https://doi.org/10.1007/978-3-031-72443-5_6

The terminology—primary acquired melanosis (PAM)—may be used by the ophthalmologist in a clinical setting to describe any form of flat acquired conjunctival pigmentation that cannot be attributed to a secondary influence. This identification should trigger a biopsy, allowing the pathologist to determine if melanocytic atypia is present (PAM with atypia) or represents conjunctival pigmentation without any melanocytic atypia (PAM without atypia). The designation of atypia is reserved for the pathologist because it is impossible to predict melanocytic atypia from clinical criteria alone.

Damato and Coupland suggested that the term "PAM" be reserved only for clinical diagnosis and offered the term "conjunctival melanocytic intraepithelial neoplasia (C-MIN) with or without atypia" for the histological terminology of these lesions, with more severe changes regarded as "melanoma in situ"[8], as was classified in the fourth edition of the WHO Classification of tumors of the eye [9]. The more general term "conjunctival melanocytic intraepithelial lesions" (C-MIL) has been used by others [10]. In a recent study comparing the results according to the three classification systems—PAM, C-MIN, and C-MIL—they had comparable accuracy of 81–83% in their ability to identify lesions with potential for recurrence [11]. In a recent paper, Jakobiec recommended that "intraepithelial melanocytic proliferation" be adopted for histopathological diagnosis [12].

The authors of this chapter consider that the hybrid nomenclature—one term for the ophthalmologist and another for the pathologist—neither adds value to the classification of the disorder nor improves the management. For the remainder of the chapter, therefore, the terminology PAM will be used in a clinical context and PAM with and without atypia when discussing pathology.

The prevalence and natural behavior of PAM are controversial. One study [13] reported the prevalence of PAM in Caucasians with no known non-European ancestry to be 36%. This number is exceptionally high compared with other studies. It is important to consider that the authors of this study included lesions that were detectable only by high-magnification slit-lamp examination, and some lesions were so small that they would not have been detected on routine clinical inspection. Furthermore, there was no histological confirmation of the diagnosis in this series.

6.2 Etiology

PAM is more prevalent in fair-complexioned individuals than in patients with dark skin tones and is almost always unilateral. If bilateral conjunctival pigmentation is encountered, the ophthalmologist should first consider either complexion-associated conjunctival pigmentation or a systemic condition associated with bilateral conjunctival pigmentation.

6.2.1 Sunlight Exposure

The importance of sun exposure in the development of PAM is not apparent. However, in one study [13], those who lived south of Washington, DC, for five or more years had a significantly higher prevalence of PAM lesions of their exposed intrapalpebral conjunctiva than those who did not. Also, patients with pinguecula or pterygium had a higher prevalence of PAM. Silvers et al. [5] noted a high incidence of solar elastosis in biopsy specimens from patients with conjunctival pigmented lesions. These facts suggest a possible role of sunlight exposure, but while they might explain PAM arising in the bulbar conjunctiva in the interpalpebral fissure, they do not account for cases in which PAM originates in the fornices and the palpebral conjunctiva.

6.2.2 Relationship to Nevi and Dysplastic Nevus Syndrome

The prevalence of PAM has been shown to increase significantly as the number of facial nevi increases [13]. Seregard et al. [14], in a case–control study, observed that ocular melanocytic lesions, including PAM, are not more common in individuals with dysplastic nevus syndrome than in the general population.

6.2.3 Cigarette Smoking

Cigarette smoking and hypertension have been observed as significant independent factors in the development of PAM [13]. No other etiological factors have been implicated in the development of PAM.

6.3 Clinical Features

Primary acquired melanosis appears clinically as a flat and variably brown conjunctival lesion, ranging from golden brown to dark chocolate in color (Figs. 6.1 and 6.2) [7]. There are no published size criteria for the clinical diagnosis of PAM [12], although in one large series [15] PAM extended circumferentially for a mean of 3 clock hours, ranging from 1 to 12 clock hours. PAM is usually monocular, although binocular cases may occur. The lesion may involve any area of the conjunctiva in a contiguous or multispotted pattern, necessitating eversion of the eyelids to examine both the upper and lower palpebral zones. PAM develops most commonly at the limbus and epibulbar intrapalpebral region and may extend into the corneal epithelium (Fig. 6.3). According to Shields et al.'s experience with 311 eyes [15], the conjunctival quadrants affected by PAM were temporal,

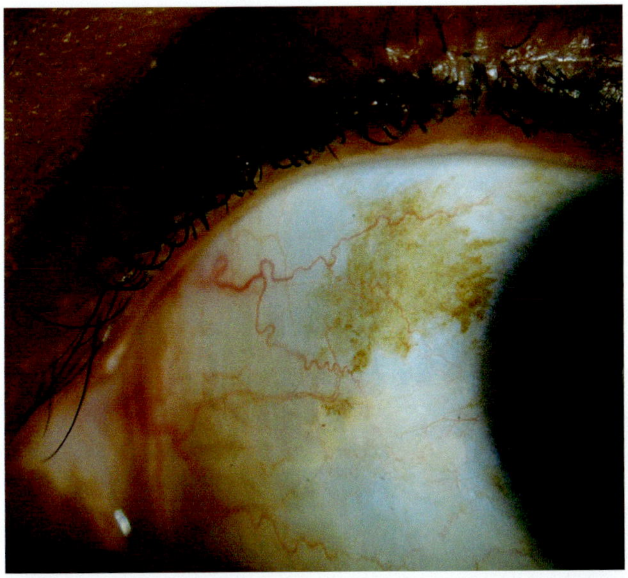

Fig. 6.1 PAM without atypia. Would the lesion be enough to make the diagnosis of PAM and justify a biopsy?

57%; inferior, 45%; nasal, 42%; and superior, 37%. In the same study, the anatomic locations of PAM included bulbar conjunctiva in 91%, limbal conjunctiva in 55%, cornea in 23%, forniceal conjunctiva in 13%, palpebral conjunctiva in 12%, and caruncle in 11%. In some patients with widespread lesions, the eyelid epidermis may also be involved [7]. PAM occurs typically in middle-aged or elderly white patients, although it may also appear in young adults, but usually not in children. In one study [16], the mean age at the time of diagnosis was 45 years and in another study this was 62 years [13]. There is no significant difference in the prevalence of PAM between males and females [13], although in one extensive study [15] 62% of patients with PAM were female.

Primary acquired melanosis lesions may remain stable for long periods of time or may grow in size. A "waxing and waning" phenomenon in which areas in the lesions darken or lighten is well known [7]. Parts of, or rarely the entire, PAM lesion can be amelanotic (PAM sine pigmento); thus, the borders of the lesion often cannot be identified, and the clinically recognized borders are misleading [16].

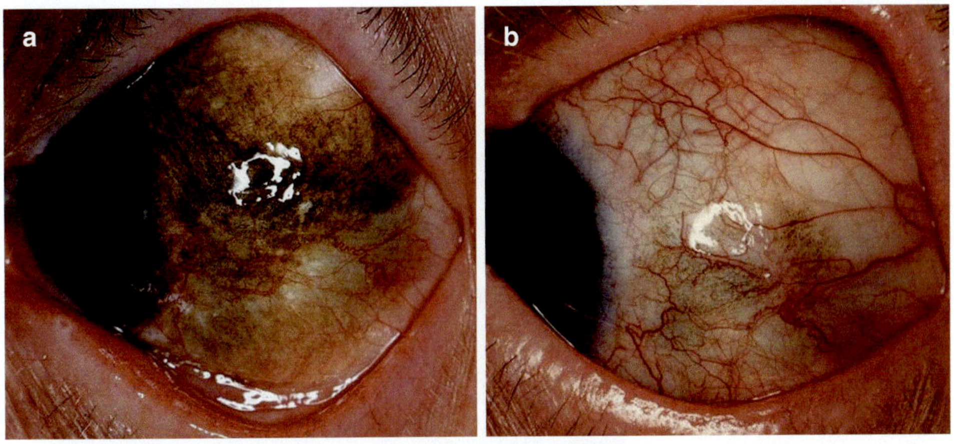

Fig. 6.2 Diffuse PAM with atypia entirely covering the temporal bulbar conjunctiva (**a**). After treatment with topical mitomycin C. Some pigmentation, probably PAM without atypia, has remained unchanged for 6 years (**b**)

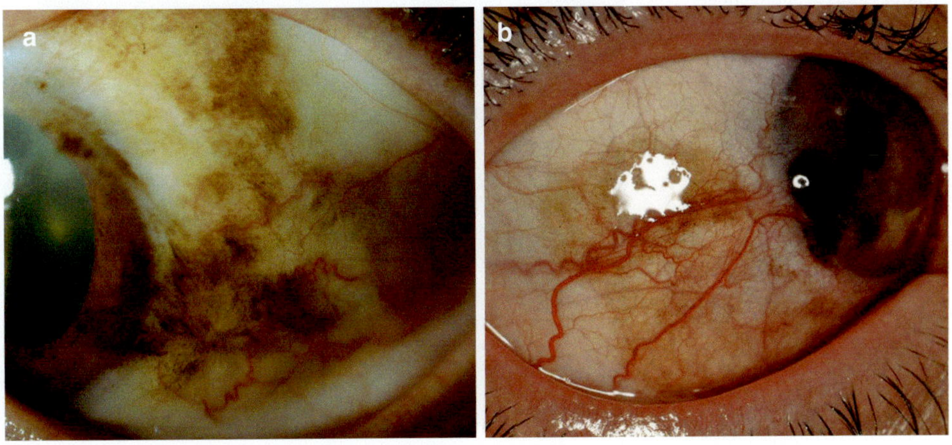

Fig. 6.3 Conjunctival PAM with atypia, with corneal involvement (**a**). Another case that has progressed to corneo-limbal melanoma (**b**)

6.4 Ancillary Studies

The clinical suspicion of PAM is based on the features described in the previous section. Because PAM lesions are flat and intraepithelial, there are no established imaging tools that can aid in the diagnosis. However, Messmer et al. [17], using in vivo confocal microscopy (OCT), could display small dendritic cells and hyperreflective granules confined to the basal epithelium in PAM without atypia and extensive networks of hyperreflective dendritic cells and hyperreflective granules and patches throughout the epithelium in all cases of PAM with atypia. Alzahrani et al. showed a thick basal epithelial hyperreflective band in all instances of PAM using OCT [18] (Fig. 6.4 and 6.5), and Shousha et al. also showed correlation between histopathological findings and ultra-high-resolution OCT [19]. A Wood's lamp may help in the detection of subclinical pigmentation but is seldom used in clinical practice [20].

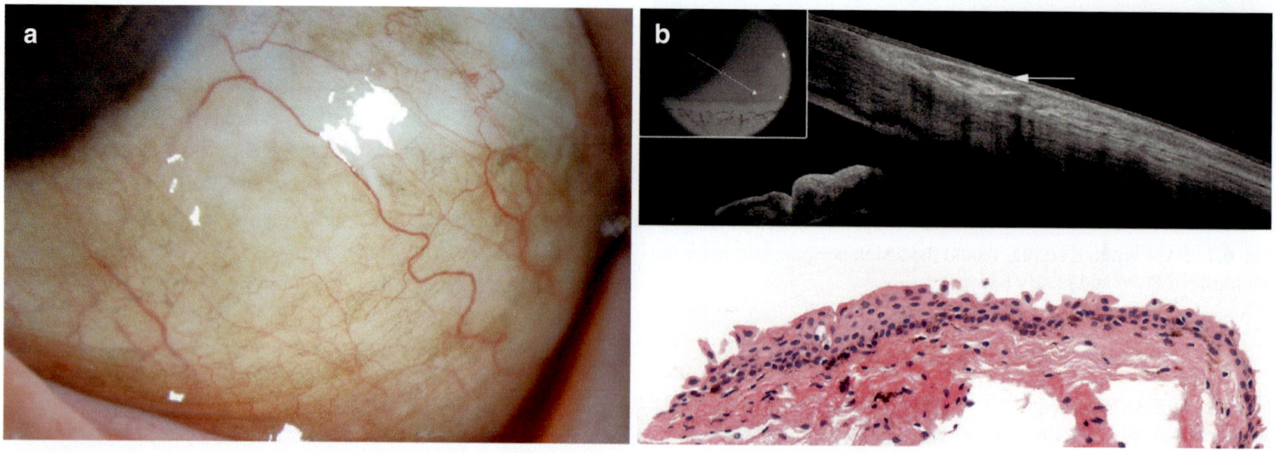

Fig. 6.4 Diffuse conjunctival PAM (**a**) without atypia. Note (arrow) basal epithelial hyper-reflective band of approximate 20 micron thickness (**b**, above) and corresponding melanotic hyperpigmentation that is restricted to the basal layer (**b**, below) (hematoxylin and eosin, original magnification, 200×). (Reprinted from Alzahrani YA, Kumar S, Abdul Aziz H, Plesec T, Singh AD. Primary Acquired Melanosis: Clinical, Histopathologic and Optical Coherence Tomographic Correlation. Ocul Oncol Pathol. 2016;2:123–7. Copyright © 2015, © 2015 S. Karger AG, Basel)

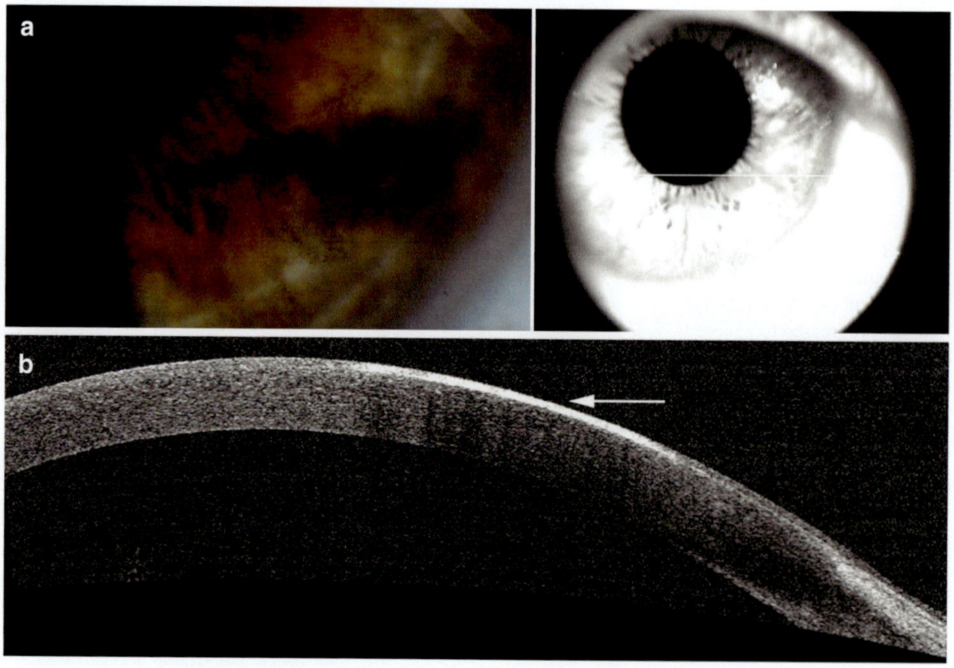

Fig. 6.5 Corneal PAM. (**a**) Clinical appearance. (**b**) Note corresponding epithelial hyper-reflective band. (Reprinted from Alzahrani YA, Kumar S, Abdul Aziz H, Plesec T, Singh AD. Primary Acquired Melanosis: Clinical, Histopathologic and Optical Coherence Tomographic Correlation. Ocul Oncol Pathol. 2016;2:123–7. Copyright © 2015, © 2015 S. Karger AG, Basel)

6.5 Histopathological Features

Histologically, PAM is divided into two major groups: PAM without atypia and PAM with atypia. Most conjunctival melanomas arise in the context of PAM with atypia. PAM with atypia is confined to the epithelium and is called by some pathologists "melanoma in situ" [1], and is thus not associated with any risk of metastasis. However, 11–46% transform to conjunctival melanoma [15, 16]. The mortality of conjunctival melanoma is approximately 25%. Therefore, a particularly effective treatment for conjunctival melanoma is through prevention by completely treating lesions showing histological evidence of PAM with atypia.

The lesion designated as PAM without atypia does not evolve into melanoma. As mentioned above, it is important to remember that there are no clinical criteria by which ophthalmologists can anticipate the histological diagnosis. For that reason, an ophthalmologist who encounters a fair-complexioned patient with a unilateral, acquired, flat patch of brown pigmentation should biopsy the lesion to allow the pathologist to classify the lesion as PAM without atypia or PAM with atypia. Because PAM is often without pigment (sine pigmento), at least partially, and in cases with more extensive disease, map biopsy is recommended, the results of which have impact on the use of topical chemotherapy [21].

6.5.1 Light Microscopy

Histologically, the detection of conjunctival epithelial pigmentation with or without melanocytic hyperplasia—but, without melanocytic atypia—qualifies a lesion to be designated as PAM without atypia (Fig. 6.6). One might think conceptually of such a lesion as an "ephilis" (freckle) or lentigo (despite the fact that there are no rete structures in the normal conjunctiva and therefore "lentigo" is difficult to identify in this location). Histologically, the detection of atypical melanocytes within the epithelium qualifies the lesion to be designated as PAM with atypia.

In rendering a diagnosis of PAM with atypia, the pathologist should take note of both cytological and architectural features. Melanocytic atypia is identified through the detection of melanocytes of different size and shape that appear to have a "disregard" (i.e., they are spatially separated from) for adjacent epithelial cells (Fig. 6.7). These atypical cells may be small and round, spindle-shaped, or even epithelioid. Architecturally, the atypical melanocytes may be distributed along the epithelial basement membrane (basilar hyperplasia pattern), may be segregated into nests that appear to be anchored along the basement membrane, or may be dispersed upward into the more superficial layers of the epithelium, either individually or as intraepithelial nests (pagetoid spread). In some areas, the atypical melanocytes may com-

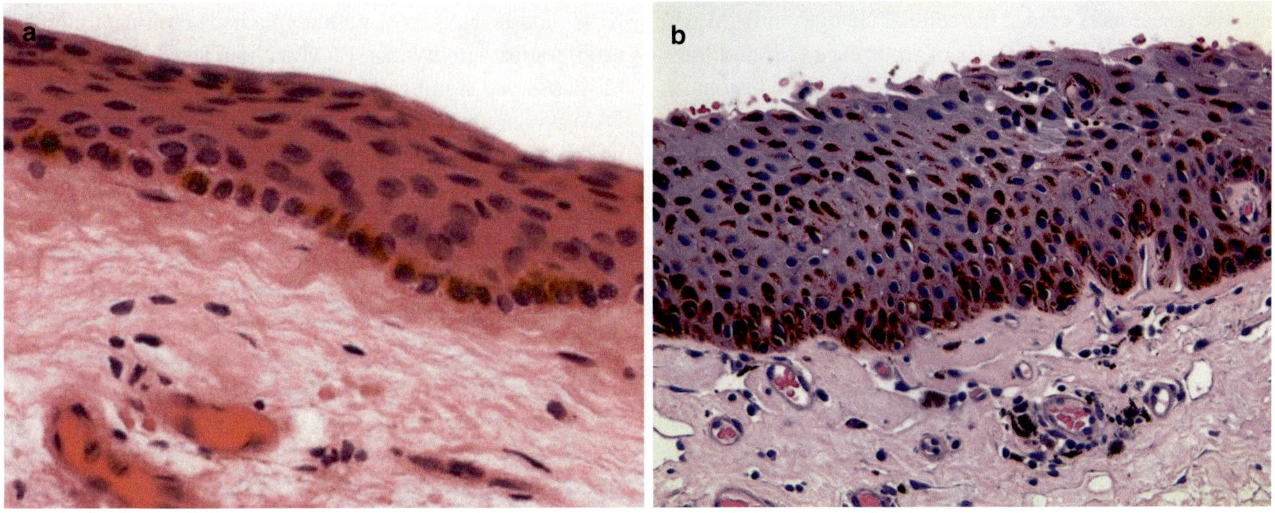

Fig. 6.6 Histological picture of conjunctival PAM without atypia, with pigmented melanocytes located only along the basal layer of the epithelium (**a**) (hematoxylin and eosin, ×20). In this case, melanin pigmentation is distributed throughout the conjunctival epithelium, yet there is no evidence of melanocytic hyperplasia or atypia. This lesion would, therefore, be designated histologically as conjunctival PAM without atypia (**b**) (hematoxylin and eosin, ×20)

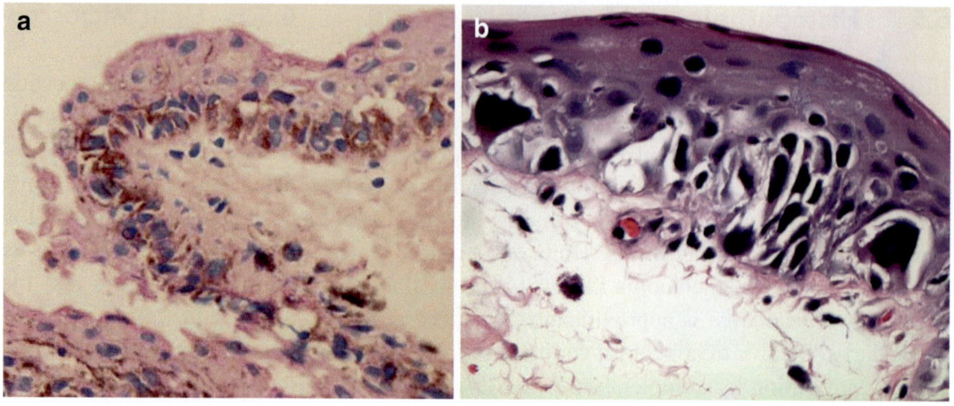

Fig. 6.7 Histological picture of conjunctival PAM with atypia, showing atypical melanocytes in the basal layers (**a**, hematoxylin and eosin, ×20). Highly atypical melanocytes populate the conjunctival epithelium singly and in nests. Note the lack of contact between these cells and the epithelium. This lesion should be designated as PAM with atypia (**b**, hematoxylin and eosin, ×40)

pletely replace the epithelium. PAM with atypia that extends into pseudoglands of Henle should not be mistaken for invasion (the lining of the pseudoglands is considered to be contiguous with the epithelium).

It is important for both pathologists and ophthalmologists to understand that junctional nevi of the conjunctiva are exceptionally rare—even in children. Therefore, the diagnosis of "junctional nevus" when rendered by a pathologist who is not experienced in ophthalmic pathology should prompt a review, especially if the lesion is not taken from a young child: the lesion is likely to represent PAM with atypia. The histological identification and differential diagnosis of PAM with atypia are among the most difficult tasks in the practice of surgical ophthalmic pathology. In two studies, the researchers graded the cellular changes in PAM with atypia and showed higher rates of recurrence [22] and transformation to melanoma [23] in the highly graded lesions.

The Conjunctiva Melanocytic Intraepithelial Lesion (C-MIL) classification has changed since its initial introduction in the fourth edition of the WHO Classification [9], where they used the term C-MIN. This publication divided C-MIN into four tiers: benign melanosis, low-grade C-MIN, high-grade C-MIN, and melanoma in situ. The fifth edition of the WHO Classification [24] combines melanoma in situ with high-grade C-MIL to yield three tiers. The histological criteria for each tier correspond to the histological criteria for diagnosing PAM without atypia ("benign melanosis" under C-MIL), PAM with mild atypia (C-MIL low grade), and PAM with severe atypia (C-MIL high grade). An international collaborative group of pathologists studied 105 biopsies from 97 patients and determined the interobserver reliability to be good using the C-MIL classification [25]. Because the histological criteria for classifying C-MIL into three categories are identical to the criteria used to stratify PAM, one can conclude that the PAM classification is also reliable and reproducible. The only difference between PAM and C-MIL is the name assigned to the classification scheme.

The authors of this chapter recommend retaining the PAM classification because it is useful clinically and histologically. Over the years, ophthalmologists have learned to clinically separate primary pigmentation from secondary pigmentation and acquired pigmentation from congenital pigmentation. Clinicians understand the need to take biopsies from lesions that are primary, acquired, unilateral, and developing in patients who do not have dark skin tones. The designation of C-MIL applies to a histological diagnosis. Some pathologists and clinicians may wish to use the two systems—PAM and C-MIL—interchangeably.

6.5.2 Immunohistochemistry

Chowers et al. [26] showed that on immunostaining for Ki-67 and PCNA, PAM with atypia had significantly higher proliferation activity than PAM without atypia. Sharara et al. [27] observed significantly higher expression of HMB-45 in PAM with atypia compared to PAM without atypia and conjunctival nevi. Jiang et al. found that Melan-A labels all melanocytes without discriminating between benign and malignant cells, while atypical melanocytes were most specifically labeled with HMB-45, whose positively increases significantly with worsening atypia [28]. However, a recent immunohistochemical study using SOX10, HMB-45, Ki-67, and P16 concluded that these stains have a limited value in distinguishing between low-grade and high-grade conjunctival melanocytic intraepithelial lesions, beyond disclosing the presence, number, and location of melanocytes within the epithelium [10]. Other pathologists may wish to use immunohistochemistry to assign lesions to the proper risk tiers: PAM with atypia low- vs. high-grade or C-MIL, low- vs. high-grade. In investigating mutations in conjunctival melanocytic lesions, none of the PAM lesions with or without atypia showed BRAF [29] or GNAQ mutations [30]. Several recent studies found PRAME (Preferentially expressed Antigen in Melanoma) to be useful for distinguishing melanoma and its probable precursors, such as PAM with high-grade atypia, from benign conjunctival melanocytic proliferation [31–33].

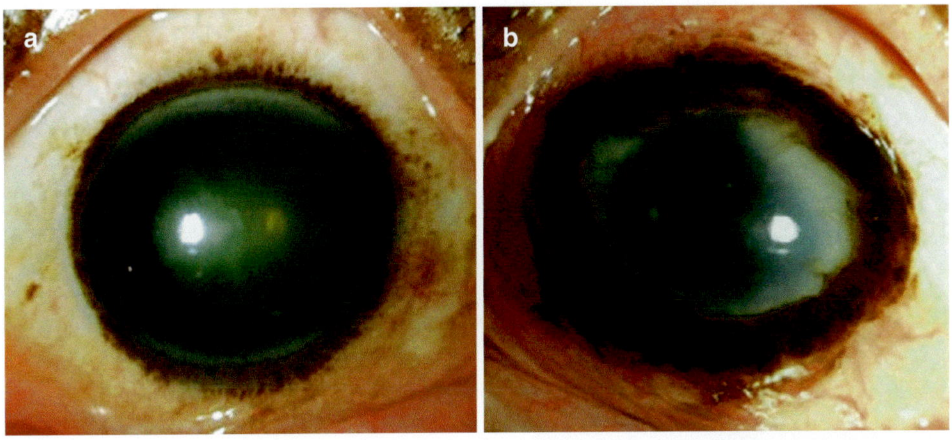

Fig. 6.8 Complexion associated melanosis in an African American patient. (**a**) Note perilimbal superficial flat pigmentation in the right eye. (**b**) The pigmentation in the left eye is more prominent because of globe shrinkage (phthisis bulbi) and because of a possible secondary effect of chronic inflammation

6.6 Differential Diagnosis

Primary acquired melanosis should be differentiated from all pigmented lesions of the conjunctiva, especially flat ones [34]. Like PAM, conjunctival nevi are always movable. The presence of cysts within the lesion supports a diagnosis of conjunctival nevus rather than PAM, although PAM may arise in the context of a nevus; therefore, the presence of cysts does not "guarantee" a diagnosis of nevus. In episcleral melanosis, as in congenital ocular melanosis or oculodermal melanosis, the pigmentation is blue-gray, nonmovable, and usually multifocal. Conjunctival melanoma is typically elevated or nodular, but in early stages, when it arises from PAM with atypia, it may appear flat.

Other melanocytic lesions of the conjunctiva include pigmentation associated with a dark skin tone that is usually bilateral and typically most intense at the limbus, fading in intensity toward the fornices (Fig. 6.8). Other conditions that can be included in a differential diagnosis are post-inflammatory melanosis and systemic conditions with flat bilateral conjunctival pigmented patches such as Addison's disease. Various benign and malignant conjunctival tumors that are usually amelanotic may be pigmented so as to simulate a conjunctival pigmented lesion, which when flat may resemble PAM.

6.7 Treatment

The management of PAM remains controversial.

6.7.1 Observation

A small minority of ophthalmologists believe that subtle PAM lesions do not meet the criteria for biopsy and recommend periodic follow-up [13]. They advise a thorough examination of the bulbar and palpebral conjunctiva and documentation of each lesion's location, size, and appearance. However, biopsy should be performed if a PAM lesion differs from the characteristic, subtle lesions, including widespread or large lesions, dark lesions, lesions of the palpebral conjunctiva, and progressive lesions.

6.7.2 Surgery

The overwhelming consensus among ophthalmic oncologists and pathologists endorses biopsy of all conjunctival lesions that meet the clinical criteria of PAM [16, 27]. Small lesions should be excised entirely, while in widespread lesions incisional biopsies should be performed at various sites of the affected conjunctiva ("map biopsies"). The specimen(s) should be examined to determine the presence or absence of cytologic atypia and, in the case of excisional biopsies, the surgical margins should also be assessed. Discordance upon clinical and pathological correlation with sample site being unaffected upon clinical examination (non-pigmented) and pathology showing melanosis with atypia is suggestive of PAM sine pigmento (Fig. 6.9 and 6.10) [21].

6.7.3 Cryotherapy

Because of the tendency for PAM with atypia to recur, with the risk of melanoma development, Brownstein et al. [35] and Jakobiec et al. [36] recommended adding cryotherapy to the surgical excision. Shields et al. [37] suggest a six-step surgical procedure for conjunctival tumors in general: alcohol corneal epitheliectomy, no-touch local removal of distinct lesions, staging conjunctival biopsy specimens, limbal peritomy, double freeze–thaw cryotherapy to the involved bulbar conjunctiva, and wound closure. This approach may be useful in widespread PAM, but not needed in every case. In the Jakobiec series [36], none of the patients treated by surgical excision and cryotherapy progressed to invasive melanoma.

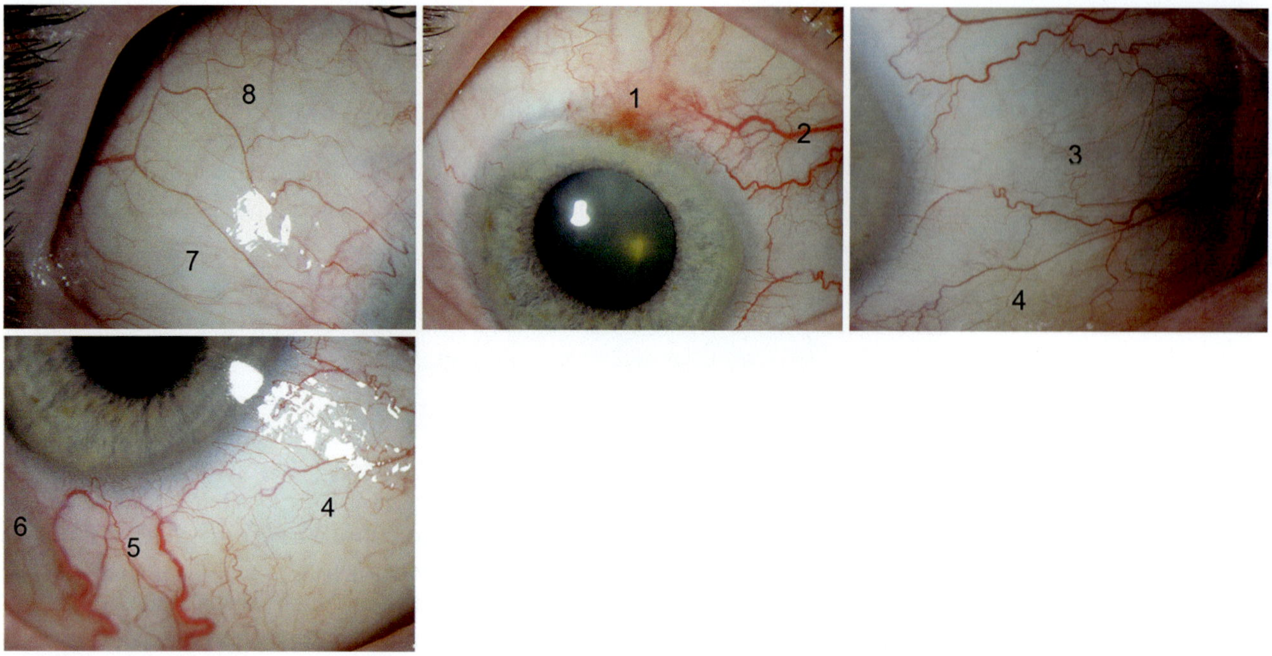

Fig. 6.9 Primary acquired melanosis sine pigmento. A middle-aged woman with prior history of conjunctival melanoma (7 years prior) presented with a noncontiguous limbal melanoma at 12:00 to 2:00 position that was excised with partial thickness scleral resection and adjuvant cryotherapy to the conjunctival margins. (Reproduced with permission from Soto H, Bowen RC, Raval V, et al. Primary acquired melanosis/melanoma: utility of conjunctival map biopsy. Br J Ophthalmol. 2022;106:605–9)

As mentioned above, in patients with PAM, clinical examination may not indicate the full extent of the intraepithelial melanocytic lesions. Additionally, the waxing-and-waning phenomenon of PAM may prevent identification of all locations of proliferating intraepithelial melanocytes that require treatment. Therefore, local excision and localized cryotherapy, even in cases of PAM that seem to be localized, may not cover the entire lesion. Furthermore, cryotherapy can cause complications such as scarring of the substantia propria, loss of eyelashes, ptosis, lax eyelids, tarsal floppiness, symblepharon, pseudopterygium, iritis, anterior-segment necrosis, macular edema, scleral melting, and cataract [35].

6.7.4 Topical Mitomycin C Chemotherapy

To cover the entire conjunctival and corneal surface, treating hidden areas of PAM and preventing the complications of cryotherapy, we originally managed a patient with widespread PAM with atypia by using mitomycin C [38]. Summarizing our experience with the first 12 consecutive patients [39], we recommended a protocol of 0.04% (0.4 mg/mL) mitomycin C drops four times daily for 2 weeks. This regimen is repeated as necessary with a pause of 2 weeks between courses, until disappearance or stabilization of the remnants of the pigmentation. At least three courses were recommended. In all patients, there was a complete or partial disappearance of pigmentation. In four patients, the pigmentation disappeared, whereas in eight patients some remnants of pigmentation remained (Fig. 6.2). In one patient, there was regrowth of the PAM, which was treated again by 0.04% mitomycin C, with success. Other groups have shown similar results in treating PAM with atypia by mitomycin C with slight differences in concentrations, duration of each cycle, and number of cycles prescribed [40–42]. All patients had conjunctival hyperemia during the treatment, and some complained of irritation, tearing, and eyelid swelling; these side effects resolved after cessation of therapy. The most severe adverse effect of this treatment is limbal stem cell deficiency (LSCD) [43]. This outcome led us to change the mitomycin C concentration to 0.03%, resulting in a similar response of the PAM and preventing LSCD.

It is important to note that treatment with mitomycin C should be applied only to intraepithelial lesions and should not be used for invasive conjunctival melanoma.

6.7.5 Topical Interferon α-2b

Interferon alpha-2b also has been shown to be effective in treating PAM with atypia in small case series [44–46], and has been used by many centers [47, 48]. However, its recent market withdrawal, supply shortage of this drug affects its availability, prevents its use [48].

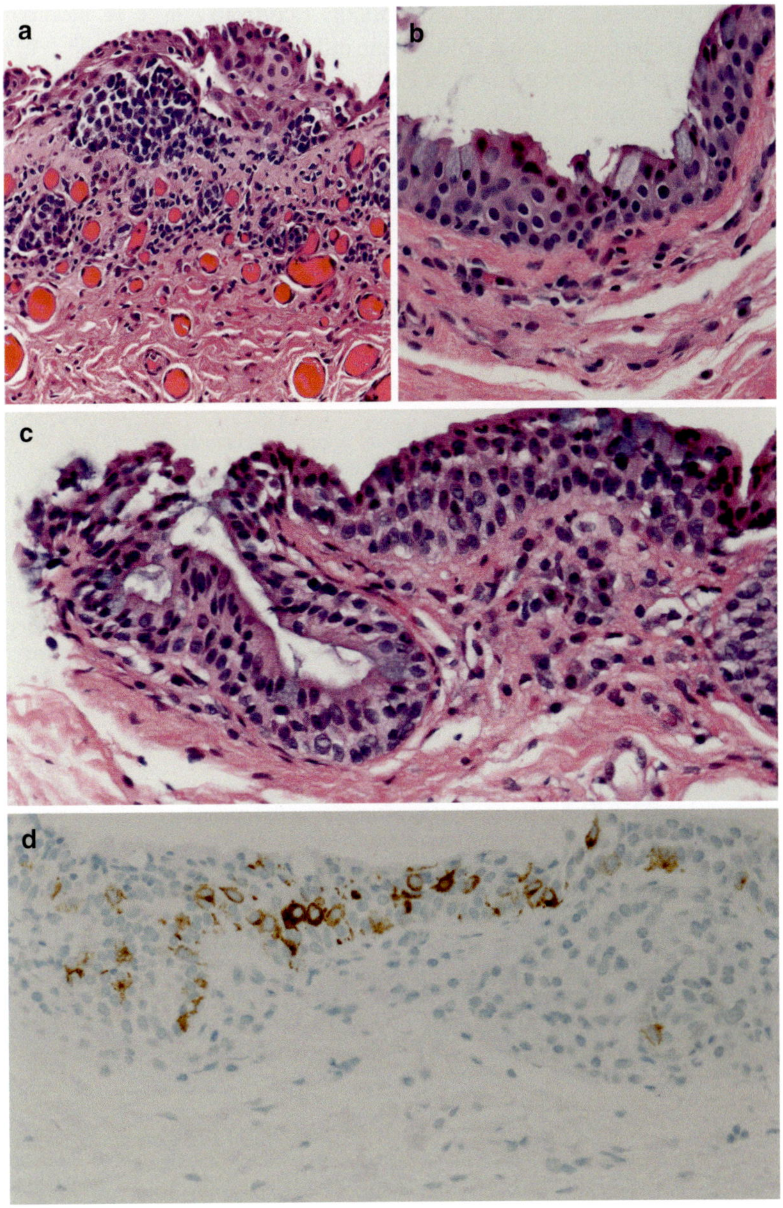

Fig. 6.10 Histopathology revealed minimally invasive melanoma with clear margins (**a**, H&E 400×; 1, diagnostic biopsy: grade 4). Map biopsies from inferior quadrants (**b**, H&E 400×; 3–7) were negative for melanosis (grade 0). Map biopsies from adjacent regions (2, superior nasal; 8, superior temporal) showed PAM with mild atypia (grade 2) (**c**, H&E 400×; D, HMB 45400×). Of note, if map biopsy was not done, PAM sine pigmento would not have been identified. (Reproduced with permission from: Soto H, Bowen RC, Raval V, et al. Primary acquired melanosis/melanoma: utility of conjunctival map biopsy. Br J Ophthalmol. 2022;106:605–9)

6.8 Prognosis

The study of the natural history of PAM in humans is not possible. A successful attempt in an animal model [49], generated by applying a 1% solution of DMBA to the conjunctiva in rabbits, showed a spectrum of disease, ranging from increased melanin production and melanocytic hyperplasia without atypia through atypical melanocyte hyperplasia of PAM.

The incidence of PAM recurrence depends on the presence or absence of atypia [16]. Recurrence after excision is rare in PAM without atypia; when this happens, it appears without cytological atypia. On the other hand, about 60% of lesions designated as "PAM with atypia" recur after excision alone; half of these recur as malignant melanoma. In one study [16], the median interval between the biopsy of PAM and the biopsy of melanoma was 2.5 years. Progression after 6 years is very rare, and progression to melanoma more than 10 years after the biopsy of PAM with atypia has not been observed. Recurrence is more likely when the lesion is incompletely excised or when the cornea is involved. Thus, when treating PAM with atypia, it is essential to treat the entire conjunctival and corneal lesion.

It is important to note that the mortality rate from conjunctival melanoma is about 25% with no difference between patients who had melanoma with PAM and those who had melanoma without PAM (Fig. 6.3) [27]. However, no mortality has been reported from PAM without transformation to melanoma. Although patients with PAM without atypia tend to be younger than patients with PAM with atypia [16], there is no evidence to indicate progression of PAM without atypia to PAM with atypia.

References

1. Ackerman AB, Sood R, Koenig M. Primary acquired melanosis of the conjunctiva is melanoma in situ. Mod Pathol. 1991;4:253–63.
2. Reese AB. Precancerous and cancerous melanosis. Am J Ophthalmol. 1966;61:1272–7.
3. Zimmerman LE. Criteria for management of melanosis. Arch Ophthalmol. 1966;76:307–8. [Letter]
4. Zimmerman LE. The histogenesis of conjunctival melanoma; the first Algernon B. Reese lecture. In: Jakobiec FA, editor. Ocular and adnexal tumors. Birmingham: Aesculapius; 1978. p. 600–30.
5. Silvers DN, Jakobiec FA, Freeman TR, et al. Melanoma of the conjunctiva: a clinicopathologic study. In: Jakobiec FA, editor. Ocular and adnexal tumors. Birmingham: Aesculapius; 1978. p. 583–99.
6. Zimmerman LE, Sobin LH. International histological classification of tumours. No. 24: histological typing of tumours of the eye and its adnexa. Geneva: World Health Organization; 1980. p. 30.
7. Jakobiec FA, Folberg R, Iwamoto T. Clinicopathologic characteristics of premalignant and malignant melanocytic lesions of the conjunctiva. Ophthalmology. 1989;96:147–66.
8. Damato B, Coupland SE. Conjunctival melanoma and melanosis: a reappraisal of terminology, classification and staging. Clin Experiment Ophthalmol. 2008;36:786–95.
9. Eberhart CG, Coupland SE, Folberg R, et al. Conjunctival melanocytic intraepithelial neoplasia. In: Grossniklaus HE, Eberhart CG, Kivela TT, editors. WHO classification of tumours of the eye. IARC: Lyon; 2018. p. 31–3.
10. Milman T, Zhang Q, Ang S, et al. Immunohistochemical profiling of conjunctival melanocytic intraepithelial lesions, including SOX10, HMB45, KI67, and P16. Am J Ophthalmol. 2021;222:148–56.
11. Milman T, Eiger-Moscovich M, Henry RK, et al. Validation of the newly proposed World Health Organization classification system for conjunctival melanocytic intraepithelial lesions: a comparison with C-MIN and PAM classification schemes. Am J Ophthalmol. 2021;223:60–74.
12. Jakobiec FA. Conjunctival primary acquired melanosis: is it time for a new terminology? Am J Ophthalmol. 2016;162:3–19.
13. Gloor P, Alexandrakis G. Clinical characterization of primary acquired melanosis. Invest Ophthalmol Vis Sci. 1995;36:1721–9.
14. Seregard S, Trampe E, Mansson-Brahme E, et al. Prevalence of primary acquired melanosis and nevi of the conjunctiva and uvea in the dysplastic nevus syndrome. A case-control study. Ophthalmology. 1995;102:1524–9.
15. Shields JA, Shields CL, Mashayekhi A, et al. Primary acquired melanosis of the conjunctiva: risks for progression to melanoma in 311 eyes. Ophthalmology. 2008;115:511–9.
16. Folberg R, McLean IW, Zimmerman LE. Primary acquired melanosis of the conjunctiva. Hum Pathol. 1985;16:129–35.
17. Messmer EM, Mackert MJ, Zapp DM, et al. In vivo confocal microscopy of pigmented conjunctival tumors. Graefes Arch Clin Exp Ophthalmol. 2006;244:1437–45.
18. Alzahrani YA, Kumar S, Abdul Aziz H, Plesec T, Singh AD. Primary acquired melanosis: clinical, histopathologic and optical coherence tomographic correlation. Ocul Oncol Pathol. 2016;2:123–7.
19. Shousha MA, Karp CL, Canto AP, et al. Diagnosis of ocular surface lesions using ultra-high-resolution optical coherence tomography. Ophthalmology. 2013;120:883–91.
20. Folberg R, McLean IW, Zimmerman LE. Conjunctival melanosis and melanoma. Ophthalmology. 1984;91:673–8.
21. Soto H, Bowen RC, Raval V, et al. Primary acquired melanosis/melanoma: utility of conjunctival map biopsy. Br J Ophthalmol. 2022;106:605–9.
22. Maly A, Epstein D, Meir K, et al. Histological criteria for grading of atypia in melanocytic conjunctival lesions. Pathology. 2008;40:676–81.
23. Sugiura M, Colby KA, Mihm MC Jr, et al. Low-risk and high-risk histologic features in conjunctival primary acquired melanosis with atypia: clinicopathologic analysis of 29 cases. Am J Surg Pathol. 2007;31:185–92.
24. Coupland SE, Milman T, Verdijk RM, Brouwer NJ. Conjunctival Melanocytic Intraepithelial Lesions. In: WHO Classification of Tumours Editorial Board. Eye tumours [Internet; beta version ahead of print]. Lyon (France): International Agency for Research on Cancer; 2023. (WHO classification of tumours series, 5th ed.; vol. 13).
25. Mudhar HS, Krishna Y, Cross S, et al. A multicenter study validates the WHO 2022 classification for conjunctival melanocytic intraepithelial lesions with clinical and prognostic relevance. Lab Invest. 2023;104:100281.
26. Chowers I, Livni N, Solomon A, et al. MIB-1 and PC-10 immunostaining for the assessment of proliferative activity in primary acquired melanosis without and with atypia. Br J Ophthalmol. 1998;82:1316–9.
27. Sharara NA, Alexander RA, Luthert PJ, et al. Differential immunoreactivity of melanocytic lesions of the conjunctiva. Histopathology. 2001;39:426–31.
28. Jiang K, Brownstein S, Lam K, Burns B, Farmer J. Usefulness of a red chromagen in the diagnosis of melanocytic lesions of the conjunctiva. JAMA Ophthalmol. 2014;132:622–9.
29. Goldenberg-Cohen N, Cohen Y, Rosenbaum E, et al. T1799A BRAF mutations in conjunctival melanocytic lesions. Invest Ophthalmol Vis Sci. 2005;46:3027–30.
30. Dratviman-Storobinsky O, Cohen Y, Frenkel S, et al. Lack of oncogenic GNAQ mutations in melanocytic lesions of the conjunctiva as compared to uveal melanoma. Invest Ophthalmol Vis Sci. 2010;51:6180–2.
31. LeBlanc RE, Miller DM, Zegans ME. PRAME immunohistochemistry is useful in the evaluation of conjunctival melanomas, nevi, and primary acquired melanosis. J Cutan Pathol. 2021;48:1442–8.
32. Mudhar HS, Milman T, Stevenson S, et al. PRAME expression by immunohistochemistry and reverse transcription quantitative PCR in conjunctival melanocytic lesions—a comprehensive clinicopathologic study of 202 cases and correlation of cytogenetics with PRAME expression in challenging conjunctival melanocytic lesions. Hum Pathol. 2023;134:1–18.
33. Huang YY, Hrycaj SM, Chan MP, et al. PRAME expression in junctional melanocytic proliferations of the conjunctiva: a potential biomarker for primary acquired melanosis/conjunctival melanocytic intraepithelial lesions. Am J Dermatopathol. 2022;44:734–40.

34. Folberg R, Jakobiec FA, Bernardino VB, et al. Benign conjunctival melanocytic lesions. Clinicopathologic features. Ophthalmology. 1989;96:436–61.
35. Brownstein S, Jakobiec FA, Wilkinson RD, et al. Cryotherapy for precancerous melanosis (atypical melanocytic hyperplasia) of the conjunctiva. Arch Ophthalmol. 1981;99:1224–31.
36. Jakobiec FA, Rini FJ, Fraunfelder FT, et al. Cryotherapy for conjunctival primary acquired melanosis and malignant melanoma. Experience with 62 cases. Ophthalmology. 1988;95:1058–70.
37. Shields JA, Shields CL, De Potter P. Surgical management of conjunctival tumors. Arch Ophthalmol. 1997;115:808–15.
38. Frucht-Pery J, Pe'er J. Use of Mitomycin C in the treatment of conjunctival primary acquired melanosis with atypia. Arch Ophthalmol. 1996;114:1261–4.
39. Pe'er J, Frucht-Pery J. The treatment of primary acquired melanosis (PAM) with atypia by topical Mitomycin C. Am J Ophthalmol. 2005;139:229–34.
40. Yuen VH, Jordan DR, Brownstein S, et al. Topical mitomycin treatment for primary acquired melanosis of the conjunctiva. Ophthalmic Plast Reconstr Surg. 2003;19:149–51.
41. Kurli M, Finger PT. Topical mitomycin chemotherapy for conjunctival malignant melanoma and primary acquired melanosis with atypia: 12 years' experience. Graefes Arch Clin Exp Ophthalmol. 2005;243:1108–14.
42. Chalasani R, Giblin M, Conway RM. Role of topical chemotherapy for primary acquired melanosis and malignant melanoma of the conjunctiva and cornea: review of the evidence and recommendations for treatment. Clin Experiment Ophthalmol. 2006;34:708–14.
43. Lichtinger A, Pe'er J, Frucht-Pery J, et al. Limbal stem cell deficiency after topical mitomycin C therapy for primary acquired melanosis with atypia. Ophthalmology. 2010;117:431–7.
44. Finger PT, Sedeek RW, Chin KJ. Topical interferon alpha in the treatment of conjunctival melanoma and primary acquired melanosis complex. Am J Ophthalmol. 2008;145:124–9.
45. Herold TR, Hintschich C. Interferon alpha for the treatment of melanocytic conjunctival lesions. Graefes Arch Clin Exp Ophthalmol. 2010;248:111–5.
46. Garip A, Schaumberger MM, Wolf A, et al. Evaluation of a short-term topical interferon α-2b treatment for histologically proven melanoma and primary acquired melanosis with atypia. Orbit. 2016;35:29–34.
47. Cid-Bertomeu P, Huerva V. Use of interferon alpha 2b to manage conjunctival primary acquired melanosis and conjunctival melanoma. Surv Ophthalmol. 2022;67:1391–404.
48. Jiang J, Bohringer D, Auw-Hadrich C, et al. Current practice in the treatment of epithelial and melanocytic tumours with interferone-alpha-2b: a survey of tertiary eye centers in Germany. Klin Monatsbl Augenheilkd. 2023;240:891–6.
49. Folberg R, Baron J, Reeves RD, et al. Animal model of conjunctival primary acquired melanosis. Ophthalmology. 1989;96:1006–13.

Conjunctival Melanoma

7

Jacob Pe'er and Robert Folberg

7.1 Introduction

Conjunctival melanoma is a rare but potentially devastating malignancy. It may arise de novo, from preexisting conjunctival nevus or primary acquired melanosis (PAM) with atypia or from a combination of nevus and PAM with atypia. All these arise from melanocytes that migrate from the neural crest to reside in the conjunctival mucosal epithelium and show similarities to cutaneous melanoma. In the medical literature, conjunctival melanoma is sometimes labeled alongside uveal melanoma as "ocular melanoma." The clinical behavior, etiologies, molecular biology, and histopathological features of conjunctival and uveal melanoma differ. Therefore, conjunctival melanoma should be approached as an entity separate from uveal melanoma [1].

7.2 Epidemiological Aspects

According to several studies, conjunctival melanoma accounts for 2–5% of ocular melanomas [2] and fewer than 3% of excisional biopsies of conjunctival lesions [3]. Cutaneous melanoma is 450–900 times more common than conjunctival melanoma, a ratio that is increasing.

Because of the rarity of conjunctival melanoma, incidence studies based on population-based data are scarce. The incidence of conjunctival melanoma ranges between 0.3 and 0.8 per million in Caucasian adults and has been rising during the last five decades [4, 5]. According to a Dutch survey, the annual incidence of conjunctival melanoma ranges between 0.28 and 0.34 per million inhabitants [6]. A Swedish study showed a significant increase in the incidence of conjunctival melanoma from 1960 to 2005, from 0.10 cases/million to 0.74/million in males and from 0.06/million to 0.45/million in females [4]. Population-based registry data from the Surveillance, Epidemiology, and End Results (SEER) program of the National Cancer Institute (NCI) of the United States show a significant increase in the incidence rate of conjunctival melanoma from 0.22 cases per million per year in 1973–1979 to 0.46 in 1990–1999 [5]. The most significant increase is for white men. Because changes in incidence coincide with those seen in cutaneous melanoma, the authors suggest a link to sunlight exposure. A study from Denmark has also shown an increase in the incidence of conjunctival melanoma between 1960 and 2012 to 0.5 per million per year, caused mainly by an increase in older patients (>65 years) [7]. A European study from 41 cancer centers showed a crude incidence of 0.46 per million and an increase with age [8]. Another recent Canadian study showed 0.32 cases per million individuals annually [9].

Population-based data indicate that a similar number of men and women develop conjunctival melanoma [6, 8], but other studies report a higher incidence in males [4, 5, 9]. Conjunctival melanoma is more common in middle-aged and older persons between the fourth and seventh decades of life [4, 6], and only a few cases in children have been reported [10]. When conjunctival melanoma develops in xeroderma pigmentosum—a rare event—younger patients are affected [11]. Conjunctival melanoma is less common in the black population and other non-white individuals [2, 5], and according to the SEER program, the overall white-to-black incidence ratio in conjunctival melanoma is 2.6:1 [12]. In a study from New Zealand, non-Europeans were diagnosed at a significantly younger age [13].

J. Pe'er (✉)
Ocular Oncology Service and Ophthalmic Pathology Laboratory, Department of Ophthalmology, Hadassah—Hebrew University Medical Center, Jerusalem, Israel
e-mail: peer@hadassah.org.il

R. Folberg
Ophthalmology and Pathology, Oakland University William Beaumont School of Medicine, Rochester, MI, USA

© The Author(s), under exclusive license to Springer Nature Switzerland AG 2024
J. Pe'er et al. (eds.), *Clinical Ophthalmic Oncology*, https://doi.org/10.1007/978-3-031-72443-5_7

7.3 Etiology and Associated Diseases

Until recently, there was no clear evidence that ultraviolet radiation is a causative factor in the development of conjunctival melanoma, even though most of these tumors develop in the sunlight-exposed bulbar conjunctiva [2, 14]. However, in recent molecular studies, mutations in the telomerase reverse transcriptase (TERT) promoter, typical of UV-induced DNA damage and identical to mutations in cutaneous melanoma, were found in bulbar conjunctival melanoma but not in uveal melanoma [15–17]. In two studies from Scandinavia, the increased incidence of conjunctival melanoma in five decades was more frequent in the bulbar conjunctiva. This may indicate etiological and genetic differences between bulbar and nonbulbar conjunctival melanoma [4, 7]. However, another work noticed no differences in gene expression of oncology-related genes between sun-exposed and nonexposed conjunctival melanoma, suggesting less influence of UV on genetic profile [18]. About 70–75% of conjunctival melanomas are associated with PAM with atypia, 7–17% with conjunctival nevus, and 8–19% develop de novo [19]. No significant association with cutaneous melanoma, dysplastic nevus syndrome, neurofibromatosis type 1, or ocular or oculodermal melanocytosis (nevus of Ota) has been observed [20].

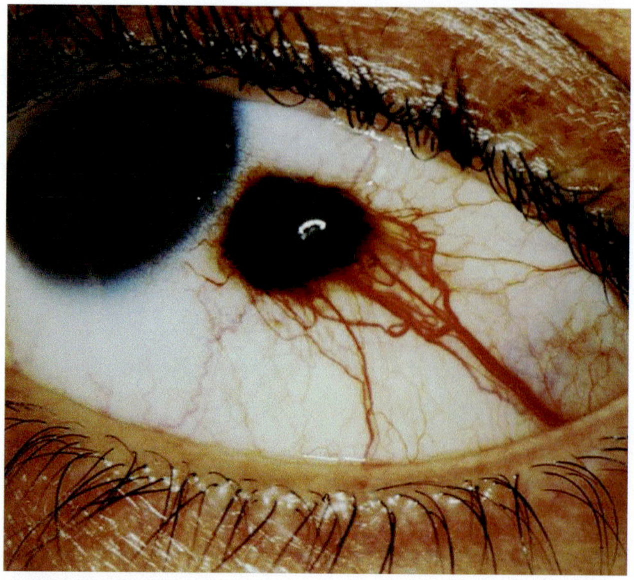

Fig. 7.1 Melanoma of the peri-limbal bulbar conjunctiva with "feeder vessels" entering the tumor

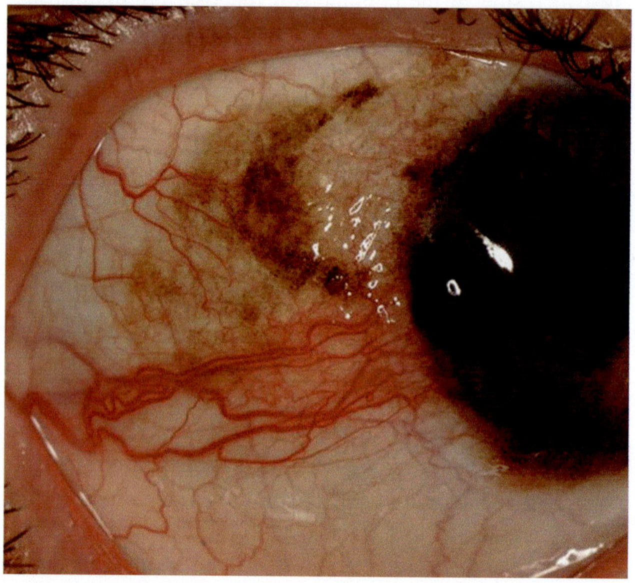

Fig. 7.2 Conjunctival PAM with atypia, which has progressed to corneal-limbal melanoma

7.4 Clinical Features

Conjunctival melanoma usually affects one eye and is typically pigmented. Amelanotic conjunctival melanoma does occur and can be mistaken clinically for squamous cell carcinoma [21]. Careful high-magnification slit-lamp examination typically reveals pigmentation flecks, even in amelanotic melanomas. Any region of the conjunctiva, including the caruncle and plica semilunaris, may be affected (Figs. 7.1, 7.2, 7.3, 7.4, 7.5, and 7.6). Most conjunctival melanomas, however, develop at the limbus (Fig. 7.7). Conjunctival nevi are very rare in the palpebral conjunctiva and fornix. Therefore, pigmented lesions in these areas should be considered suspicious for melanoma and excised. In vivo confocal microscopy [22], ultrasound biomicroscopy [23], and high-resolution optical coherence tomography (HR-OCT) [24] serve as additional diagnostic tools in differentiating conjunctival melanoma from other conjunctival melanocytic lesions (Fig. 7.8).

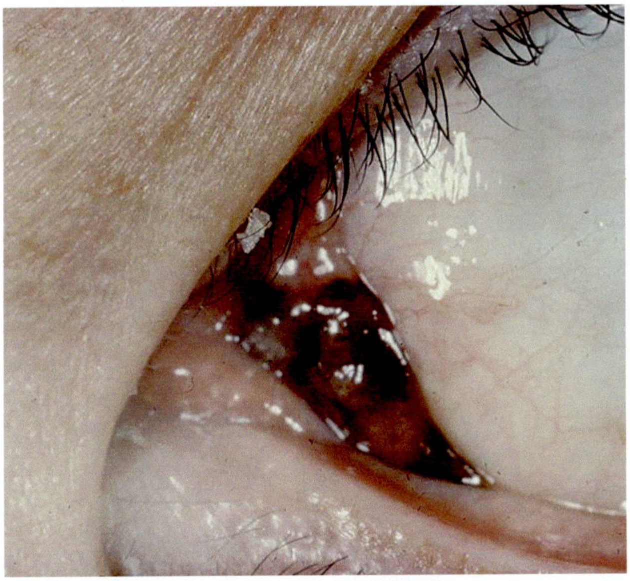

Fig. 7.3 Melanoma of the plica semilunaris

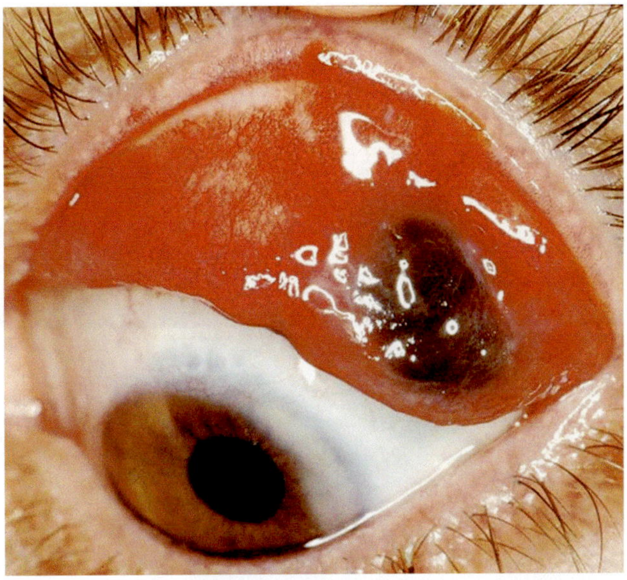

Fig. 7.4 Melanoma of the upper palpebral conjunctiva

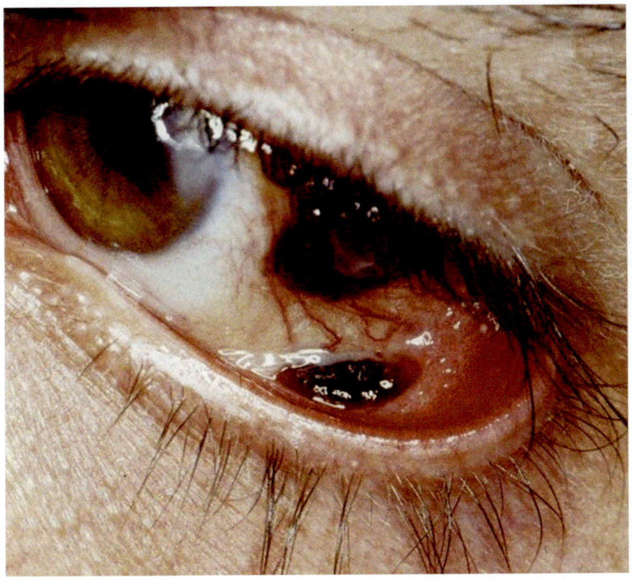

Fig. 7.5 Multifocal melanoma arising from PAM with atypia, with a tumor in the bulbar conjunctiva and a tumor in the lower fornix

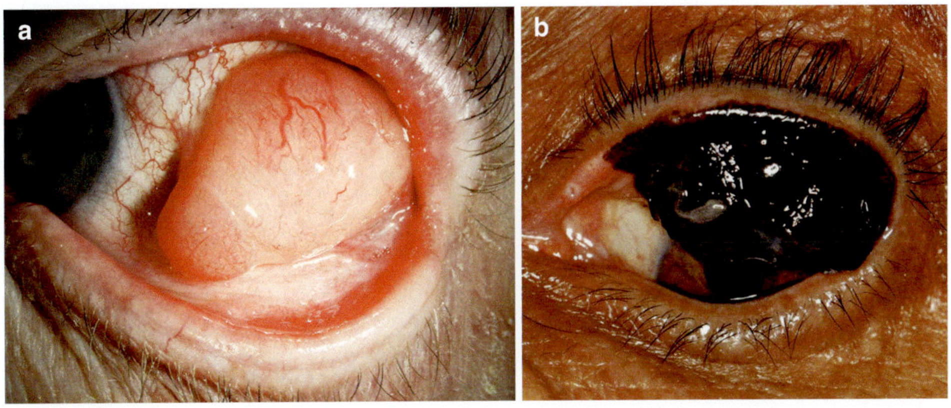

Fig. 7.6 Large amelanotic conjunctival melanoma (**a**). Extensive conjunctival melanoma involved the entire upper palpebral conjunctiva, which could be seen only upon inversion of the upper eyelid (**b**). As bulbar conjunctiva was not involved, there was a delay in diagnosis

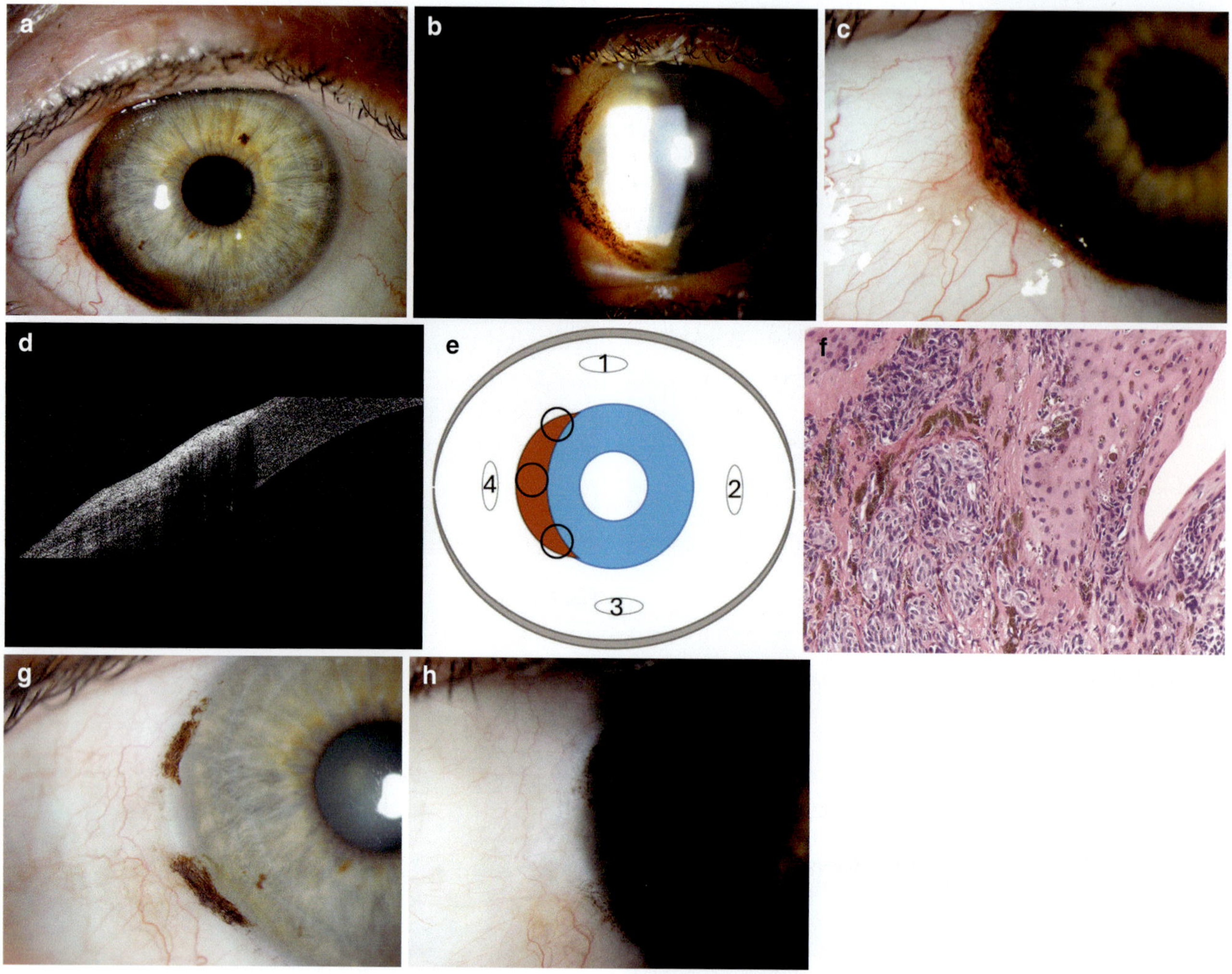

Fig. 7.7 A 65-year-old woman presented with new-onset pigmentation in the right eye. Examination showed superficial speckled pigmentation at limbus from 6:30 to 11:0 with 2 mm extension onto corneal surface at 6:30 (**a–c**). AS OCT shows thickened stroma with hyperreflectivity (**d**). Conjunctival primary melanosis with melanoma in situ was suspected. Main tumor biopsies that comprised of a 2.5 mm circular disc (**e**, circle) that included conjunctival limbus and adjacent corneal epithelium from temporal, superotemporal, and inferotemporal limbus were confirmatory for PAM with severe atypia (melanoma in situ) (**f**, H&E 200×), whereas map biopsies (oval) of the bulbar conjunctiva were negative. Because of localized nature of the melanoma, we elected to treat her with EPB (45 Gy in 50.5 h to the depth of 2.0 mm). Note marked improvement 3 months after EPB (**g**) with progressive rarefaction of pigmentation at 42 months (**h**). She remained free of local recurrence and metastasis over the duration of the follow-up. (Courtesy Arun D. Singh, MD (Clinical) and Gabriella Yeaney, MD (Pathology), Cleveland Clinic, Cleveland, Ohio)

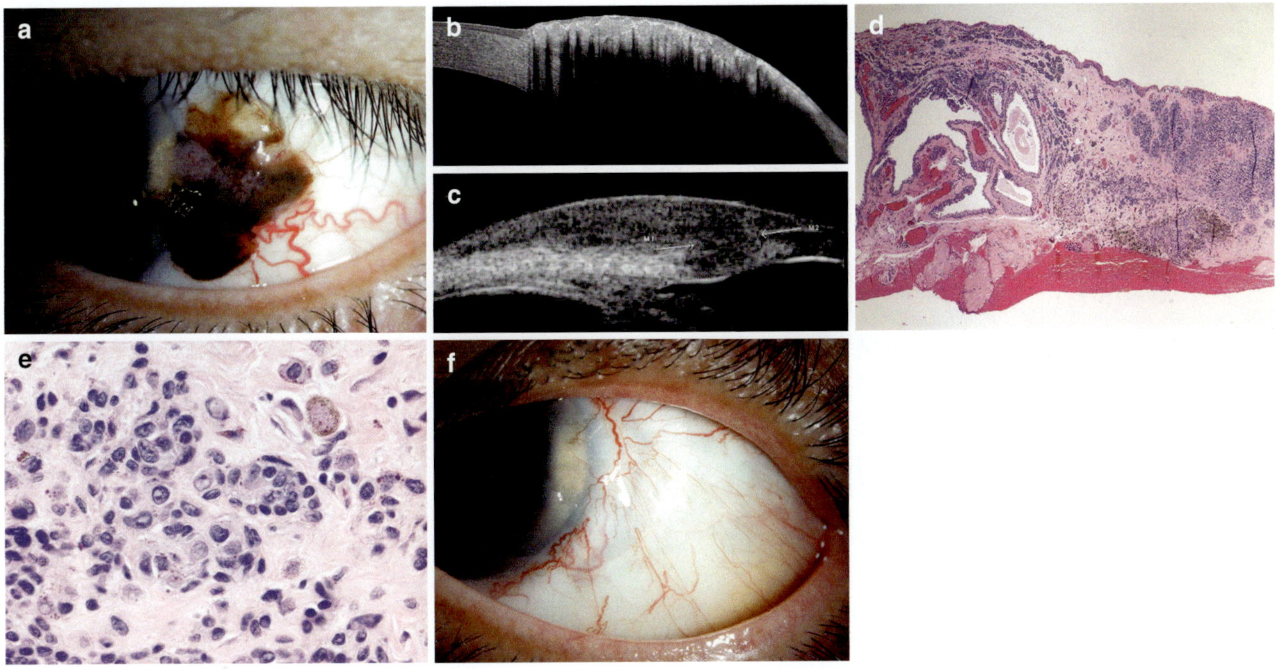

Fig. 7.8 Conjunctiva melanoma. Malignant transformation of a conjunctival nevus. Partially melanocytic mass (8.0 × 6.0 × 2.0 mm) with feeder and intrinsic vessels, and corneal involvement (**a**). AS OCT showed subepithelial mass with pigment-induced shadowing artifact (**b**). Note that deep margin not visible by OCT showed full-thickness corneoscleral invasion by UBM (**c**, arrows). The patient underwent excision (including corneal epitheliectomy using absolute alcohol) with adjuvant cryotherapy. Intraoperative observations confirmed adherence to the cornea and sclera at 3 o'clock. The lesion was excised parallel to Bowman layer and scleral plane. Further deep dissection was not performed due to concern of corneal perforation (to be managed by episcleral plaque brachytherapy [EPB]). Repair (10 mm vertical and 12 mm horizontal) was done with conjunctival autograft. Histopathology (**d**, H&E 20×) revealed asymmetry, lack of maturation at base (**e**, H&E 600×) and atypical cells with macronucleoli, and epithelial cysts consistent with melanoma arising in conjunctival nevus. The deep (scleral margin) was positive. After allowing 4 weeks for healing, EPB was performed (45 Gy to the depth of 3 mm over 72 h). Then, 23 months later, the patient underwent uncomplicated surgery (20/20) for radiation-induced cataract. He has remained free of local recurrence and distant metastasis over 48 months of surveillance (**f**). (Courtesy: Arun D. Singh, MD (Clinical) and Gabriella Yeaney, MD (Pathology), Cleveland Clinic, Cleveland, Ohio)

7.5 Variants

7.5.1 Conjunctival Melanoma Associated with PAM

Microinvasive melanoma arising in PAM with atypia can be difficult to identify clinically; therefore, one should search carefully for subtle placoid thickening within the area of PAM. The more dramatic clinical evidence for melanoma development from PAM is the sudden emergence of one or more nodules in flat lesions (Fig. 7.9) [25, 26]. Multifocal melanomas are usually associated with PAM with atypia and may appear simultaneously or sequentially in different parts of the conjunctiva [25, 26]. Melanoma with PAM may also involve the adjacent eyelid skin [19]. (For details on PAM, see Chap. 6.)

7.5.2 Conjunctival Melanoma Associated with Nevus

Conjunctival melanoma arising from a nevus, or de novo, appears clinically as a solitary pigmented or nonpigmented smooth vascularized nodule, commonly in the limbal area. Rarely are these lesions pedunculated (Fig. 7.10) [2].

7.5.3 Primary Melanoma of the Cornea

Primary melanoma of the cornea is uncommon, although several cases have been reported [2]. Many of these cases represent examples of corneal invasion from a limbal melanoma (Fig. 7.11). It is important to remember that Bowman layer is a barrier to the invasion of the corneal stroma. Therefore, pigmented neoplasms affecting the cornea are usually superficial to Bowman layer unless this tissue has been violated by previous surgery.

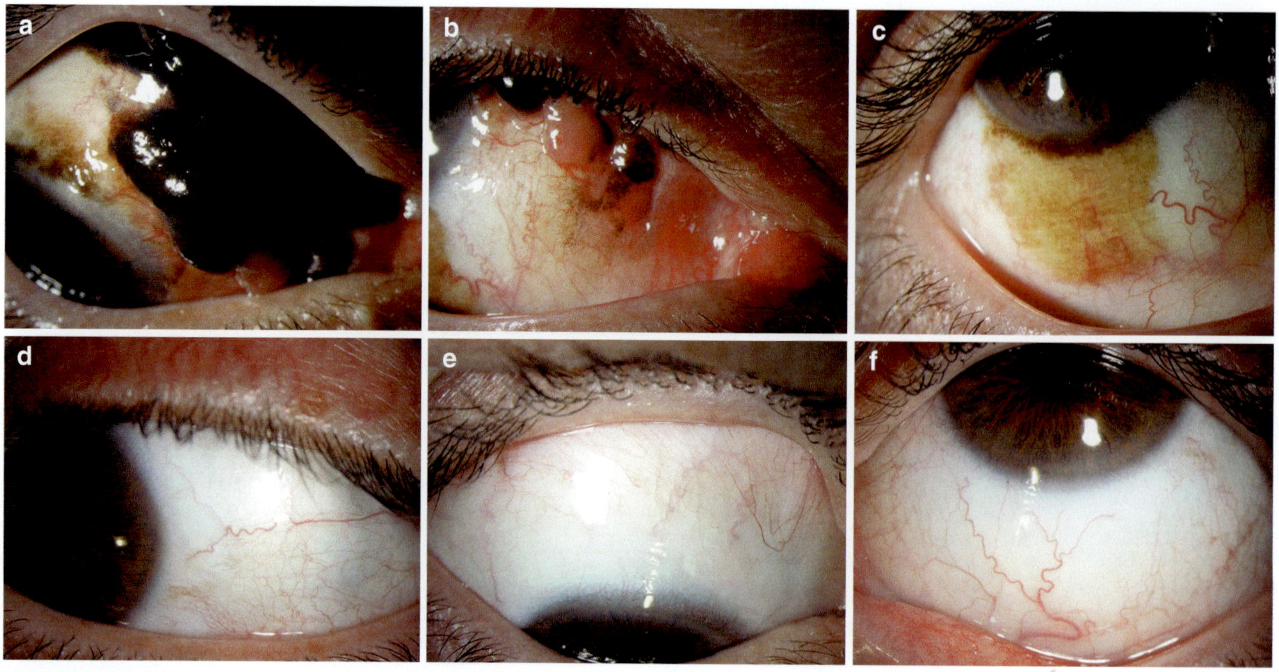

Fig. 7.9 Conjunctiva melanoma. Malignant transformation of primary acquired melanosis (PAM). Partially melanocytic mass (**a, b**) with diffuse PAM (**c**). The patient underwent excision with adjuvant cryotherapy. Intraoperative observations confirmed lack of adherence to the sclera. The conjunctiva was ballooned with lidocaine and epinephrine mixture. 2 mm beyond the visible margin of the conjunctiva, the conjunctival incision was made extending from superotemporal to the nasal bulbar region and extending inferiorly and then curving back toward the limbus from 12 to 4 o'clock position. The lesion was superficial to the Tenon's, and therefore, the underlying Tenon's was spared. Very slow careful dissection was performed maintaining the encapsulation of the melanoma and pigmentation. The underlying tissues did not have any pigmentation. The wound was 40 mm horizontal × 18 mm vertical. Double freeze–thaw cryotherapy was applied to the conjunctival margins. Amniotic membrane graft was placed over the medial bulbar region, particularly covering the muscle insertion. Additional map biopsy samples were also obtained. Histopathology revealed melanoma arising in a background of melanosis with severe atypia/melanoma in situ (main tumor) and melanosis with severe atypia (melanoma in situ) of the inferior conjunctiva. After allowing 4 weeks for healing, four cycles of topical mitomycin (0.04%) were prescribed. The patient remained free of local recurrence but developed metastasis to the brain, liver, and lymph nodes 22 months after the initial presentation (**d, e, f**). (Courtesy: Arun D. Singh, MD (Clinical) and Gabriella Yeaney, MD (Pathology), Cleveland Clinic, Cleveland, Ohio)

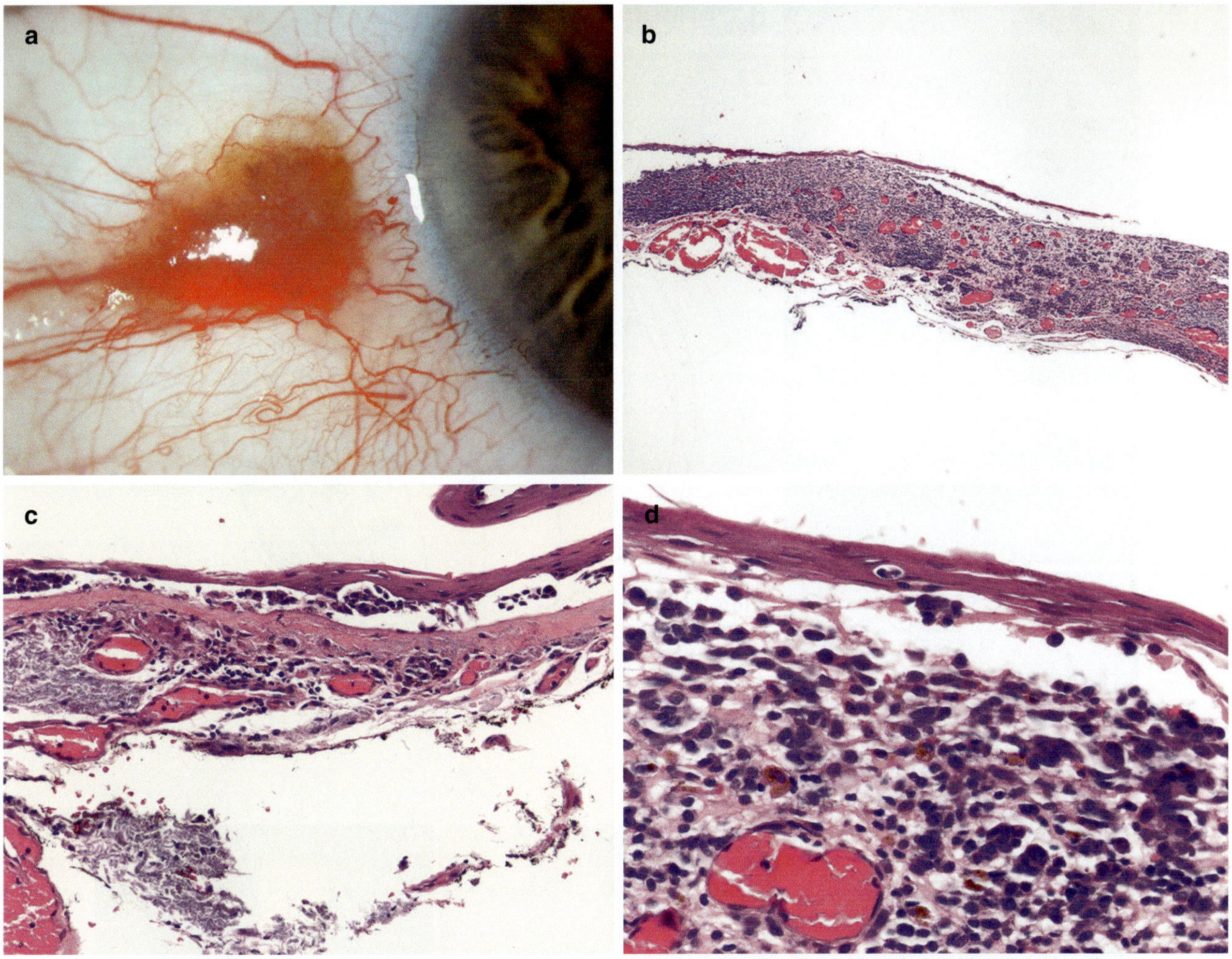

Fig. 7.10 Conjunctiva melanoma. Malignant transformation of nevus. The lesion had been present since age 13 years with more redness in recent months. Tan-colored mass (8.0 × 5.0 mm) with trace of inherent pigment (**a**). The patient underwent excision with adjuvant cryotherapy. Intraoperative observations confirmed lack of adherence to the sclera. Double freeze–thaw cryotherapy was applied to the conjunctival margins. The wound was 12 mm horizontal × 9 mm vertical and could be close primarily without the use of graft. On histopathology, the bulk of the lesion was composed of a stromal proliferation of banal-appearing melanocytes (**b**, H&E 40×) with associated cyst formation and maturation toward the base (**c**, H&E 200x), consistent with conjunctival nevus. However, there was intraepithelial nesting, epithelioid morphology, and increased atypia, diagnostic of melanoma in situ (**d**, H&E 400×). (Courtesy: Arun D. Singh, MD (Clinical) and Gabriella Yeaney, MD (Pathology), Cleveland Clinic, Cleveland, Ohio)

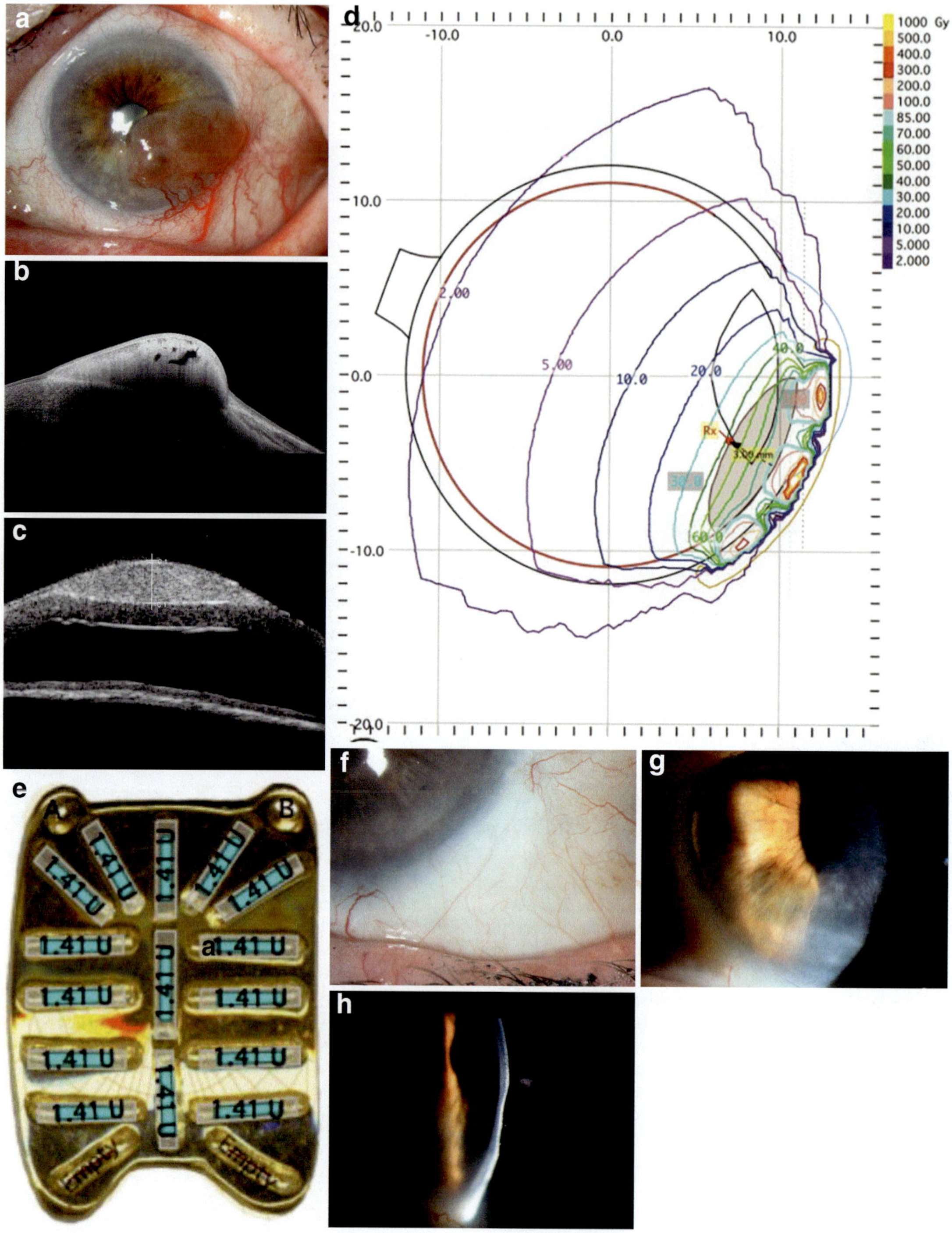

Fig. 7.11 An 81-year-old woman was referred for evaluation of a pyogenic granuloma of the left eye. Examination revealed primary acquired melanosis (PAM) with multifocal of melanoma. The temporal bulbar melanoma was less conspicuous (5.0 × 3.0 × 1.0 mm) than the corneal melanoma (7.5 × 5.6 × 1.1 mm) with feeder vessels (**a**). Anterior-segment OCT (**b**) and UBM did not suggest extension into corneal stroma (**c**). Both conjunctival and corneal melanoma were excised as a single tumor combined with alcohol corneal epitheliectomy, cryotherapy to the conjunctival margins, and map biopsies. Total excision was 12 × 7 mm in size that was repaired with Tenon closure and postoperative use of 16 mm Kontur bandage soft lens (Kontur Kontact Lens, Co., Inc. Hercules, CA, USA). Intraoperatively, there was no involvement of the sclera or the underlying muscle. However, there was evidence of superficial corneal stromal involvement at 6 o'clock position for approximately 3 mm × 3 mm area requiring superficial lamellar keratectomy (approximately 10%). Histopathology confirmed invasive melanoma with negative corneal and conjunctival epithelium but deep margin was positive. Map biopsies were negative for PAM elsewhere. Allowing for 4 weeks of healing, episcleral/corneal plaque brachytherapy was performed with plaque being centered over the area of corneal stromal involvement. 45 Gy was delivered over 72 h (**d**) using an I-125 source using EP 917 plaque (**e**, IsoAid, Port Richey, FL, USA). The patient remained free from local recurrence (**f**) and metastasis at 2.5-year follow-up visit with visual acuity of 20/40 (**f**) and only slight corneal stromal opacity (**g**) and corneal thinning (**h**). (Courtesy: Arun D. Singh, MD (Clinical) and Gabriella Yeaney, MD (Pathology), Cleveland Clinic, Cleveland, Ohio)

7.6 Differential Diagnosis

Any conjunctival pigmented lesion may simulate conjunctival melanoma.

7.6.1 Conjunctival Nevus

Conjunctival nevi may be elevated and dark, and in the absence of cysts (typical of compound conjunctival nevi), it may be challenging to differentiate the nevus from melanoma by clinical examination alone [26]. Most conjunctival nevi are noticed in childhood and adolescence. Therefore, any newly elevated pigmented conjunctival lesion that develops in adulthood should be viewed with suspicion. Conjunctival nevi almost always emerge in the bulbar conjunctiva and caruncle. Therefore, any pigmented lesion in the palpebral conjunctiva or fornix should be considered suspicious for melanoma [26].

7.6.2 Epithelial Tumors (Nonmelanocytic)

Nonmelanocytic epithelial tumors such as squamous papilloma, conjunctival intraepithelial neoplasia, and invasive squamous cell carcinoma may acquire melanin in darkly complexioned individuals [27].

7.6.3 Intraocular Tumors

Epibulbar extension of uveal melanoma or melanocytoma should also be considered in the differential diagnosis of conjunctival melanoma [28]. In these cases, the trans-scleral nature of the lesion can be identified by high-frequency ocular ultrasound.

7.6.4 Miscellaneous Lesions

Staphyloma, subconjunctival hematoma, foreign body, and hematic cyst may also be confused clinically with conjunctival melanoma [2]. The rare occurrence of metastatic cutaneous melanoma to the conjunctiva has been reported [29].

7.7 Histopathological Features

7.7.1 Light Microscopy

The definitive diagnosis of conjunctival melanoma is made by histopathological examination. Most cases can be diagnosed with confidence by light microscopy (Fig. 7.12). Four types of atypical melanocytes have been described in conjunctival melanoma: small polyhedral, spindle, balloon, and round epithelioid cells with eosinophilic cytoplasm [26]. Intraepithelial PAM with atypia may be a precursor to invasive melanoma. Therefore, PAM with atypia often appears alongside a focus of invasive melanoma (Fig. 7.13). Any basement membrane breaching by atypical melanocytes in

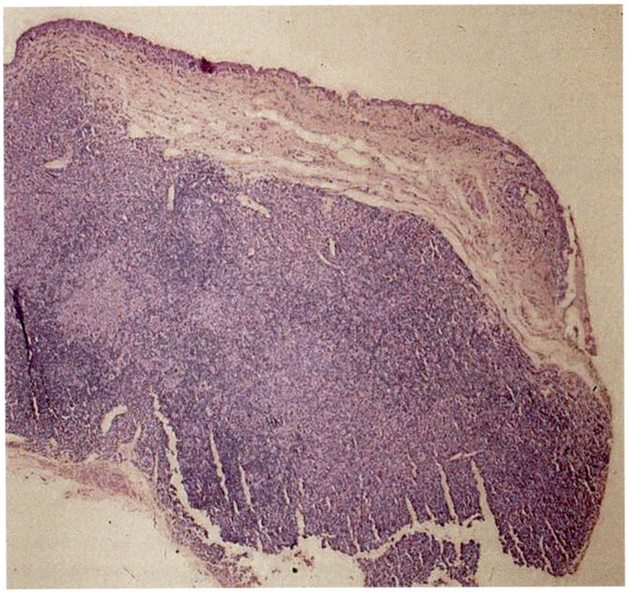

Fig. 7.12 Low-magnification histological picture showing thick conjunctival melanoma involving the specimen's margin (hematoxylin and eosin; original magnification ×4)

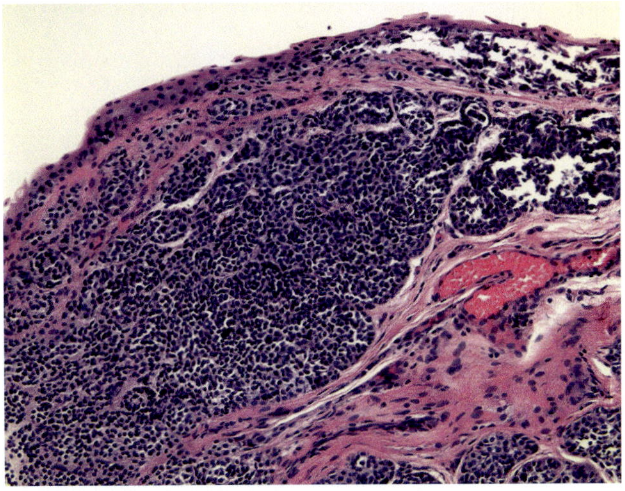

Fig. 7.13 This photomicrograph illustrates conjunctival melanoma arising in the context of PAM with atypia. Note the lack of maturation or architectural organization from top to bottom and the presence of atypical intraepithelial melanocytes that do not appear to be cohesive or to have any architectural relationship with the epithelial cells (hematoxylin and eosin; original magnification ×20)

PAM with atypia should be considered invasive melanoma. The presence of atypical melanocytes within the epithelium of subepithelial cysts represents PAM with atypia and not invasive melanoma. Cysts and solid epithelial inclusions found frequently in compound conjunctival nevi may confuse pathologists without experience in ophthalmic pathology, who can mistake these benign findings for malignancy.

7.7.2 Immunohistochemistry and Molecular Pathology

If in doubt, immunohistochemical stains such as HMB-45, MELAN-A, and SOX-10, either individually or in a cocktail, can demonstrate the presence of melanocytes [30–32], and Ki-67 proliferation index may help to differentiate melanoma from nevi [33]. BRAF mutations are found in about a third to half of conjunctival melanoma cases, and similar to cutaneous melanoma, the most common BRAF mutation is V600E [34–37]. BRAF mutations are seldom encountered in uveal melanomas. Conversely, GNAQ mutations occur in uveal melanomas and are not found in conjunctival melanomas [38]. TERT promoter mutations with a UV signature are found in 32–41% of conjunctival melanomas [14–16]. NRAS mutations, NF1 mutations, and ATRX loss may also be found in these tumors [37, 39]. PRAME expression by immunohistochemistry helps distinguish melanoma and PAM with high-grade atypia from benign melanocytic conjunctival lesions [40, 41]. Expression of programmed cell death protein-1 (PD-1) and programmed death-ligand 1 (PD-L1) [42, 43], as well as specific micro-RNA [44], are reported in conjunctival melanoma. All these markers may have therapeutic implications.

7.7.3 Histopathological Prognostic Factors

Several histopathological features indicate a poor prognosis in patients with conjunctival melanoma. The significant prognostic factor predictive of metastasis is the depth of invasion, measured with an ocular micrometer from the top of the epithelium to the deepest point of invasion. The other important histological prognostic factors are pagetoid spread, mixed cell tumors versus spindle cell tumors, histological evidence of lymphatic invasion, increased lymphangiogenic activity, high number of mitotic figures, and high cell proliferation index using immunohistochemical stains such as PCNA or Ki-67 [2, 19, 45, 46]. PD-L1 expression, TERT promoter mutations, and ATRX loss correlate with poor prognosis [47–49]. BRAF mutation is of limited use for prognosis in conjunctival melanoma [36, 37]. Ulceration in conjunctival melanoma is also a critical histopathological predictor for adverse outcomes [45, 50]. The presence of PAM with atypia does not appear to be a prognostic indicator [19].

7.8 Clinical Course

7.8.1 Local Recurrence

Local recurrence of conjunctival melanoma has been reported in 56–65% of the patients, and nearly half of these patients develop more than one recurrence [2, 4, 6, 51]. The mean interval between the first treatment and the first recurrence is about 2.5 years. Some authorities report that patients treated by surgical excision alone have more recurrences than those receiving adjuvant therapy such as cryotherapy or brachytherapy. Still, it is unknown if this recommendation applies to surgical resections with clear margins. For example, patients with multifocal disease, usually originating in PAM with atypia, are prone to develop recurrences because it can be challenging to ensure a clear resection margin. Other risk factors for developing recurrence are melanoma in locations other than the limbus and involvement of surgical margins [51]. Therefore, the pathologist's report should specifically comment on the tumor involvement of surgical margins. Other risk factors that were found in a large study are older age, history of prior conjunctival surgery, and advanced AJCC T-subcategory [52]. Local recurrences are managed as the primary melanoma.

7.8.2 Local Spread

Conjunctival melanoma can spread locally in the conjunctiva and metastasize to regional lymph nodes and systemically [53]. "In-transit" metastases of conjunctival melanoma, which are believed to represent local lymphatic spread within the conjunctiva, have been described (Figs. 7.14 and 7.15) [54, 55]. Dissemination of melanoma cells at the time of tumor excision has also been reported. Spread of conjunctival melanoma through the nasolacrimal duct to the nasal cavity and paranasal sinuses has been attributed to the shedding of exfoliated melanoma cells in the tear film, by direct extension, and as regional hematogenous metastases [2]. Epistaxis or epiphora may indicate extension and recurrence of the conjunctival melanoma in the nasolacrimal system [56]. Rarely does conjunctival melanoma invade the eyeball or extend directly into the orbit [2, 57].

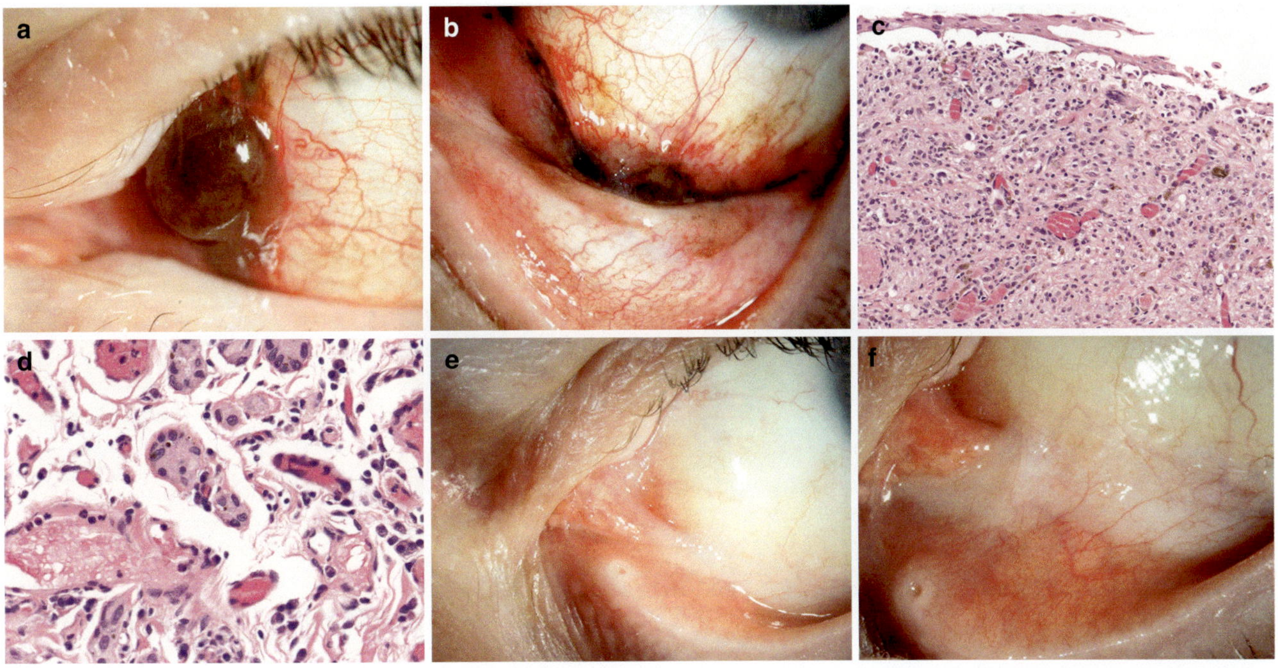

Fig. 7.14 Conjunctival melanoma with lymphovascular invasion. In addition to melanocytic nodular lesion in plica (**a**, 6.0 × 5.0 × 2.0 mm), there was pigmentation along the inferior fornix with central nodularity (**b**). Intraoperatively, after the globe had been rotated superotemporally with a 6-0 vicryl traction suture was placed at inferotemporal limbus, the lesion appeared to be localized to the plical conjunctiva and inferior forniceal conjunctiva without extension or involvement into deeper structures such as the sclera or muscle. Incision with 2 mm margins was started at the plica and extended into the inferior fornix around the lesion. A tissue plane for dissection was created freeing it off from the underlying uninvolved Tenon's with a monopolar cautery needle. Three additional map biopsies were obtained (superior, temporal, and superonasal bulbar conjunctiva). Following double freeze–thaw cryotherapy to the conjunctival margins, the 20 × 10 mm area of exposed Tenon's was left to heal by secondary intention. Histopathology of the main tumor revealed a nodule composed of fascicles of atypical cells with prominent nucleoli, patchy pigmentation, chronic inflammation, and mitotic activity (**c**, H&E 200×). Immunohistochemical stains (MelanA positive, Ki-67 index 15%; PRAME positive; BRAF V600E negative [wt]) were also performed. PRAME-positive melanoma cells focally present at the margin. Satellite nodules were suspicious for vascular invasion (**d**, H&E 400×). Only one map biopsy (superonsal was positive for PAM). After allowing 4 weeks for healing, four cycles of topical mitomycin (0.04%) were prescribed for positive margins. Sentinel lymph node biopsy was not done due to the presence of vascular invasion. He was started on adjuvant pembrolizumab. After allowing 4 weeks for healing, four cycles of topical mitomycin (0.04%) were prescribed. Note the absence of pigmentation 9 months after the completion of MMC (**e**, **f**) with progressive rarefaction. He has remained free of local recurrence and metastasis over 9 months of surveillance. (Courtesy: Arun D. Singh, MD (Clinical) and Gabriella Yeaney, MD (Pathology), Cleveland Clinic, Cleveland, Ohio)

7.8.3 Regional and Distant Metastasis

Conjunctival melanoma can metastasize to any organ in the body. In about half of the patients with metastases, regional lymph node metastases are detected before systemic disease [51, 58]. Other common locations are the brain, liver, and lung [51]. It is essential, however, to emphasize that in conjunctival melanoma the most common primary locations of the metastases are the regional parotid (preauricular) and submandibular lymph nodes. This reflects a significant difference between conjunctival and uveal melanoma, which tends to disseminate almost exclusively to the liver, at least initially. Therefore, ophthalmologists should be specific when referring patients with conjunctival melanoma to oncologists and must avoid applying the general term "ocular melanoma" lest the oncologist assumes, incorrectly, that the first target for metastasis is likely to be the liver as is the case with uveal melanoma.

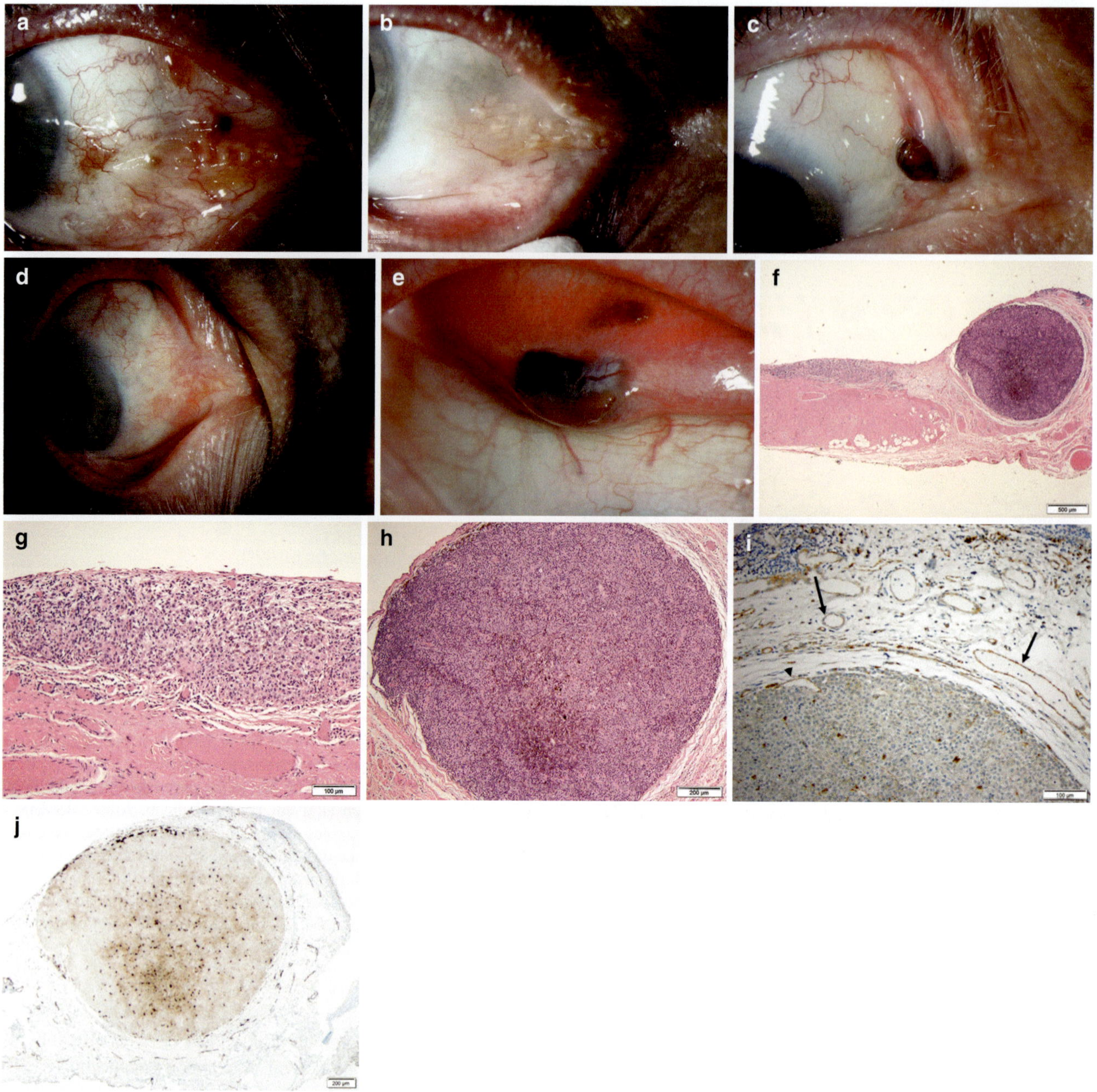

Fig. 7.15 A patient presented with an incompletely excised invasive conjunctival melanoma arising from the right caruncle (**a**). Clinical appearance at 9 months after wide-margin excision, partial thickness scleral dissection, adjuvant cryotherapy, and topical mitomycin (**b**). Despite clear margins in histopathology, there was local recurrence at 36 months with nodular-shaped pigmented mass at the caruncle area (**c**), which was excised. At 48 months, the caruncular area remained clear of tumor recurrence (**d**); however, the right upper tarsal conjunctiva showed multifocal nodular pigmented lesions that were also excised and treated with adjuvant cryotherapy (**e**). Low-magnification (10×) (**f**) and high-magnification (40×) (**g**, **h**) H&E histological images of the excised right upper tarsal conjunctival lesions showing two distinct micronodules with clear lateral and deep margins. CD31 highlights small vessels within the tumor (arrowhead) and in the surrounding substantia propria but no circumferential vessel wall around the nodule (**i**). D2-40 confirms there is no lymphovascular wall around the satellite nodule. Several small vessels in the substantia propria appear compressed by the expanding neoplasm (**j**). (Reproduced with permission from: Echegaray JJ, Yeaney G, Chen R, Singh AD. Conjunctival Melanoma Angiotropic Microsatellitosis: A Mechanism of Local Extravascular Migratory Metastasis. Ocul Oncol Pathol. 2020 Aug;6(4):287–292)

7.9 Treatment

7.9.1 Surgery

The primary treatment of conjunctival melanoma is surgical excision of the entire tumor. Most authorities recommend an excision margin of 3–5 mm, but this is not always feasible. Complete tumor excision should always be combined with adjuvant therapy (Fig. 7.16). When deep limbal and scleral involvement is suspected, lamellar scleral excision should be considered [59]. In one center, they used a complete circumferential peripheral and deep margin assessment ("slow Mohs") surgical technique [60]. When the cornea is involved, some surgeons use absolute alcohol to devitalize corneal epithelial cells adjacent to a limbal melanoma before excision [59]. Areas of PAM with atypia, either around the excised melanoma or distant from it, must be treated because these lesions can give rise to recurrent melanomas. The PAM can be treated by surgery, cryotherapy, brachytherapy, and topical chemotherapy using mitomycin C or immunotherapy using interferon alpha 2b or 2a (see Chap. 6).

7.9.2 Cryotherapy

Cryotherapy to the surgical margins and to the surgical bed, using a double freeze–thaw cycle, is the usual form of adjunctive therapy [25]. However, it should not be used as a primary treatment modality.

7.9.3 Radiotherapy

Conjunctival melanoma is not radio-sensitive; therefore, brachytherapy should not be used as the sole treatment modality [61]. However, brachytherapy has been advocated as a supplemental therapy, usually using gamma radiation (Iodine-125) or beta radiation, (Ru-106 or Sr-90) applicators (Fig. 7.17). It has been reported to be superior to cryotherapy as adjuvant therapy after surgical excision [61–66]. Proton beam radiotherapy has also been advocated in treating extensive conjunctival melanoma as an alternative to exenteration [67, 68].

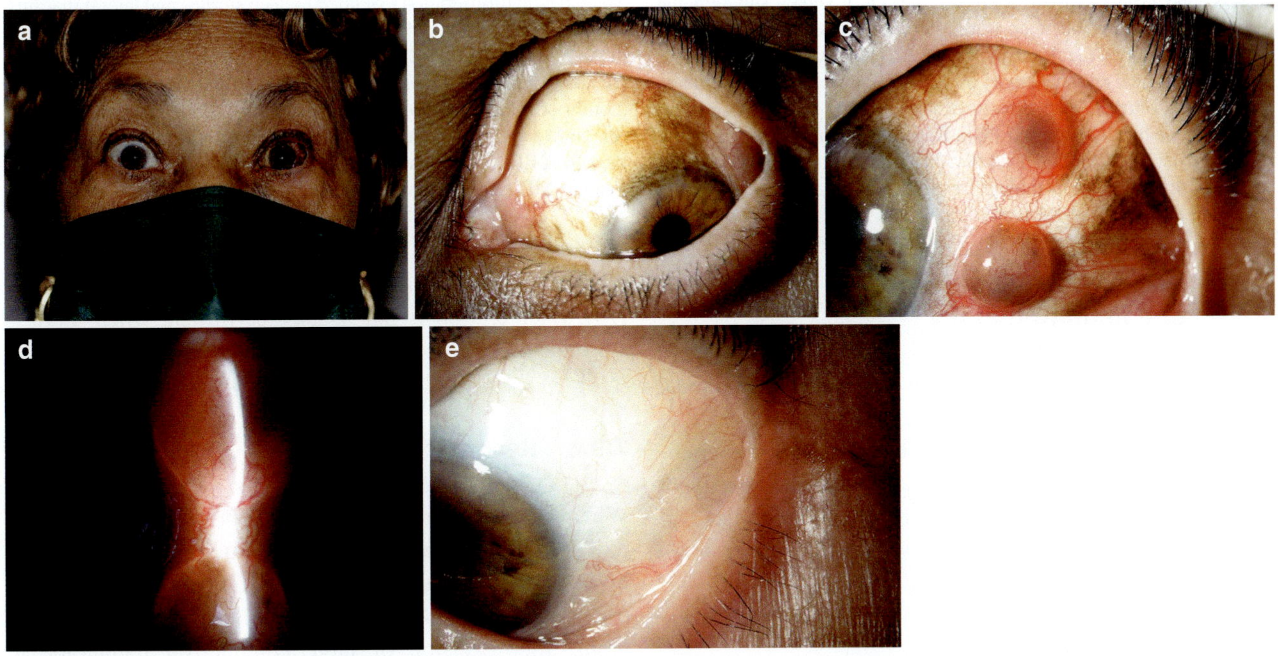

Fig. 7.16 A 90-year-old African American woman (**a**) presented with a foreign body sensation in the left eye. She had been diagnosed to have conjunctival cysts. On examination, there was diffuse conjunctival superficial speckled pigmentation in all quadrants (**b**) with two nodular lesions in the temporal bulbar conjunctiva with feeder vessels (**c**). The nodules were mobile and almost translucent (**d**). Excision with map biopsy and cryotherapy was planned. Two conjunctiva lesions were excised by an incision 2 mm outside the visible margin and dissected to the level of the sclera. Double freeze–thaw cryotherapy was applied to the conjunctival margins at the resection site and areas of pigmentation. The conjunctival defect (9 mm vertically and 7 mm horizontally) was closed by mobilizing the Tenon's to cover the defect. Histopathology revealed invasive melanoma arising in a background of PAM with severe atypia (melanoma in situ) with deep and lateral margins free of melanocytic proliferation. Map biopsies (superior, lateral, inferior, nasal) were positive for PAM with severe atypia. After allowing 4 weeks for healing, four cycles of topical mitomycin (0.04%) were prescribed, which had to be discontinued after two cycles due to corneal toxicity. She remained free of local recurrence and metastasis for 30 months after the initial presentation (**e**). Note the absence of any residual of pigmentation

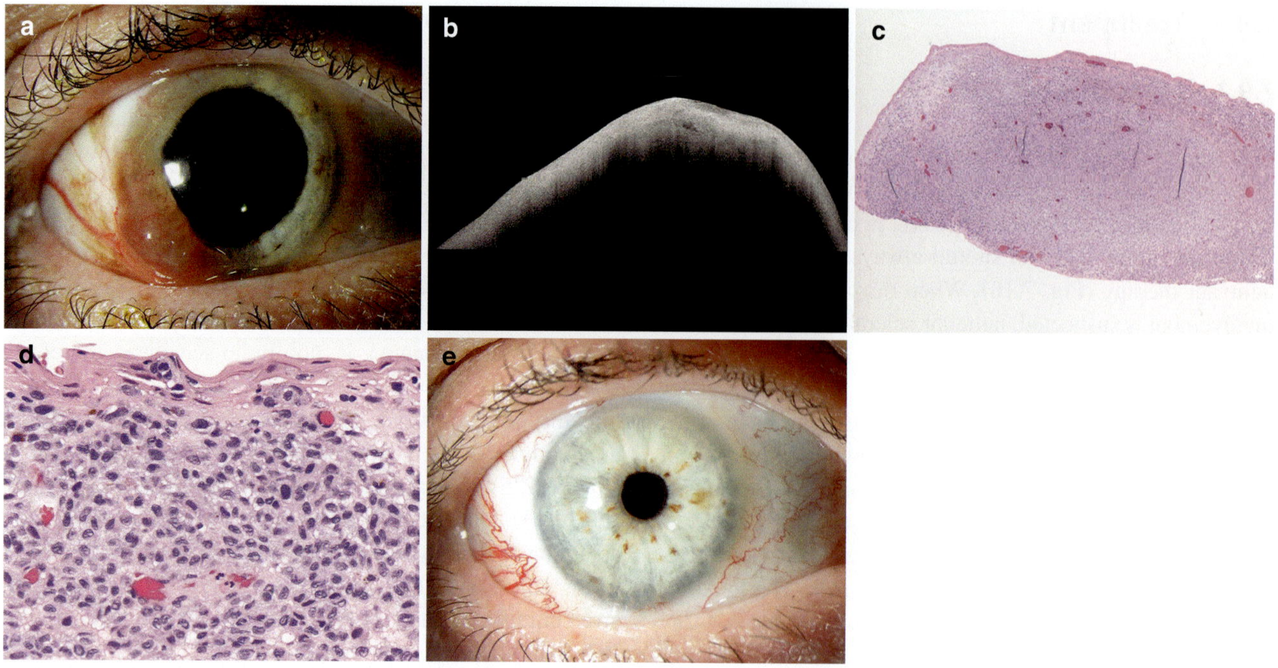

Fig. 7.17 Amelanotic conjunctiva melanoma arising in PAM. Amelanotic mass (8.0 × 5.0 × 2.0 mm) with feeder and intrinsic vessels, and corneal involvement (**a**). AS OCT shows subepithelial mass without discernible deep margin (**b**). The patient underwent partial excision up to the level of the sclera and Bowman membrane (including corneal epitheliectomy using absolute alcohol) and adjuvant cryotherapy. Further deep dissection was avoided with planned episcleral plaque brachytherapy [EPB]). Repair (10 mm vertical and 5 mm horizontal) was done with amniotic graft and bandage contact lens (Kontur 20 mm). Histopathology revealed an expansile melanocytic neoplasm replacing the substantia propria (**c,** H&E 20×) with mitotic activity and pagetoid nests in the epithelial layer (**d,** H&E 400×), consistent with invasive melanoma, 1.5 mm in greatest thickness. Melanocytic proliferation extended to deep surface and lateral margins. After allowing 4 weeks for healing, EPB was performed (45 Gy to the depth of 3.0 mm over 72 h). Sentinel lymph node biopsy was negative. He has remained free of local recurrence and distant metastasis over 60 months of surveillance with visual acuity of 20/20 after cataract surgery (**e**). Note avascular conjunctiva surrounded by telangiectatic vessels at the site of EPB. (Courtesy: Arun D. Singh, MD (Clinical) and Gabriella Yeaney, MD (Pathology), Cleveland Clinic, Cleveland, Ohio)

7.9.4 Topical Chemotherapy and Immunotherapy

In recent years, topical mitomycin C [69–71] and topical interferon alpha-2b [72–74] have been used successfully as adjuvant treatment to surgical excision in treating conjunctival malignant melanoma (Fig. 7.18). Topical treatment should not be used as the primary treatment for conjunctival melanoma.

7.9.5 Orbital Exenteration

Previously, orbital exenteration was the preferred treatment for conjunctival melanoma and PAM. However, a literature review has failed to demonstrate the advantages of such mutilating radical surgery over a conservative approach in treating conjunctival melanoma [75]. Therefore, exenteration of the orbit, including the eyelids to include the palpebral and forniceal conjunctiva, is currently performed only as a palliative treatment for very advanced disease. Because of the progressive disease, survival after exenteration is low [76]. Exenteration is not usually performed when there is systemic metastatic disease.

7.9.6 Reconstruction

When wide excision is performed, reconstruction of the conjunctiva is often needed. Such reconstruction can be achieved by transplanting mucosal tissue from the mouth or the contralateral conjunctiva. The successful use of amniotic membrane after excision of large conjunctival melanoma to prevent conjunctival scars and symblepharon has been described [77].

7.9.7 Regional and Distant Metastasis

Regional lymph node metastasis is associated with a poor prognosis [60]. Patients with regional metastases tend to live longer than those with systemic metastases. Regional metas-

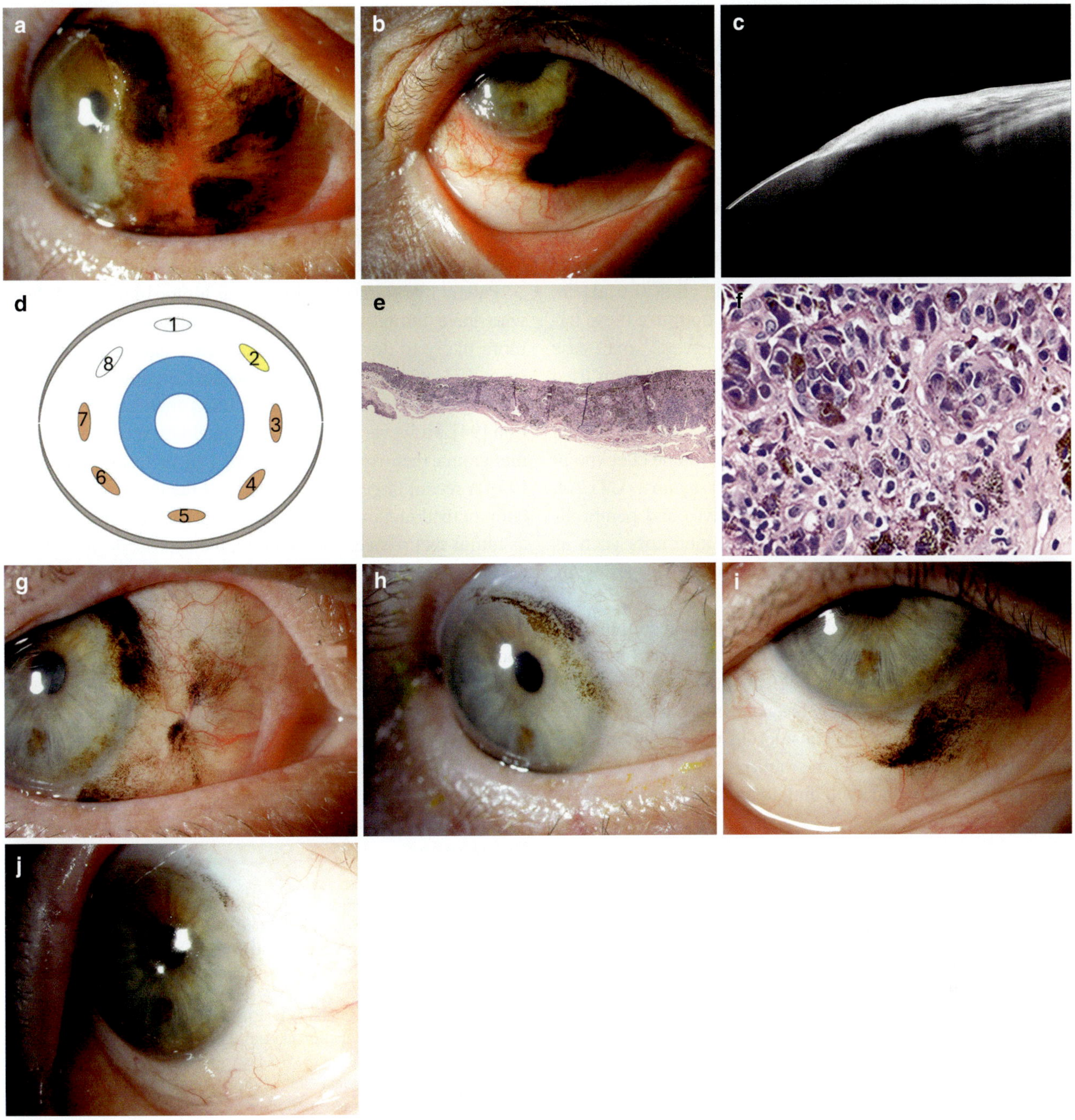

Fig. 7.18 Conjunctiva melanoma. Malignant transformation of primary acquired melanosis (PAM). Extensive conjunctival and corneal involvement (**a, b**). AS OCT shows thickened stroma with hyperreflectivity (**c**). Multiple areas of conjunctival pigmentation were noted in all four quadrants; therefore, we elected to perform map biopsy with adjuvant cryotherapy. In total, eight samples were obtained. Each sample was approximately 3 mm × 2 mm in size and included only conjunctival epithelium. Where possible, pigmented tissue was included in the sample, which were labeled (1–8) in a clockwise manner starting at 12 o'clock (**d,** white, normal epithelium; light brown, PAM with low-grade atypia; dark brown, PAM with severe atypia [melanoma in situ]). Histopathology revealed PAM with atypia (melanoma in situ) at multiple sites (**e**, H&E 40×. **f**, H&E 600×). After allowing 4 weeks for healing, four cycles of topical mitomycin (0.04%) were prescribed, which had to be discontinued after two cycles due to corneal toxicity. Note marked improvement 3 months after the completion of MMC (**g, h**) with progressive rarefaction of pigmentation at 6 months (**i**). He remained free of local recurrence and metastasis over 60 months of surveillance (**j**). (Courtesy: Arun D. Singh, MD (Clinical) and Gabriella Yeaney, MD (Pathology), Cleveland Clinic, Cleveland, Ohio)

tases can be treated by lumpectomy and adjuvant radiotherapy [60]. Disseminated conjunctival melanoma has been treated with systemic chemotherapy, mainly dacarbazine, with a possible combination of interferon or interleukin 2. However, the results are poor, and the life expectancy is a few months.

In recent years, there has been impressive progress in treating systemic metastases of cutaneous melanoma by biological drugs. Because of the similarities between conjunctival and cutaneous melanoma, such treatment has been suggested for conjunctival melanoma, and clinical trials are currently ongoing to further evaluate and optimize these targeted therapies and immunotherapy, and several small case series have been published. The drugs that have been tried for targeted therapy are BRAF and MEK inhibitors, such as vemurafenib (zelboraf) and dabrafenib (tafinlar), and recently encorafenib (braftovi) [78–81]. Immune checkpoint inhibitors such as ipilimumab (yervoy) against CTLA4, PD-1 inhibitors such as nivolumab (opdivo) and pembrolizumab (keytruda) [82, 83], and PDL-1 inhibitors such as avelumab (bavencio) and atezolizumab (tecentriq) are being studied [84].

These drugs have been used for metastatic conjunctival melanoma as a single agent and in various combinations. The experience with these biological drugs is encouraging but still limited. In using these drugs for metastatic conjunctival melanoma, one should consider the adverse effects that may affect any organ, sometimes seriously, and may result in treatment cessation and switching to another therapy [20].

7.9.8 Sentinel Lymph Node Biopsy

In the past two decades, some ophthalmic oncologists have advocated preoperative lymphoscintigraphy and sentinel lymph node biopsy (SLNB) to evaluate the metastatic status of patients with conjunctival melanoma [85–88], although other experts identify little if any advantage to this approach (see Vol 2 Chapter 12 for details). A recent study found a significant association between positive SLN and worse disease-specific survival and emphasized the importance of SLNB for prognosis in patients with conjunctival melanoma and selecting high-risk patients for adjuvant drug treatment [89].

7.9.9 Prognosis

The conjunctival melanoma-related mortality rate is 12–19% in 5 years and 23–30% in 10 years [1, 3, 4, 40, 48, 72]. There are many risk factors for metastatic spread of conjunctival melanoma; the most important ones are tumor thickness of nodular tumor and tumor location. Unfavorable tumor locations with a high risk of metastatic spread are nonlimbal or nonbulbar conjunctival sites such as palpebral conjunctiva, fornices, plica semilunaris, caruncle, and eyelid margins, and orbital invasion [38, 90].

The risk of metastasis increases with tumor thickness, from 0.8 to 4.0 mm [2, 51, 58, 91]. There is a continuous worsening in prognosis with increasing tumor thickness without any critical threshold. However, thin lesions (less than 0.8 mm in thickness) seldom give rise to metastasis unless lymphatic involvement is identified.

Patients who undergo incisional tumor biopsy and those who have tumor excision without adjuvant treatment are more likely to develop local recurrence and metastatic diseases [92, 93]. A significantly worse outcome is shown in patients with low tumor pigmentation than high pigmentation [94]. However, the level of pigmentation of conjunctival melanoma recurrence is not related to metastases or death [95]. A recent large study showed that the tumor origin of the conjunctival melanoma did not affect clinical outcomes such as tumor recurrence, exenteration, metastasis, or death [96].

The American Joint Committee on Cancer Staging (AJCC, seventh edition), based on TNM classification, was found to be predictive of local control and systemic spread of conjunctival melanoma [97–99]. A multicenter international study showed that the eighth edition of the AJCC tumor staging [100] was related to the risk of local recurrence of conjunctival melanoma after treatment [101], and can be used to estimate metastasis and mortality rates [102] accurately.

References

1. Rodrigues M, Koning L, Doupland SE, et al. So close, yet so far: discrepancies between uveal and other melanomas. A position paper from UM cure 2020. Cancers. 2019;11:1032.
2. Seregard S. Conjunctival melanoma. Surv Ophthalmol. 1998;42(4):321–50.
3. Grossniklaus HE, Green WR, Luckenbach M, et al. Conjunctival lesions in adults. A clinical and histopathologic review. Cornea. 1987;6(12):78–116.
4. De Woolf-Rouendaal D. Conjunctival melanoma in The Netherlands: a clinico-pathological and follow-up study (thesis), vol. 9. Katwijk: All in BV; 1990. p. 177.
5. Triay E, Bergman N, Nilsson B, et al. Time trends in the incidence of conjunctival melanoma in Sweden. Br J Ophthalmol. 2009;93(11):1524–8.
6. Yu GP, Hu DN, McCormick S, et al. Conjunctival melanoma: is it increasing in the United States? Am J Ophthalmol. 2003;135(6):800–6.
7. Larsen AC. Conjunctival malignant melanoma in Denmark: epidemiology, treatment and prognosis with special emphasis on tumorigenesis and genetic profile. Acta Ophthalmol. 2016;94:1–27.
8. Virgili G, Parravano M, Gatta G, et al. Incidence and survival of patients with conjunctival melanoma in Europe. JAMA Ophthalmol. 2020;138:601–8.
9. Ghazawi FM, Darwich R, Le M, et al. Incidence trends of conjunctival malignant melanoma in Canada. Br J Ophthalmol. 2020;104:23.

10. Taban M, Traboulsi EI. Malignant melanoma of the conjunctiva in children: a review of the international literature 1965-2006. J Pediatr Ophthalmol Strabismus. 2007;44(5):277–82.
11. Vasanthapuram VH, Kaliki S. Conjunctival melanoma in patients with xeroderma pigmentosum: a series of four cases. Int Ophthalmol. 2020;40:1143–6.
12. Hu DN, Yu G, McCormick SA, et al. Population-based incidence of conjunctival melanoma in various races and ethnic groups and comparison with other melanomas. Am J Ophthalmol. 2008;145(3):418–23.
13. Lim JZ, Misra SL, Gokul A, et al. Conjunctival melanoma in Aotearoa—New Zealand: a 21-year analysis of incidence and survival. Asia Pac J Ophthalmol. 2023;12:273–8.
14. Pane AR, Hirst LW. Ultraviolet light exposure as a risk factor for ocular melanoma in Queensland, Australia. Ophthalmic Epidemiol. 2000;7(3):159–67.
15. Griewank KG, Murali R, Schilling B, et al. TERT promoter mutations in ocular melanoma distinguish between conjunctival and uveal tumours. Br J Cancer. 2013;109:497–501.
16. Koopmans AE, Ober K, Dubbink HJ, et al. Prevalence and implications of TERT promoter mutation in uveal and conjunctival melanoma and in benign and premalignant conjunctival melanocytic lesions. Invest Ophthalmol Vis Sci. 2014;55:6024–30.
17. Swaminathan SS, Field MG, Sant D, et al. Molecular characteristics of conjunctival melanoma using whole-exome sequencing. JAMA Ophthalmol. 2017;135:1434–7.
18. Mikkelsen LH, Maag E, Klarskov Andersen M, et al. The molecular profile of mucosal melanoma. Melanoma Res. 2020;30:533–42.
19. Folberg R, McLean IW, Zimmerman LE. Malignant melanoma of the conjunctiva. Hum Pathol. 1985;16(2):136–43.
20. Brouwer NJ, Verdijk RM, Heegaard S, et al. Conjunctival melanoma: new insights in tumour genetics and immunology, leading to new therapeutic options. Prog Retin Eye Res. 2022;86:100971.
21. Gallo B, Thaung C, Hay G, et al. Invasive conjunctival melanoma mimicking ocular surface squamous neoplasia: a case series. Br J Ophthalmol. 2021;105:775–8.
22. Messmer EM, Mackert MJ, Zapp DM, et al. In vivo confocal microscopy of pigmented conjunctival tumors. Graefes Arch Clin Exp Ophthalmol. 2006;244(11):1437–45.
23. Ho VH, Prager TC, Diwan H, et al. Ultrasound biomicroscopy for estimation of tumor thickness for conjunctival melanoma. J Clin Ultrasound. 2007;35(9):533–7.
24. Nanji AA, Sayyad FE, Galor A, Dubovy S, Karp CL. High-resolution optical coherence tomography as an adjunctive tool in the diagnosis of corneal and conjunctival pathology. Ocul Surf. 2015;1:226–35.
25. Jakobiec FA, Rini FJ, Fraunfelder FT, et al. Cryotherapy for conjunctival primary acquired melanosis and malignant melanoma. Experience with 62 cases. Ophthalmology. 1988;95(8):1058–70.
26. Jakobiec FA, Folberg R, Iwamoto T. Clinicopathologic characteristics of premalignant and malignant melanocytic lesions of the conjunctiva. Ophthalmology. 1989;96(2):147–66.
27. Folberg R, Jakobiec FA, Bernardino VB, et al. Benign conjunctival melanocytic lesions. Clinicopathologic features. Ophthalmology. 1989;96(4):436–61.
28. Rummelt V, Naumann GO, Folberg R, et al. Surgical management of melanocytoma of the ciliary body with extrascleral extension. Am J Ophthalmol. 1994;117(2):169–76.
29. Kiratli H, Shields CL, Shields JA, et al. Metastatic tumours to the conjunctiva: report of 10 cases. Br J Ophthalmol. 1996;80(1):5–8.
30. Heegaard S, Jensen OA, Prause JU. Immunohistochemical diagnosis of malignant melanoma of the conjunctiva and uvea: comparison of the novel antibody against melan-a with S-100 protein and HMB-45. Melanoma Res. 2000;19(4):350–4.
31. Sharara NA, Alexander RA, Luthert PJ, et al. Differential immunoreactivity of melanocytic lesions of the conjunctiva. Histopathology. 2001;39(4):426–31.
32. Iwamoto S, Burrows RC, Grossniklaus HE, et al. Immunophenotype of conjunctival melanomas: comparisons with uveal and cutaneous melanomas. Arch Ophthalmol. 2002;129(12):1625–9.
33. Jakobiec FA, Bhat P, Colby KA. Immunohistochemical studies of conjunctival nevi and melanomas. Arch Ophthalmol. 2010;128(2):174–83.
34. Goldenberg-Cohen N, Cohen Y, Rosenbaum E, et al. T1799A BRAF mutations in conjunctival melanocytic lesions. Invest Ophthalmol Vis Sci. 2005;46(9):3027–30.
35. Lake SL, Jmor F, Dopierala J, et al. Multiplex ligation-dependent probe amplification of conjunctival melanoma reveals common BRAF V600E gene mutation and gene copy number changes. Invest Ophthalmol Vis Sci. 2011;52(8):5598–604.
36. Griewank KG, Westekemper H, Murali R, et al. Conjunctival melanomas harbor BRAF and NRAS mutations and copy number changes similar to cutaneous and mucosal melanomas. Clin Cancer Res. 2013;19:3143–52.
37. Larsen AC, Dahl C, Dahmcke CM, et al. BRAF mutations in conjunctival melanoma: investigation of incidence, clinicopathological features, prognosis and paired premalignant lesions. Acta Ophthalmol. 2016;94:463–70.
38. Dratviman-Storobinsky O, Cohen Y, Frenkel S, et al. Lack of oncogenic GNAQ mutations in melanocytic lesions of the conjunctiva as compared to uveal melanoma. Invest Ophthalmol Vis Sci. 2010;51(12):6180–2.
39. Scholz SL, Cosgarea I, Süßkind D, et al. NF1 mutations in conjunctival melanoma. Br J Cancer. 2018;118:1243–7.
40. Mudhar HS, Milman T, Stevenson S, et al. PRAME expression by immunohistochemistry and reverse transcription quantitative PCR in conjunctival melanocytic lesions—a comprehensive clinicopathologic study of 202 cases and correlation of cytogenetics with PRAME expression in challenging conjunctival melanocytic lesions. Hum Pathol. 2023;134:1–18.
41. Sekoranja D, Hawlina G, Pizem J. PRAME expression in melanocytic lesions of the conjunctiva. Histopathology. 2021;79:989–96.
42. Cao J, Brouwer NJ, Richards KE, et al. PD-L1/PD-1 expression and tumor-infiltrating lymphocytes in conjunctival melanoma. Oncotarget. 2017;8:54722–34.
43. Cao J, Brouwer NJ, Jordanova ES, et al. HLA class I antigen expression in conjunctival melanoma is not associated with PD-L1/PD-1 status. Invest Ophthalmol Vis Sci. 2018;59:1005–15.
44. Larsen AC, Mikkelsen LH, Borup R, et al. MicroRNA expression profile in conjunctival melanoma. Invest Ophthalmol Vis Sci. 2016;57:4205–12.
45. Esmaeli B, Roberts D, Ross M, et al. Histologic features of conjunctival melanoma predictive of metastasis and death (an American ophthalmological thesis). Trans Am Ophthalmol Soc. 2012;110:64–73.
46. Briceño CA, Elner VM, Demirci H. Lymphangiogenic and chemotactic factors in conjunctival melanoma. Ophthalmic Plast Reconstr Surg. 2016;32:428–33.
47. Van Ipengurg JA, van den Bosch QCC, Paridaens D, et al. ATRX loss in the development and prognosis of conjunctival melanoma. Int J Mol Sci. 2023;24:12988.
48. Lassalle S, Nahon-Esteve S, Frouin E, et al. PD-L1 expresssion in 65 conjunctival melanomas and its association with clinical outcome. Int J Mol Sci. 2020;21:9147.
49. Van Ipenburg JA, Naus NC, Dubbink HJ, et al. Prognostic value of TRET promoter mutations in conjunctival melanomas in addition to clinicopathologic features. Br J Ophthalmol. 2021;105:1454–61.

50. Savar A, Esmaeli B, Ho H, et al. Conjunctival melanoma: local-regional control rates, and impact of high-risk histopathologic features. J Cutan Pathol. 2011;38(1):18–24.
51. Shields CL, Shields JA, Gunduz K, et al. Conjunctival melanoma: risk factors for recurrence, exenteration, metastasis and death in 150 consecutive patients. Arch Ophthalmol. 2000;118(11):1497–507.
52. Vaidya S, Dalvin LA, Yaghy A, et al. Conjunctival melanoma: risk factors for recurrent or new tumor in 540 patients at a single ocular oncology center. Eur J Ophthalmol. 2021;31:2675–85.
53. Mudhar HS, Rennie IG. Local conjunctival metastases from primary conjunctival melanoma: clinico-pathological correlation and implications. Br J Ophthalmol. 2013;97(1):33–9.
54. Heindl LM, Hofmann-Rummelt C, Adler W, et al. Prognostic significance of tumor-associated lymphangiogenesis in malignant melanomas of the conjunctiva. Ophthalmology. 2011;118(12):2351–60.
55. Barnhill RL, Lemaitre S, Lévy-Gabrielle C, et al. Satellite in transit metastases in rapidly fatal conjunctival melanoma: implications for angiotropism and extravascular migratory metastasis (description of a murine model for conjunctival melanoma). Pathology. 2016;48:166–76.
56. Missotten GS, Gambrelle J, de Wolff-Rouendaal D, et al. Epistaxis or epiphora as a sign for extension of a conjunctival melanoma. A series of six patients with nasolacrimal recurrence. Br J Ophthalmol. 2010;94(10):1328–31.
57. Sandinha T, Russell H, Kemp E, et al. Malignant melanoma of the conjunctiva with intraocular extension: a clinicopathological study of three cases. Graefes Arch Clin Exp Ophthalmol. 2007;245(3):431–6.
58. Tuomaala S, Kivela T. Metastatic pattern and survival in disseminated conjunctival melanoma: implications for sentinel lymph node biopsy. Ophthalmology. 2004;111(4):816–21.
59. Shields JA, Shields CL, DePotter P. Surgical management of conjunctival tumors. The 1994 Lynn B. McMahan lecture. Arch Ophthalmol. 1997;115(6):808–15.
60. Osemwota O, Mudigonda T, Philip C, et al. Conjunctival melanoma treated with complete circumferential peripheral and deep margin assessment ("slow Mohs") surgery: dermatologic surgery. Dermatologic Surg. 2021;47:286–8.
61. Lommatzsch PK, Lommatzsch RE, Kirsch I, et al. Therapeutic outcome of patients suffering from malignant melanoma of the conjunctiva. Br J Ophthalmol. 1990;74(10):615–9.
62. Krause L, Ritter C, Wachtlin J, et al. Recurrence rate following adjuvant strontium-90 brachytherapy after excision of conjunctival melanoma. Klin Monatsbl Augenheilkd. 2008;225(7):649–52.
63. Damato B, Coupland SE. An audit of conjunctival melanoma treatment in Liverpool. Eye (Lond). 2009;23(4):801–9.
64. Karim R, Conway RM. Conservative resection and adjuvant plaque brachytherapy for early-stage conjunctival melanoma. Clin Experiment Ophthalmol. 2011;39(4):293–8.
65. Cohen VM, Papastefanou VP, Liu S, Stoker I, Hungerford JL. The use of strontium-90 Beta radiotherapy as adjuvant treatment for conjunctival melanoma. J Oncol. 2013;2013:349162.
66. Brouwer NJ, Marinkovic M, Peters FP, et al. Management of conjunctival melanoma with local excision and adjuvant brachytherapy. Eye. 2021;35:490–8.
67. Wuestemeyer H, Sauerwein W, Meller D, et al. Proton radiotherapy as an alternative to exenteration in the management of extended conjunctival melanoma. Graefes Arch Clin Exp Ophthalmol. 2006;244(4):438–46.
68. Scholz SL, Herault J, Stang A, et al. Proton radiotherapy in advanced malignant melanoma of the conjunctiva. Graefes Arch Clin Exp Ophthalmol. 2019;257:1309–18.
69. Krause L, Mladenova A, Bechrakis NE, et al. Treatment modalities for conjunctival melanoma. Klin Monatsbl Augenheilkd. 2009;226(12):1012–6.
70. Kurli M, Finger PT. Topical mitomycin chemotherapy for conjunctival malignant melanoma and primary acquired melanosis with atypia: 12 years' experience. Graefes Arch Clin Exp Ophthalmol. 2005;243(11):1108–14.
71. Ditta LC, Shildkrot Y, Wilson MW. Outcomes in 15 patients with conjunctival melanoma treated with adjuvant topical mitomycin C: complications and recurrences. Ophthalmology. 2011;118(9):1754–9.
72. Finger PT, Sedeek RW, Chin KJ. Topical interferon alfa in the treatment of conjunctival melanoma and primary acquired melanosis complex. Am J Ophthalmol. 2008;145(1):124–9.
73. Garip A, Schaumberger MM, Wolf A, et al. Evaluation of a short-term topical interferon α-2b treatment for histologically proven melanoma and primary acquired melanosis with atypia. Orbit. 2016;35:29–34.
74. Kikuchi I, Kase S, Ishijima K, Ishida S. Long-term follow-up of conjunctival melanoma treated with topical interferon alpha-2b eye drops as adjunctive therapy following surgical resection. Graefes Arch Clin Exp Ophthalmol. 2017;255:2271–6.
75. Tatla T, Hungerford J, Plowman N, et al. Conjunctival melanoma: the role of conservative surgery and radiotherapy in regional metastatic disease. Laryngoscope. 2005;115(5):817–22.
76. Baum SH, Westekemper H, Bechrakis NE, et al. Conjunctival and uveal melanoma: survival and risk factors following orbital exenteration. Eur J Ophthalmol. 2022;32:612–9.
77. Dalla Pozza G, Ghirlando A, Busato F, et al. Reconstruction of conjunctiva with amniotic membrane after excision of large conjunctival melanoma: a long-term study. Eur J Ophthalmol. 2005;15(4):446–50.
78. Cao J, Heiijkants RC, Jochemsen AG, et al. Targeting of the MAPK and AKT .pathways in conjunctival melanoma shows potential synergy. Oncotarget. 2016;8:58021–36.
79. Mor JM, Heindl LM. Systemic BRAF/MEK inhibitors as a poten tial treatment option in metastatic conjunctival melanoma. Ocul Oncol Pathol. 2017;3:133–41.
80. Dagi Glass LR, Lawrence DP, Jakobiec FA, Freitag SK. Conjunctival melanoma responsive to combined systemic BRAF/MEK inhibitors. Ophthalmic Plast Reconstr Surg. 2017;33:e114–6.
81. Miura S, Onishi M, Watabe D, et al. Conjunctival malignant melanoma treated successfully with BRAF inhibitor: encorafenib plus binimetinib. Dermatol Online J. 2022;28:1.
82. Ford J, Thuro BA, Thakar S, Hwu WJ, Richani K, Esmaeli B. Immune checkpoint inhibitors for treatment of metastatic melanoma of the orbit and ocular adnexa. Ophthalmic Plast Reconstr Surg. 2017;3:e82–5.
83. Kini A, Fu R, Compton C, Miller DM, Ramasubramanian A. Pembrolizumab for recurrent conjunctival melanoma. JAMA Ophthalmol. 2017;135:891–2.
84. Sa HS, Daniel C, Esmaeli B. Update of immune checkpoint inhibitors for conjunctival melanoma. J Ophthalmic Vis Res. 2022;17:405–12.
85. Amato M, Esmaeli B, Ahmadi MA, et al. Feasibility of preoperative lymphoscintigraphy for identification of sentinel lymph node in patients with conjunctival and periocular skin malignancies. Ophthalmic Plast Reconstr Surg. 2003;19(2):102–6.
86. Savar A, Ross MI, Prieto VG, et al. Sentinel lymph node biopsy for ocular adnexal melanoma: experience in 30 patients. Ophthalmology. 2009;116(11):2217–23.
87. Cohen VM, Tsimpida M, Hungerford JL, Jan H, Cerio R, Moir G. Prospective study of sentinel lymph node biopsy for conjunctival melanoma. Br J Ophthalmol. 2013;97:1525–9.
88. Aziz HA, Gastman BR, Singh AD. Management of Conjunctival Melanoma: critical assessment of sentinel lymph node biopsy. Ocul Oncol Pathol. 2015;1:266–73.

89. Esmaeli B, Rubin ML, Xu S, et al. Greater tumor thickness, ulceration, and positive sentinel lymph node biopsy are associated with worse prognosis in patients with conjunctival melanoma: Implications for future AJCC classifications.
90. Bas Z, Dockery PW, Lally SE, et al. Conjunctival melanoma in 430 cases: Comperative analysis of the impact of orbital invasion on tumor recurrence, metastasis, and death. Ophthalmic Plast Reconstr Surg. 2023;39:49–57.
91. Paridaens AD, Minassian DC, McCartney AC, et al. Prognostic factors in primary malignant melanoma of the conjunctiva: a clinicopathological study of 256 cases. Br J Ophthalmol. 1994;78(4):252–9.
92. Larsen AC, Dahmcke CM, Dahl C, et al. A retrospective review of conjunctival melanoma presentation, treatment, and outcome and an investigation of features associated with BRAF mutations. JAMA Ophthalmol. 2015;133:1295–303.
93. Brouwer NJ, Marinkovic M, van Duinen SG, Bleeker JC, Jager MJ, Luyten GPM. Treatment of conjunctival melanoma in a Dutch referral Centre. Br J Ophthalmol. 2017;102:1277.
94. Brouwer NJ, Konstantinou EK, Marinkovic M, et al. Lack of pigmentation in conjunctival melanoma is associated with light iris and worse prognosis. Br J Ophthalmol. 2019;103:332–7.
95. Brouwer NJ, Marinkovic M, Luyten GP, et al. Pigmentation of conjunctival melanoma recurrence and outcome. Graefes Arch Clin Exp Ophthalmol. 2019;257:1783–8.
96. Pacheo RR, Yaghy A, Dalvin LA, et al. Conjunctival melanoma: outcomes based on tumour origin in 629 patients at a single ocular oncology Centre. Eye. 2022;36:603–11.
97. Edge SB, Byrd DR, Compton CC, Fritz AG, Greene FL, Trotti A. Malignant melanoma of the conjunctiva. In: AJCC cancer staging manual. 7th ed. New York: Springer; 2010. p. 539–6.
98. Yousef YA, Finger PT. Predictive value of the seventh edition American joint committee on cancer staging system for conjunctival melanoma. Arch Ophthalmol. 2012;139(5):599–606.
99. Shields CL, Kaliki S, Al-Dahmash SA, et al. American joint committee on cancer (AJCC) clinical classification predicts conjunctival melanoma outcomes. Ophthalmic Plast Reconstr Surg. 2012;28(5):313–23.
100. Coupland SE, Barnhill R, Conway RM, et al. Conjunctival melanoma. In: AJCC cancer staging manual. 8th ed. Chicago: Springer; 2018. p. 795–803.
101. Jain P, Finger PT, Fili M, et al. Conjunctival melanoma treatment outcomes in 288 patients: a multicenter international data-sharing study. Br J Ophthalmol. 2021;105:1358–64.
102. Jain P, Finger PT, Damato B, et al. Multicenter, international assessment of the eighth edition of the American joint committee on cancer staging manual for conjunctival melanoma. JAMA Ophthalmol. 2019;137:905–11.

Conjunctival Stromal Tumors

8

Jacob Pe'er and Shahar Frenkel

8.1 Introduction

The conjunctival stroma contains various tissue elements such as vascular, fibrous, and neural; naturally, benign and malignant tumors may originate from these types of tissue (Table 8.1). However, conjunctival stromal tumors are rare. This chapter describes the salient features of conjunctival stromal tumors according to their tissue of origin.

8.2 Vascular Tumors

Vascular tumors of the conjunctiva are uncommon, and with the exception of Kaposi's sarcoma, most are benign lesions that have no malignant potential. According to one large series [1], the most common conjunctival vascular lesions are lymphangioma/lymphangiectasia and pyogenic granuloma.

Table 8.1 Classification of stromal tumors of the conjunctiva

Category	Subtypes	
Vascular tumors	Pyogenic granuloma	Racemose malformation
	Capillary hemangioma	Hemangiopericytoma
	Cavernous hemangioma	Kaposi's sarcoma
	Acquired sessile hemangioma	Lymphangiectasia
	Varix	Lymphangioma
	Malignant hemangioendothelioma	
Fibrous tumors	Fibroma	Nodular fasciitis
	Benign fibrous histiocytoma	Malignant fibrous histiocytoma
Neural tumors	Neurofibroma (localized)	Neurofibroma (diffuse)
	Schwannoma (neurilemoma)	Granular cell tumor
	Neurothekeoma	Merkel cell carcinoma
Histiocytic tumors	Xanthoma	Juvenile xanthogranuloma
	Reticulohistiocytoma	
Myxoid tumors	Myxoma	
Myogenic tumors	Rhabdomyosarcoma	Leiomyosarcoma
Lipomatous tumors	Lipoma	Herniated orbital fat
	Liposarcoma	
Lymphoproliferative tumors	Benign reactive lymphoid hyperplasia	Lymphoma
	Leukemic infiltrates	
Choristomas	Dermoid	Dermolipoma
	Osseous choristoma	Lacrimal gland choristoma
	Complex choristoma	
Metastatic tumors		
Secondary tumors		

J. Pe'er (✉) · S. Frenkel
Ocular Oncology Service and Ophthalmic Pathology Laboratory, Department of Ophthalmology, Hadassah—Hebrew University Medical Center, Jerusalem, Israel
e-mail: peer@hadassah.org.il

© The Author(s), under exclusive license to Springer Nature Switzerland AG 2024
J. Pe'er et al. (eds.), *Clinical Ophthalmic Oncology*, https://doi.org/10.1007/978-3-031-72443-5_8

8.2.1 Pyogenic Granuloma

The term "pyogenic granuloma" is a misnomer since it is neither pyogenic nor granulomatous. It is granulation tissue, although some consider it a polypoid form of acquired capillary hemangioma [2]. Pyogenic granuloma is a fibrovascular response to tissue insults such as surgical or nonsurgical trauma or inflammation, although spontaneous pyogenic granulomas have also been reported. Pyogenic granuloma is commonly observed in the conjunctiva after chalazion surgery, strabismus surgery, excision of conjunctival lesions, and in the anophthalmic socket following enucleation, and is considered an aberrant wound-healing response.

8.2.1.1 Clinical Features

Pyogenic granuloma has been reported in every part of the conjunctiva and even in the limbus and the cornea, mostly following a corneal epithelial defect [3]. Pyogenic granuloma appears as a fleshy, elevated, red, often pedunculated, richly vascularized mass (Fig. 8.1a).

8.2.1.2 Histopathological Features

Pyogenic granuloma is composed of granulation tissue with marked chronic inflammation with lymphocytes, plasma cells, neutrophils, and proliferation of small, mostly capillary-sized blood vessels (Fig. 8.1b).

8.2.1.3 Treatment

Pyogenic granuloma often responds to topical corticosteroids when diagnosed early, but many cases require surgical excision. In 2014, Millsop et al. were the first to report on the use of topical 0.5% timolol gel for the treatment of pyogenic granuloma on the skin [4]. The first report of this treatment on the ocular surface was by Oke et al. in 2017 in a report of four children treated with topical timolol 0.5% bid for at least 21 days [5]. Since then, there have been numerous reports asserting the efficacy and safety of this treatment modality.

8.2.2 Capillary Hemangioma

Capillary hemangioma usually appears during early infancy and is very rare in adults. Like its counterpart in the skin, it may grow over several months and then regress spontaneously within several years.

8.2.2.1 Clinical Features

Capillary hemangioma is a distinct or diffuse red, elevated conjunctival lesion that can occur anywhere in the conjunctiva. It can be an isolated lesion or in association with an eyelid or orbital capillary hemangioma (Fig. 8.2a).

8.2.2.2 Histopathological Features

Similar to capillary hemangiomas in other locations, it shows numerous capillary channels and proliferation of endothelial cells (Fig. 8.2b).

8.2.2.3 Treatment

Usually, no treatment is needed, and the child should only be observed. There are rare cases, especially when the lesion is large and potentially amblyogenic, in which surgical excision or local or systemic corticosteroids are employed [1, 6]. The experience in treating conjunctival capillary hemangioma by beta-blockers is still limited and showed a response to topical timolol in one baby and a failure to respond to oral propranolol in another baby [7].

8.2.3 Cavernous Hemangioma

Cavernous hemangioma presents as a red or blue multiloculated lesion in the deep conjunctival stroma in children and adolescents (Fig. 8.3a) [6]. This lesion is usually isolated but may be associated with syndromes [1]. It may cause a recurrent subconjunctival hemorrhage [8]. Histologically, similar to such lesions in other locations, it is composed of large blood-filled spaces lined by endothelial cells and separated by fibrous septa (Fig. 8.3b). It can be managed by a surgical excision.

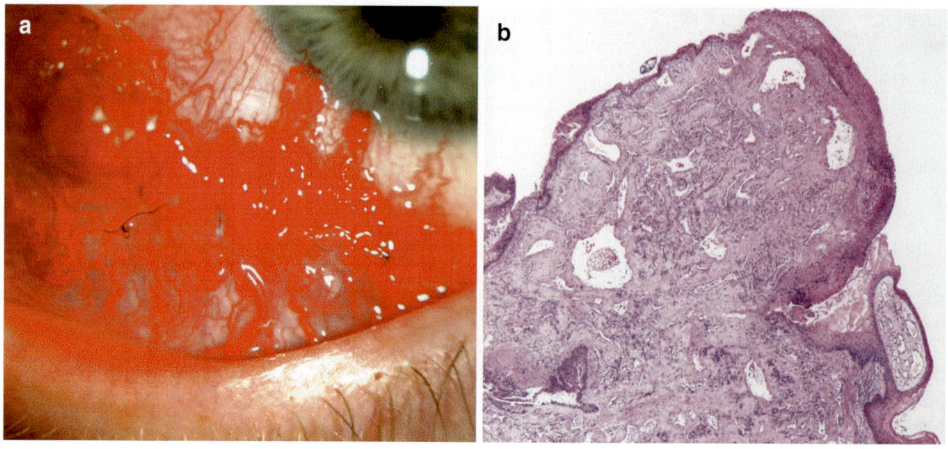

Fig. 8.1 Pyogenic granuloma. A 31-year-old man with a 3-week history of a rapidly growing recurrent conjunctival vascular growth in the inferonasal conjunctival fornix. (**a**) Clinical picture: note prominent vascularity. (**b**) Histopathology shows a polypoid lesion with lobular pattern of capillary proliferation. The vessels are variably dilated (Original magnification ×4)

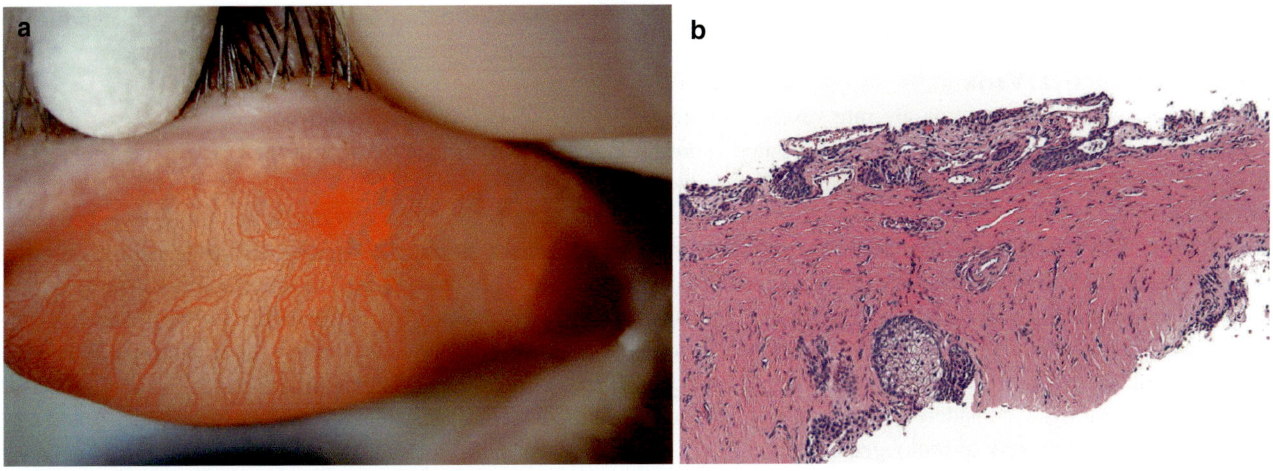

Fig. 8.2 Capillary hemangioma. (**a**) Color photograph of a circumscribed vascular conjunctival lesion overlying the upper tarsus. (**b**) On histopathology examination, the tarsal conjunctival stroma revealed numerous thin-walled capillary-type vessels, most of which contained red blood cells within their lumen (H&E ×10)

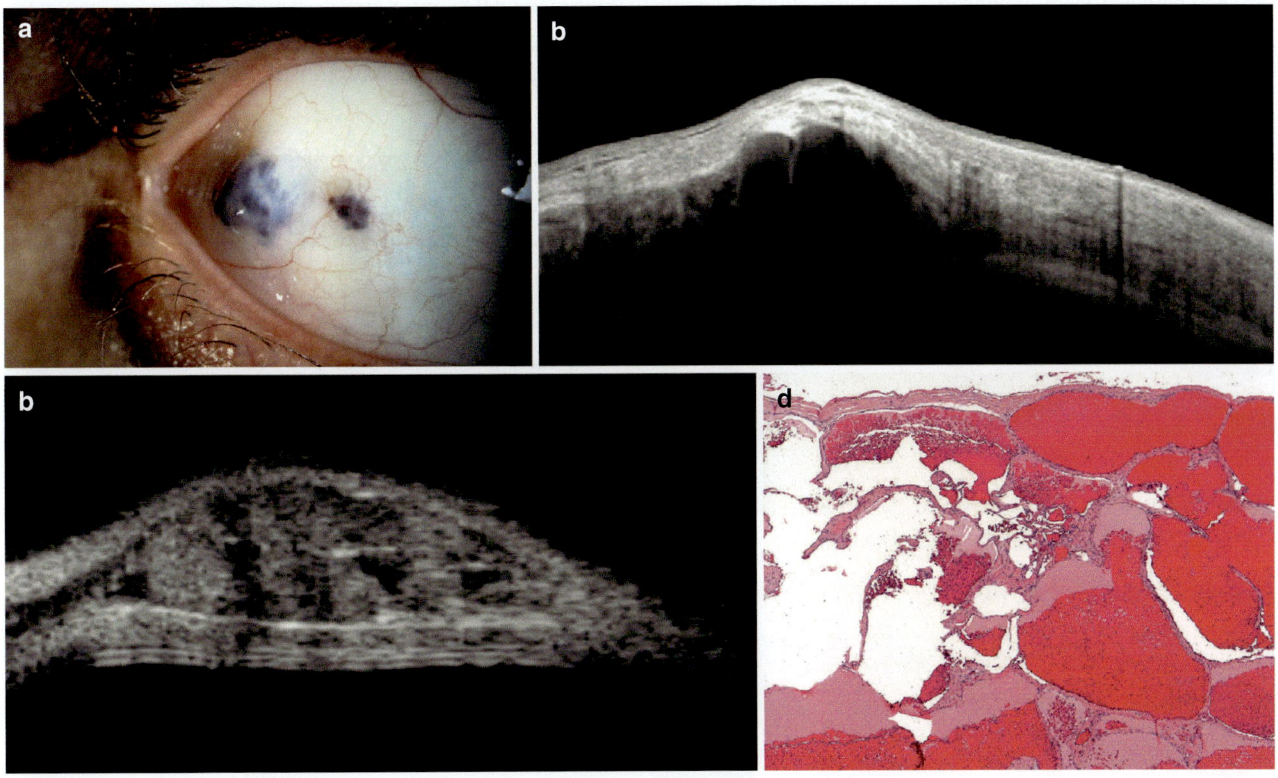

Fig. 8.3 Cavernous hemangioma. (**a**) A clinical picture of a clustered "grapelike" lesions involving the temporal conjunctiva was observed on slit-lamp examination. (**b**) On OCT, there were clear spaces located into the subepithelial layer of the conjunctiva. (**c**) Ultrasonography showed two well-defined lesions with many low reflective intrinsic cystic-like pockets. (**d**) Large, well-circumscribed vascular proliferation of thin-walled veins that completely replaced the conjunctival stroma. Most of the lumina were engorged with blood (H&E ×4)

8.2.4 Acquired Sessile Hemangioma

Shields et al. [9] described vascular lesions of adults that consist of a sessile network of convoluted blood vessels immediately beneath the conjunctival epithelium, usually on the bulbar conjunctiva. Histologically, the lesion comprises of 2–3 layers of dilated congested blood vessels that are otherwise of normal appearance. There are no systemic associations. Since most of these lesions remain stable and have no known complications, they should be managed by observation. Successful treatment with topical timolol was reported [10].

8.2.5 Varix and Racemose Hemangioma

8.2.5.1 Conjunctival Varix

Varix and racemose hemangioma are rare vascular malformations of the conjunctiva. Varix is a mass of dilated venous channels that may range from a single channel to complex venous channels. Many of them are anterior extensions of orbital varix. The color ranges from blue-red to black [1]. It is usually movable and not fixed to the sclera. Thrombosis is frequent. Some consider it to be in the spectrum of lymphangioma. Management should be conservative by observation and symptomatic treatment. When it is symptomatic, surgical excision should be considered, although the surgeon should bear in mind the risk of prolonged bleeding [1, 3].

8.2.5.2 Conjunctival Racemose Hemangioma

Conjunctival racemose hemangioma is a lesion of dilated arteries and veins communicating directly without a capillary bed between them. It appears as a loop of dilated vessels in the conjunctival stroma (Fig. 8.4). It should be managed conservatively by observation. Wyburn–Mason syndrome should be ruled out in such cases [6], with a dilated fundus examination and imaging of the brain vasculature.

8.2.6 Hemangiopericytoma

Hemangiopericytoma is very rare in the conjunctiva. It appears as an elevated pedunculated red mass (Fig. 8.5). Histologically, it is a solid tumor composed of spindle-shaped pericytes and small blood vessels [11, 12]. Treatment is by complete surgical excision with tumor-free margins, and although there have been no reports on malignant transformation of conjunctival hemangiopericytoma, the potential exists in other locations. Therefore, close follow-up is recommended.

8.2.7 Kaposi's Sarcoma

Prior to the AIDS era, Kaposi's sarcoma, in general, and in the conjunctiva in particular, was a rare tumor that mainly affected elderly and immunosuppressed patients. Since the eruption of

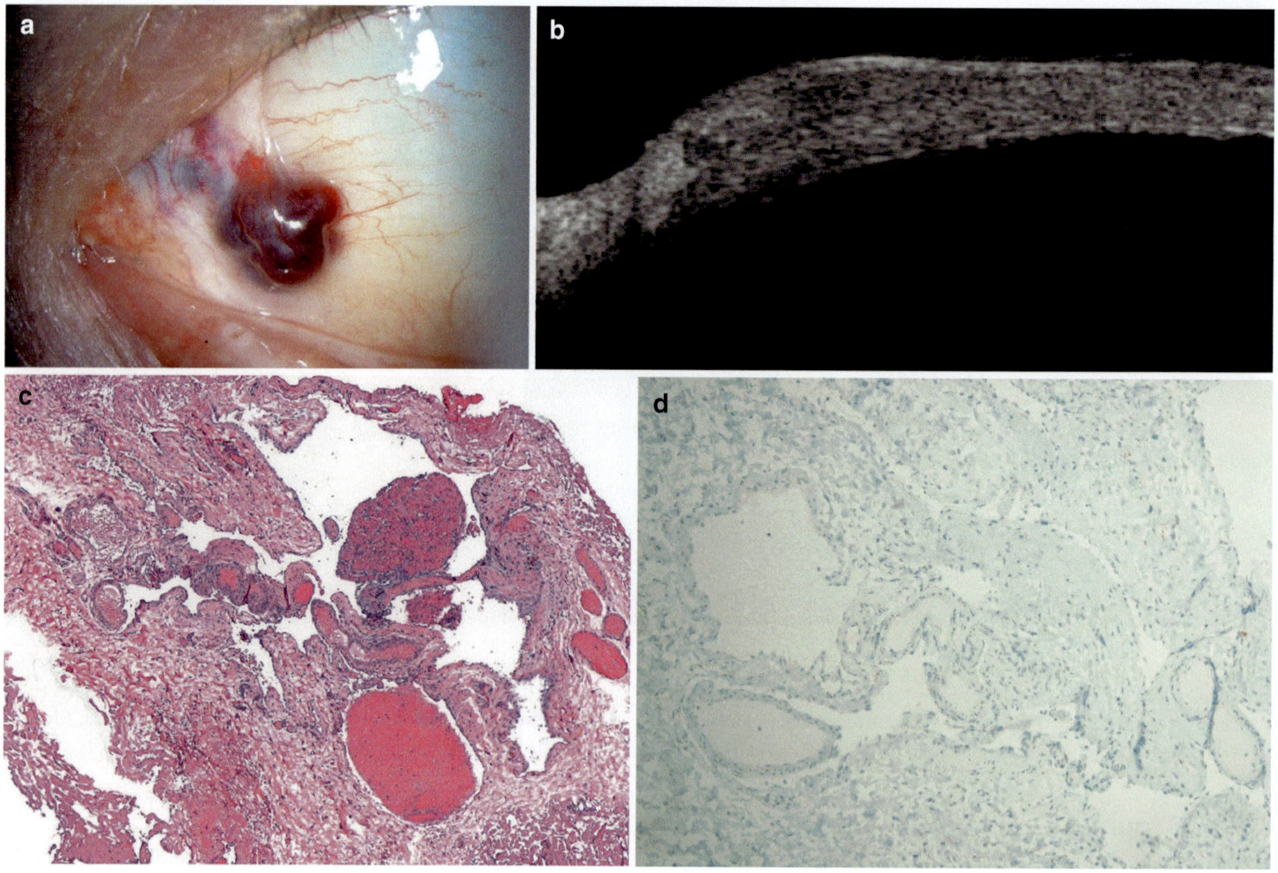

Fig. 8.4 Racemose hemangioma. (**a**) A multilobulated vascular lesion was identified in the medial canthal region that was extending posteriorly along the anterior margin of the caruncle. (**b**) The lesion consisted of highly reflective portions with well-defined, low reflective channels on ultrasonography. (**c**) Vascular proliferation composed of a mixture of thick-walled arteries and thin-walled veins within a fibrotic conjunctival stroma (H&E, ×4). (**d**) The endothelial cells were negative for lymphatic marker D2-40 (×10)

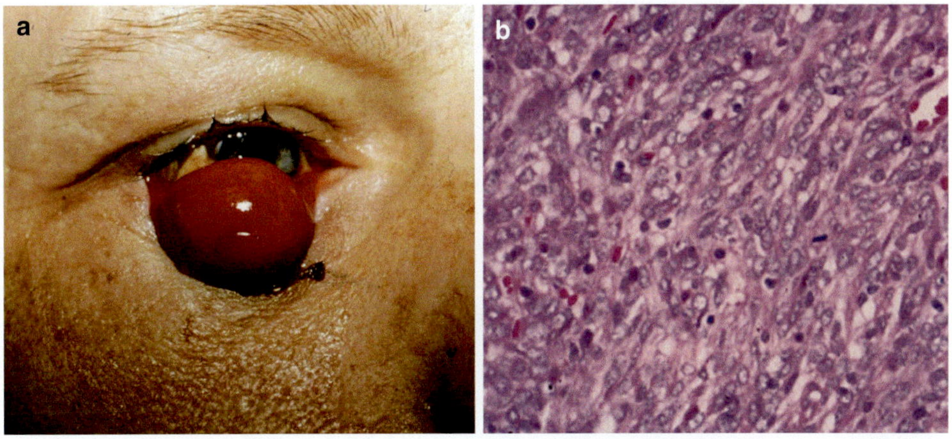

Fig. 8.5 Hemangiopericytoma. (**a**) The patient at presentation showing a large ovoid conjunctival lesion that protruded over her right lower lid. (**b**) Histopathology shows relatively solid tumor composed of spindle-shaped cells and inconspicuous small blood vessels) (hematoxylin eosin, ×450). (Reprinted from Grossniklaus et al. [11]. With permission from Elsevier)

the AIDS epidemic, this malignant tumor has been diagnosed much more frequently in AIDS patients. Sometimes conjunctival Kaposi's sarcoma is the first sign of AIDS [13, 14]. However, in recent years, it has been diagnosed less frequently because of the more effective treatment of AIDS in developed countries.

8.2.7.1 Clinical Features

Kaposi's sarcoma appears as a single isolated or multiple confluent red painless conjunctival masses.

8.2.7.2 Histopathological Features

The tumors are composed of malignant spindle-shaped cells with elongated oval nuclei, well-formed capillary channels, and vascular slits containing blood but no definite endothelial lining.

8.2.7.3 Treatment

Localized tumors can be excised surgically, with or without the addition of cryotherapy. However, Kaposi's sarcoma is responsive to chemotherapy and low-dose radiation therapy [15]. Giant conjunctival Kaposi's sarcoma in HIV-positive patients responded with complete remission to highly active antiretroviral therapy and systemic chemotherapy [16]. Treatments using intralesional interferon alpha-2b [17], intralesional mitomycin C [18], or topical timolol [19] have been reported.

8.3 Lymphangiectasia and Lymphangioma

8.3.1 Lymphangiectasia

When lymphatic channels in the conjunctiva are dilated and prominent, the condition is called lymphangiectasia.

8.3.1.1 Clinical Features

Conjunctival lymphangiectasia can either be unilateral or bilateral with focal or diffuse bulbar chemosis [20]. As a result of the communication with conjunctival veins, these dilated channels may be filled with blood and, if so, are termed "hemorrhagic lymphangiectasia" (lymphangiectasia hemorrhagica conjunctivae of Leber) [21]. The surrounding conjunctiva appears edematous, and occasionally, an associated subconjunctival hemorrhage is present. This phenomenon can occur spontaneously or after trauma or inflammation (Fig. 8.6). Congenital cases have been reported.

8.3.1.2 Histopathological Features

The lesion shows markedly dilated lymphatics, which may be filled with blood, partially surrounded by scattered inflammatory cells. The phenomenon is intermittent, with resolution of the channels' congestion and the chemosis between episodes.

8.3.1.3 Treatment

Usually, no treatment is required, although surgical excision without or with amniotic membrane transplant or conjunctival autograft has been described [20]. Recently, treatment of symptomatic conjunctival lymphangiectasia by liquid nitrogen cryotherapy [22], high-frequency radio-wave electrosurgery, and limited surgical drainage has been reported [23, 24]. A case of conjunctival lymphangiectasia fully resolved after subconjunctival injection of bevacizumab was reported [25]. A recent case series of 16 eyes treated by bleomycin sclerotherapy showed excellent response [26].

8.3.2 Conjunctival Lymphangioma

Conjunctival lymphangioma is a benign tumor of the lymphatic vessels that usually appear in the first decade of life. It can occur as an isolated conjunctival lesion but more often represents a superficial component of an orbital lymphangioma.

8.3.2.1 Clinical Features

Conjunctival lymphangioma appears as a multiloculated lesion composed of dilated cystic spaces. These spaces may contain clear fluid, but often, parts of them contain blood and are called "chocolate cysts." Inflammation in the area, such as an upper respiratory tract infection, causes

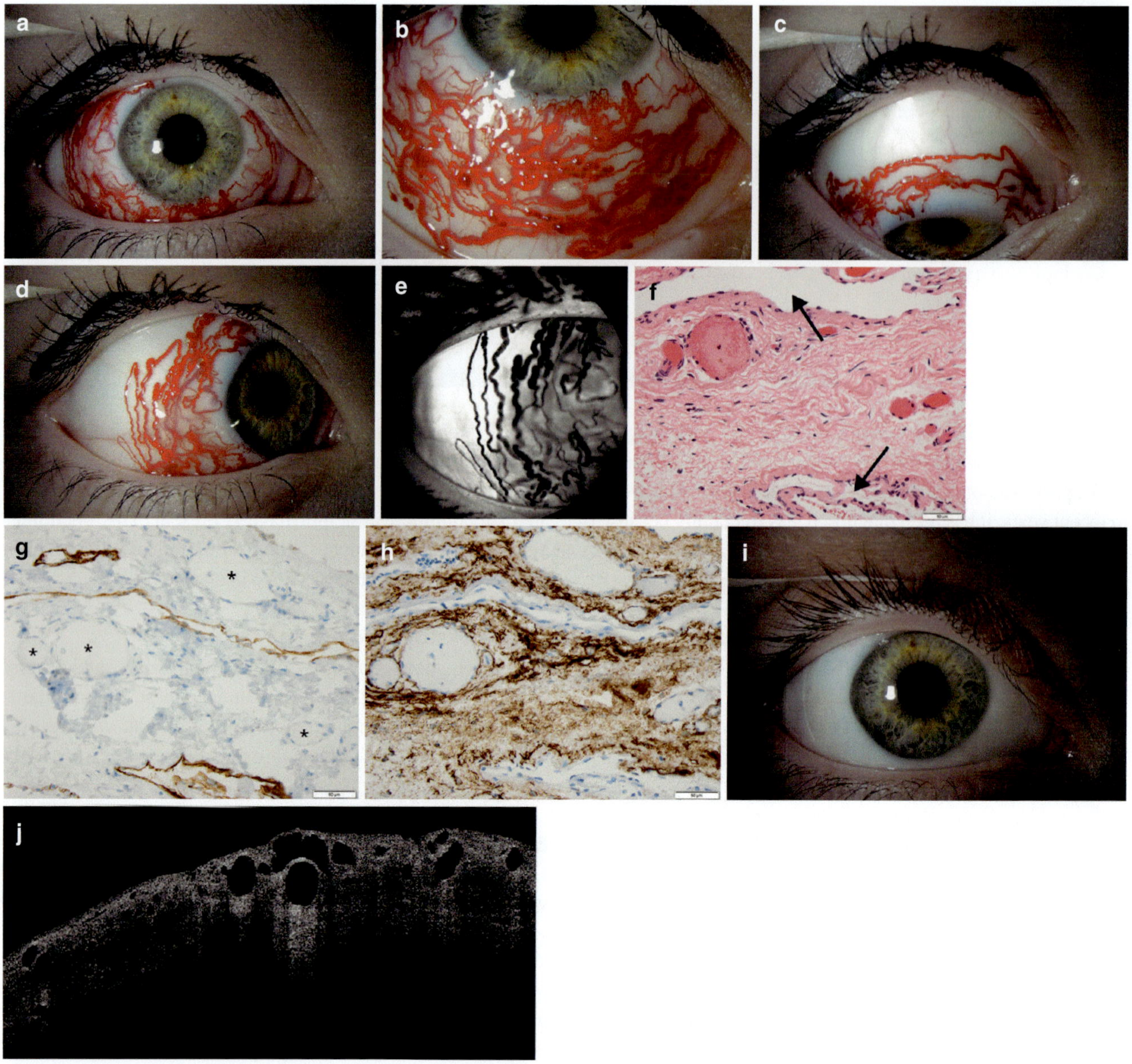

Fig. 8.6 Lymphangiectasia. (**a–d**) Slit-lamp photograph demonstrating the appearance of prominent circumferential vessels. (**e**) FA image demonstrating a complete absence of hyperfluorescence in the lesion. (**f**) Histopathology confirmed dilated tortuous empty channels (top and bottom, arrows) next to normal vessels containing blood. Stroma is free of inflammation. Bar represents 50 mm (hematoxylin and eosin). (**g**) Immunohistochemistry for D2-40/podoplanin highlights lymphatics. Dilated channels are lined by D2-40-positive endothelium. Note the negative blood vessels in the background (*). (**h**) Immunohistochemistry for CD34, a marker of fibroblasts and the vascular endothelium, shows that dilated channels are CD34 negative (consistent with lymphatics). Blood vessels show mild CD34 positivity and background stromal cells are positive. (**i**) Slit-lamp photograph demonstrating appearance 4 months after surgical drainage. (**j**) Anterior-segment OCT demonstrating dilated conjunctival lymphatic channels. (Reprinted from Goshe et al. [23]. With permission from Wolters Kluwer Health, Inc.)

congestion and dilation of the spaces. Because of the common connection of the conjunctival part to an orbital part, dilatation of the lymphangioma cysts may cause proptosis of the eye.

8.3.2.2 Histopathological Features

Conjunctival lymphangioma shows dilated lymphatic channels filled with lymph and/or blood, lined by endothelium, and separated by thin walls.

8.3.2.3 Treatment

Treatment of lymphangioma is difficult, and surgical excision or radiotherapy usually does not eradicate the tumor. Carbon dioxide laser [27] and brachytherapy [28] have been used for treating conjunctival lymphangioma, with partial success. When dilatation of the spaces raises the orbital pressure and threatens the optic nerve, percutaneous drainage of blood may offer temporary relief. Drainage and sclerotherapy have been offered as a safe and effective treatment [29–31].

8.4 Fibrous Tumors

8.4.1 Fibroma

8.4.1.1 Clinical Features

Fibroma of the conjunctiva is rare [32]. It is generally a slowly progressing acquired white stromal tumor in adults and may range from a well-circumscribed lesion to a multinodular lesion. One case of malignant fibrosarcoma has also been reported [33].

8.4.1.2 Histopathological Features

The tumor is composed of compact fibroblasts and collagen. Rare variants such as elastofibroma oculi, giant cell angiofibroma, and solitary fibrous tumor have been described [34].

8.4.1.3 Treatment

Conjunctival fibroma is treated by complete surgical excision.

8.4.2 Benign and Malignant Fibrous Histiocytoma

Fibrous histiocytoma (FH) of the conjunctiva can be benign, locally aggressive, or malignant [35]. Malignant FH is also known as undifferentiated pleomorphic sarcoma [36]. FH generally occurs in adults, but a case of benign FH and a case of malignant FH in a child with xeroderma pigmentosum have also been reported [37, 38].

8.4.2.1 Clinical Features

Conjunctival FH appears as an amelanotic mass that can range from a well-circumscribed mass to a diffuse one. It often presents in the limbus (Fig. 8.7). In a review of 42 cases [39], 25 cases showed the presence of limbal FH, 12 were conjunctival, 4 were caruncular, 1 corneal, 27 were benign, and 15 were malignant FH.

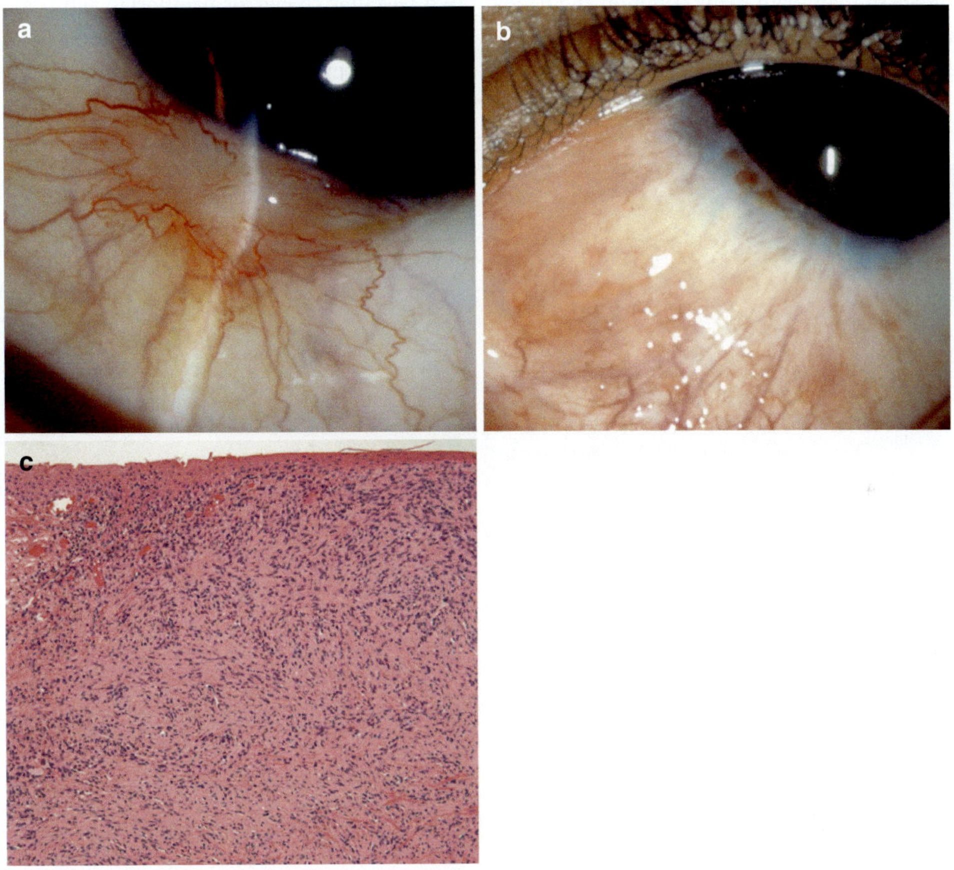

Fig. 8.7 Conjunctival fibrous histiocytoma (FH). A 10-year-old black boy presented with a limbal lesion that was excised about 2 months previously. (**a**) Clinical picture of the recurred lesion. Further excision with cryotherapy was performed. For yet another recurrence, excision was repeated. (**b**) Histopathology revealed a moderately cellular spindle cell lesion composed of bland spindle cells arranged in a vaguely storiform configuration. Entrapped collagen bundles are witnessed at the periphery of the lesion, and there are scattered inflammatory cells, mostly lymphocytes (hematoxylin and eosin-stain ×40). A final diagnosis of benign fibrous histiocytoma (extension to margin) was made. Repeat cryotherapy was performed to the surgical site. (**c**) Over a 6-year follow-up, there was no recurrence and the patient maintained normal visual acuity. (Courtesy of David Meisler, MD and Thomas Plesec, MD, Cleveland Clinic, Ohio)

8.4.2.2 Histopathological Features

FH shows a mixture of spindle-shaped fibroblasts, often arranged in a storiform pattern and lipid-laden histiocytes. Conjunctival FH with benign histological appearance may show a malignant clinical course. Malignant FH of the conjunctiva shows marked pleomorphism, atypical spindle cells, multinucleated giant cells, and many mitotic figures. Malignant FH is accepted as originating from primitive mesenchymal cells with the capacity to differentiate along either or both histiocytes and fibroblasts [40]. Malignant FH can metastasize to regional lymph nodes and hematogenously to distant organs, causing death.

8.4.2.3 Treatment

While benign FH can be treated by complete surgical excision, malignant FH should be treated by radical surgery with tumor-free margins. While the recurrence rate of benign FH is not common and can be treated by re-excision and immunotherapy, recurrence of malignant FH is common and needs aggressive surgical options, including enucleation, exenteration, and radical dissection of regional lymph nodes [39].

8.4.3 Nodular Fasciitis

Nodular fasciitis is a benign, rare nodular tumor of unknown cause that can occur at any age.

8.4.3.1 Clinical Features

Nodular fasciitis appears as a solitary white episcleral enlarging nodule at the limbus or over the sclera anterior to the insertion of one of the rectus muscles and can cause discomfort or pain [41] (Fig. 8.8). The nodule may grow quickly and show signs of inflammation. It is thought to originate from the Tenon's capsule [42].

8.4.3.2 Histopathological Features

The lesion tends to be round or oval and is not encapsulated. It is composed of bundles of fibroblasts that vary in configuration from spindle to stellate. There is a variable amount of intercellular myxoid ground substance interspersed with slit-like vascular spaces or capillaries and scanty infiltration of chronic inflammatory cells. Numerous mitotic figures can lead to its being misdiagnosed as a sarcoma [43].

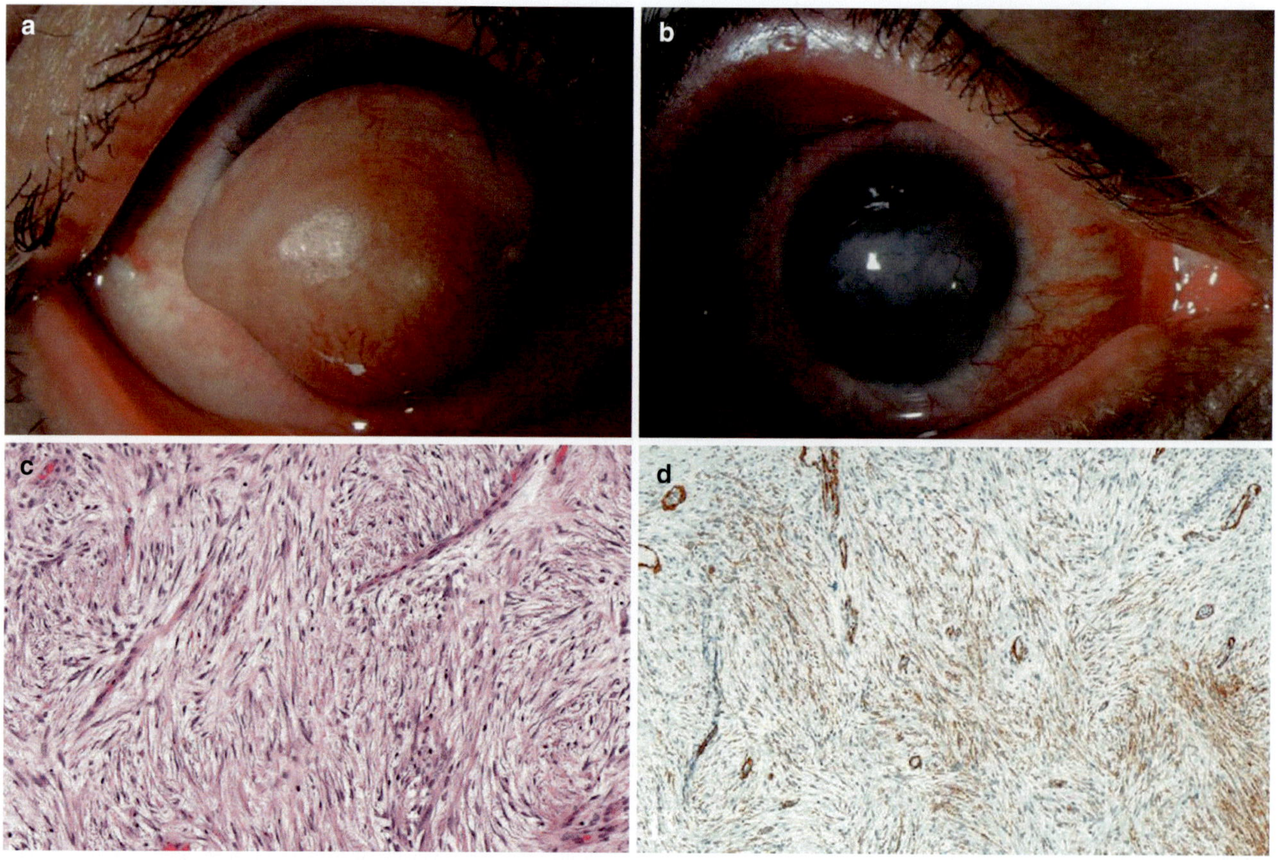

Fig. 8.8 Nodular fasciitis. Preoperative (**a**) and postoperative (**b**) appearance on slit-lamp examination. (**c**) Histopathology shows spindle cell proliferation composed of regular delicate cells with pale chromatin and small nucleoli arranged in short, irregular fascicles (hematoxylin and eosin, ×200). (**d**) Smooth muscle actin (SMA) stain of spindle cells with variable positivity, consistent with myofibroblastic differentiation. (Reprinted from McClintic et al. [41]. With permission from Wolters Kluwer Health, Inc.)

8.4.3.3 Treatment

The prognosis is excellent and complete excision is usually sufficient therapy, although recurrence can occur.

8.5 Neural Tumors

8.5.1 Neurofibroma

Neurofibroma is a peripheral nerve sheath tumor that can occur in the conjunctival stroma as a solitary circumscribed, or as a diffuse or plexiform, tumor [44]. The solitary type usually is not associated with systemic disease, while the latter is generally associated with neurofibromatosis type 1 (von Recklinghausen's disease).

8.5.1.1 Clinical Features

The solitary neurofibroma is an amelanotic, translucent, gelatinous circumscribed growing mass [45], while the plexiform neurofibroma is diffuse.

8.5.1.2 Histopathological Features

Neurofibroma demonstrates benign proliferation of Schwann cells, axons, and endoneural fibroblasts, which may be difficult to differentiate from other spindle cell tumors.

8.5.1.3 Treatment

Solitary tumors are usually treated by complete surgical excision. Plexiform neurofibroma may be difficult to excise completely. In such cases, debulking of the tumor is performed.

8.5.2 Neurilemmoma (Schwannoma)

Neurilemmoma (schwannoma) of the conjunctiva is a benign rare ocular tumor that can arise from any part of the conjunctiva—bulbar, forniceal, or palpebral [46].

8.5.2.1 Clinical Features

Neurilemmoma (schwannoma) appears as a pink-yellow elevated mass in the conjunctival stroma.

8.5.2.2 Histopathological Features

The tumor is the result of a proliferation of Schwann cells of a peripheral nerve sheath and is composed of spindle cells that may be arranged in an Antoni A pattern (where nuclei are arranged in a column) or an Antoni B pattern (where the cells are loosely arranged).

8.5.2.3 Treatment

Conjunctival neurilemmoma is treated by complete excision within the tumor capsule. Incomplete excision may lead to recurrence. Malignant schwannoma has not been recorded in the conjunctiva.

8.5.3 Granular Cell Tumor

Conjunctival granular cell tumor, known also as myoblastoma, is a very rare benign tumor of disputed origin [47, 48]. After being thought of striated muscle origin, the recent suggestion is that it is of neural derivation, probably from Schwann cells.

8.5.3.1 Clinical Features

The tumor appears as a pink, elevated, smooth mass of the conjunctival stroma, indistinguishable from other well-circumscribed tumors.

8.5.3.2 Histopathological Features

The tumor is composed of groups and cords of cells with small round to oval nuclei and voluminous cytoplasm containing fine eosinophilic granules.

8.5.3.3 Treatment

The tumor should be completely excised.

8.5.4 Neurothekeoma

Neurothekeomas are rare, benign, superficial soft-tissue tumors that most commonly occur on the head and neck. They affect females more often than males, usually in the second and early third decades. Neurothekeoma of the conjunctiva is very rare [49, 50].

8.5.4.1 Clinical Features

Clinically, neurothekeoma presents as a well-circumscribed, pink, red, or brown mass.

8.5.4.2 Histopathological Features

Neurothekeoma may present variable histological patterns, including myxoid, cellular, or mixed type, based primarily on the amount of myxoid matrix present. Contrary to the similar nerve sheath myxoma, neurothekeoma fails to react to S100 immunostaining.

8.5.4.3 Treatment

The tumor should be treated by complete excision.

8.5.5 Merkel Cell Carcinoma

Merkel cell carcinoma is a rare, highly malignant neuroendocrine neoplasm that arises from Merkel cells are specialized neuroendocrine receptors of touch located in the eyelid. Its occurrence in the conjunctiva is very rare [51, 52]. Recent studies have implicated polyomavirus in the pathogenesis of Merkel cell carcinoma [53].

8.5.5.1 Clinical Features

The tumor appears as a reddish, painless, rapidly growing solitary nodule. It usually occurs in older patients. Local recurrence is common, and it may present with lymph nodes and systemic metastasis.

8.5.5.2 Histopathological Features

Histologically, the tumor cells are seen to grow in interconnecting sheets and cords (trabecular pattern). The individual cells are uniformly round with scant cytoplasm, large oval nuclei, prominent nucleoli, and abundant mitotic figures. In addition to synaptophysin, CD56, chromogranin, and non-specific enolase, the tumor cells are also immunoreactive to low molecular weight cytokeratin 20 (CK20), a marker of Merkel cells, which is considered a diagnostic feature.

8.5.5.3 Treatment

Because of the aggressive behavior and common recurrence, surgical excision must include free margins. Sentinel lymph node biopsy and adjuvant radiotherapy should be considered.

8.6 Histiocytic Tumors

8.6.1 Xanthoma

Conjunctival xanthoma appears as a yellow subepithelial mass on the epibulbar surface. In the case of xanthoma disseminatum, in which multiple lesions are found, lesions have been described in the limbus of both eyes [54]. Histopathologically, the lesion shows subepithelial infiltrate of lipid-laden histiocytes, eosinophils, and Touton giant cells. Cases of atypical fibroxanthoma of the conjunctiva have also been reported [55].

8.6.2 Xanthogranuloma

8.6.2.1 Clinical Features

Conjunctival involvement in juvenile xanthogranuloma usually occurs as a solitary orange-pink stromal mass, usually near the limbus (Fig. 8.9) [56]. Sometimes, associated systemic findings may not be present [56]. Bilateral conjunctival xanthogranuloma in adults has also been recorded [57].

8.6.2.2 Histopathological Features

The lesions show typical findings of histiocytes and Touton giant cells; in addition, lymphocytes, plasma cells, and eosinophils can be found. Immunohistochemical stainings are positive for CD68 (histiocytic marker) and negative for CD1a and S-100 (Langerhans cell markers) [58].

8.6.2.3 Treatment

Most lesions are treated by excision. When xanthogranuloma is suspected clinically, it may be observed for spontaneous resolution or can be treated by topical or systemic corticosteroids. In resistant cases, brachytherapy has been successfully applied.

8.6.3 Reticulohistiocytoma

8.6.3.1 Clinical Features

Reticulohistiocytoma is a rare benign conjunctival lesion that usually occurs as an isolated skin nodule or as part of a systemic disorder known as "multicentric reticulohistiocytosis." The cases reported on the ocular surface were of a sin-

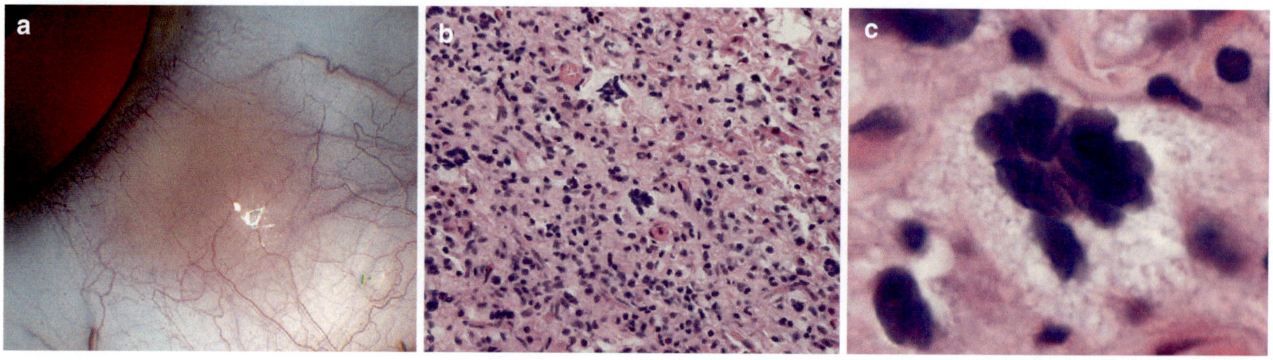

Fig. 8.9 Juvenile xanthogranuloma. (**a**) A 3-year-old girl was referred by her pediatrician for evaluation of a "red spot" in her right eye. As there was no response to topical steroids, excisional biopsy was performed. (**b**) On histopathology, there was a submucosal infiltrate consisting foamy histiocytes, lymphocytes, and typical Touton giant cells (hematoxylin and eosin. ×40 magnification). (**c**) The giant cells have a characteristic wreath of nuclei in the central part of the cell surrounded by foamy cytoplasm (oil immersion. ×100 magnification). Dermatologic evaluation was negative

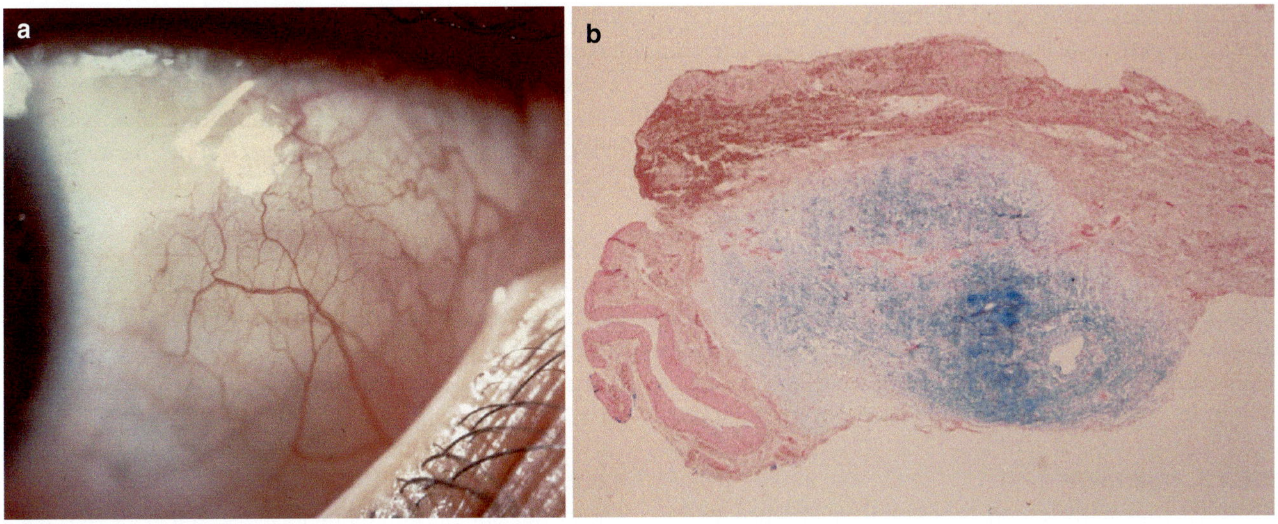

Fig. 8.10 Conjunctival myxoma. (**a**) Clinical appearance as a cyst-like mass in the nasal bulbar conjunctiva of the right eye. (**b**) Histologically, myxoma is a mass of very loose connective tissue in the conjunctival stroma containing abundant hyaluronidase-sensitive mucopolysaccharides that stain positively with Alcian blue (Original magnification ×4)

gle, painless mass localized to the cornea and limbus without systemic disease [59].

8.6.3.2 Histopathological Features

The lesions are composed predominantly of large mononuclear and a few multinucleated cells with finely granular "ground glass" cytoplasm and large nuclei with prominent nucleoli.

8.6.3.3 Treatment

The lesions are treated by complete excision.

8.7 Myxoid Tumors (Myxoma)

8.7.1 Clinical Features

Conjunctival myxoma is a rare benign stromal tumor that occurs in adults. It appears as a slow-growing, asymptomatic, freely movable, usually unilateral solitary lesion in any part of the conjunctiva but primarily located in the temporal bulbar conjunctiva [60–62] (Fig. 8.10a). The lesion may appear pink or fleshy in color. Eyelid and conjunctival myxoma may be associated with Carney complex, a disease with systemic association, which can cause significant morbidity and mortality (Chap. 16).

8.7.2 Histopathological Features

The tumors are well-circumscribed, located in the conjunctival substantia propria, and covered by conjunctival epithelium. They are hypocellular and composed of stellate- and spindle-shaped cells, some with small intracytoplasmic and intranuclear vacuoles that represent dilated cisternae of rough-surfaced endoplasmic reticulum. The stroma contains abundant mucoid material, which stains positively for hyaluronidase-sensitive mucopolysaccharides, and sparse reticulin and delicate collagen fibers (Fig. 8.10b). Scattered mast cells are found in many lesions [60, 61]. Immunohistochemistry demonstrates positivity for vimentin and CD34 and negativity for S100, SMA, SOX10, and GLUT1 [61]. Some pathologists refer to conjunctival myxoma as part of a more general conjunctival myxoid lesions entity [63, 64].

8.7.3 Treatment

Simple surgical excision is curative.

8.8 Myogenic Tumors

8.8.1 Rhabdomyosarcoma

Rhabdomyosarcoma (RMS) is the most common childhood primary orbital malignancy, but the occurrence of this tumor in the conjunctiva alone, without orbital involvement, is rare.

8.8.1.1 Clinical Features

Rhabdomyosarcoma appears as a pink, rapidly growing conjunctival vascular mass. The initial clinical manifestation of the tumor may be a noninflamed pedicle of soft tissue, but occasionally, swelling and erythema precede visible tumor formation [65].

8.8.1.2 Histopathological Features

Most conjunctival rhabdomyosarcomas are of the embryonal type, and as a submucosal tumor, some call it "botryoid" rhabdomyosarcoma (sarcoma botryoides) [65, 66]. Prognosis used to rely on the histopathological type of the tumor. Recently, the weight has shifted to the gene fusion status of forkhead box protein O1 (FOXO1). The European Paediatric Soft Tissue Sarcoma Study Group (EpSSG) found that the FOXO1 fusion status in patients with lymph node-positive (N1) alveolar rhabdomyosarcoma is a powerful predictor of prognosis [67]. The fusion status will be used to stratify these patients in the next EpSSG RMS study, and treatment will be intensified in patients with fusion-positive tumors.

8.8.1.3 Treatment

Complete surgical excision is recommended when this is possible without affecting ocular function. In most cases, the treatment also includes chemotherapy and radiotherapy. Recently, overexpression of the MET gene in orbital RMSs suggested the potential of multi-kinase inhibitors targeting MET as a new therapeutic modality [68].

8.8.2 Leiomyosarcoma

Leiomyosarcoma is a malignant mesenchymal neoplasm with smooth muscle differentiation. Although it is considered one of the most common soft-tissue sarcomas, it rarely affects the eye and is extremely rare in the conjunctiva [69–73].

8.8.2.1 Clinical Features

Leiomyosarcoma of the conjunctiva is diagnosed in adults and seems to originate in the limbus in most reported cases, with corneal invasion in some cases. Clinically, it can be indistinguishable from other tumors in this location, so a biopsy is essential.

8.8.2.2 Histopathological Features

The tumor is comprised of spindle cell proliferation forming rough bundles and fascicles, with prominent cytologic atypia and mitotic figures. Immunostainings are positive for muscle markers such as smooth muscle actin (SMA), desmin, and HHF35 (pan muscle actin).

8.8.2.3 Treatment

The tumor should be completely resected with free margins. Because of frequent recurrence and tumor aggressiveness, adjuvant brachytherapy is recommended. Extended enucleation or exenteration was needed in advanced cases [71–73].

8.8.3 Other Myogenic Tumors

Some other myogenic tumors of the conjunctiva, such as infantile myofibroma [74] and myofibrosarcoma [75], have been very rarely recorded (Fig. 8.11).

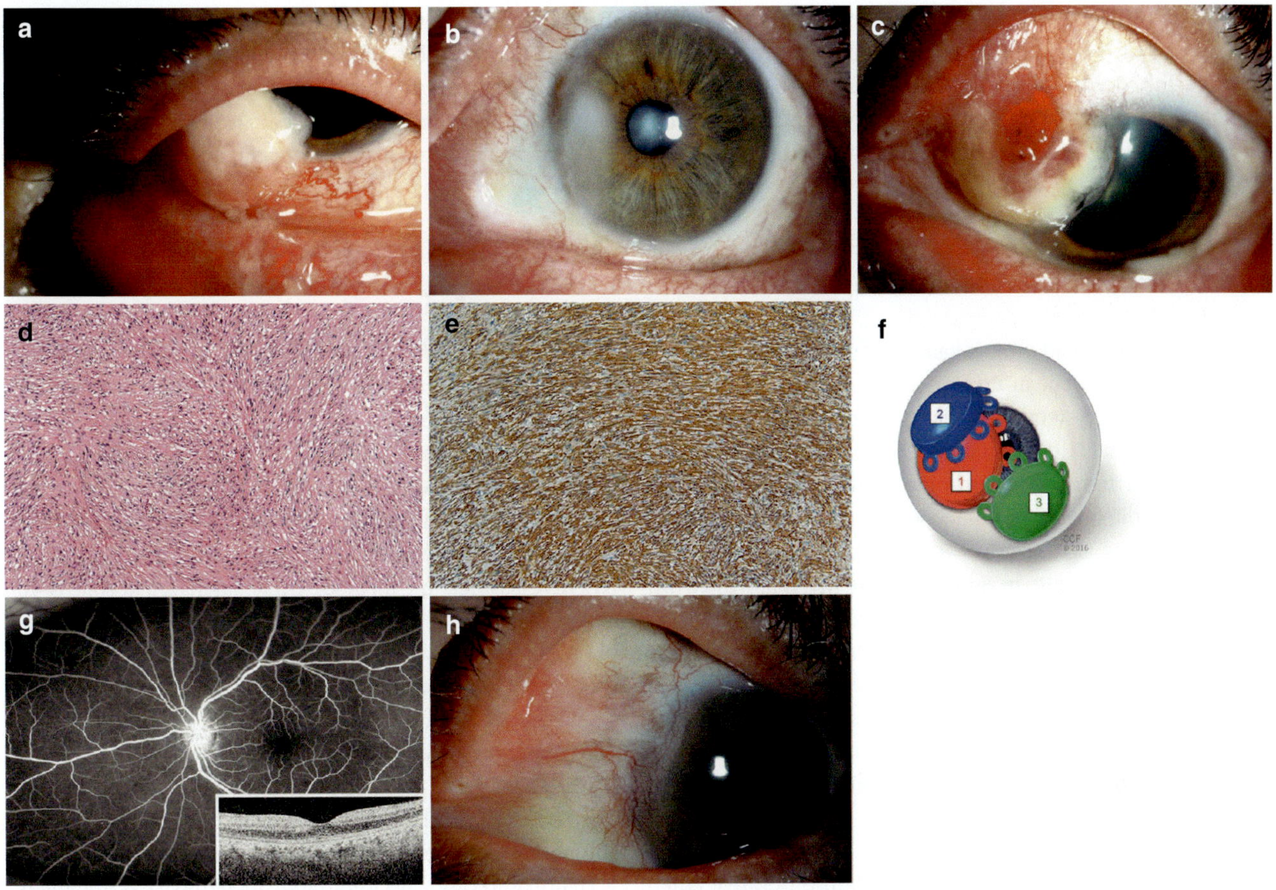

Fig. 8.11 Myofibrosarcoma. (**a**) Slit-lamp appearance at presentation. (**b**) Outcome after excision, cryotherapy to the conjunctival margins, and first episcleral brachytherapy. (**c**) Superior marginal recurrence. (**d**) Histopathological examination revealed cells with spindle nuclei in a fascicular patter with poorly defined eosinophilic cytoplasm (hematoxylin and eosin, ×100 magnification). (**e**) Immunoreactivity to smooth muscle actin (SMA) was positive (×100 magnification) and negative to H-caldesmon, desmin, myoglobin, S-100, melan A, HMB45, AE1/3 and CAM5.2 (not shown). (**f**) Five years after initial presentation, slit-lamp photo of area treated with triple episcleral brachytherapy. (**g**) Position of episcleral plaques. A planned dose of 85 Gy at a depth of 3 mm was used for the first and second plaque and 60 Gy at a depth of 4 mm was used for the third plaque. (**h**) Note the absence of radiation retinopathy on wide-field fluorescein anagram and by OCT (**h**, inset). (Reprinted from Platt et al. [75]. With permission from Wolters Kluwer Health, Inc.)

8.9 Lipomatous Tumors

True lipomatous tumors of the conjunctiva are very rare. On the other hand, herniated orbital fat under the conjunctiva is not rare and may be mistaken for a lipomatous tumor. Dermolipoma is discussed later in this chapter.

8.9.1 Lipoma

Conjunctival lipoma occurs in adults and appears as a yellow-pink stromal mass. Histopathologically, they are usually of the pleomorphic type and show variable-sized adipocytes surrounded by stellate cells. The stroma shows loose myxoid connective tissue. Floret giant cells and nuclear pyknosis were described in this tumor. Mitotic activity is absent [76, 77].

8.9.2 Liposarcoma

Liposarcoma of the conjunctiva shows clinical features similar to lipoma. Histopathologically, the tumor reveals numerous neoplastic cells containing stellate and hyperchromatic nuclei [78]. The cytoplasm of these cells contains vacuoles resembling lipid droplets, and signet-ring-type cells can be observed. The stroma may be myxomatous. The tumor is treated by complete surgical excision. A case of conjunctival liposarcoma showing multiple recurrences and metastatic disease was reported [79].

8.10 Lymphoproliferative Tumors

The conjunctival lymphoid tumors may be subdivided into benign reactive lymphoid hyperplasia (BRLH), atypical lymphoid hyperplasia, and the most common conjunctival lymphoma [80]. The conjunctival lymphoid tumors belong to the group of lymphoid tumors that affect the orbit and the eyelids—the ocular adnexal lymphoma (OAL) [81, 82]. Ocular adnexal lymphomas represent only 2% of all extranodal lymphomas, with primary conjunctival lymphomas accounting for 25–30% of them [81].

8.10.1 Clinical Features

Conjunctival lymphoid tumors can occur as an isolated lesion of the conjunctiva, but in up to one-third of patients, it is a manifestation of systemic lymphoma, which can be present simultaneously with the conjunctival disease or during follow-up. Lymphoid tumors may involve additional ocular sites, mainly the orbit, but the simultaneous involvement of the eyelid and uvea has also been reported [83]. Most conjunctival lymphoid tumors occur in adults, commonly manifested in individuals aged 60–70 years [84], but occurrence in children has also been found [85]. An association between conjunctival lymphoma and *Chlamydophila psittaci* [86] or *Helicobacter pylori* [87] has also been reported. However, it appears that bacterial involvement in the pathogenesis of conjunctival lymphoma is linked to the geographic location [88].

8.10.1.1 Symptoms

Most patients diagnosed as having lymphoproliferative conjunctival lesions are symptomatic at the time of diagnosis. Symptoms include the presentation of a conjunctival mass or irritation, and, less commonly, ptosis, epiphora, blurred vision, proptosis, and diplopia. Some of the patients are asymptomatic [83].

8.10.1.2 Signs

The lymphoproliferative tumors of the conjunctiva appear as a diffuse, slightly elevated pink mass, resembling smoked salmon in color; hence, it is termed "salmon patch" (Fig. 8.12). Most conjunctival lymphoid tumors are located at the bulbar conjunctiva and fornix, usually hidden by the eyelid in the superior and inferior quadrants and not in the horizontal exposed parts of the bulbar conjunctiva or the limbus. Some of these tumors appear in the caruncle or plica semilunaris but almost never appear in the palpebral conjunctiva.

8.10.2 Histopathological Features

As it is not possible to differentiate between benign and malignant conjunctival lymphoid tumors by clinical examination, a biopsy is needed to establish the diagnosis. The vast majority of conjunctival lymphomas are non-Hodgkin's B-cell lymphoma, mostly of low grade; [80, 84] T-cell lymphoma is extremely rare in the conjunctiva [89]. The major lymphoma subtypes, according to the Revised European and American Lymphoma (REAL) classification, include extranodal marginal zone B-cell lymphoma (EMZL), which is by far the most common type, followed by follicular lymphoma (FL), and the more malignant mantle cell lymphoma (MCL) and diffuse large B-cell lymphoma (DLBCL). Additional rare types include plasmacytoma and lymphoplasmacytic lymphoma/immunocytoma [79, 80, 83]. A few cases of conjunctival involvement showing similar salmon-patch lesions, with Rosai–Dorfman disease [90] and multiple myeloma [91], were also reported.

Histopathology with immunohistochemistry is not always enough to differentiate between benign reactive and malignant proliferation of lymphocytes, mandating the use of molecular analyses with PCR for B cell clonality [85].

8.10.3 Treatment

Systemic evaluation should be performed to exclude the presence of systemic lymphoma, which is common in DLBCL and MCL [84]. A localized unilateral lesion can be treated, as first-line, by intralesional injections of anti-CD20 monoclonal anti-

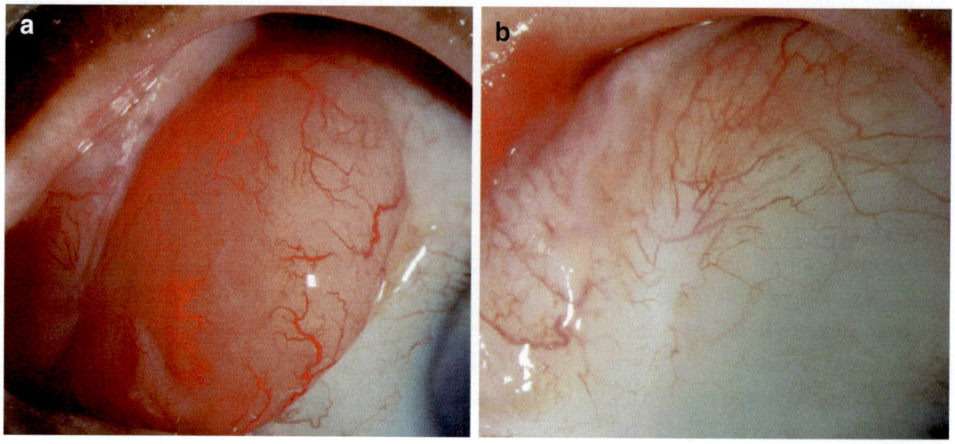

Fig. 8.12 Conjunctival lymphoma. (**a**) A typical infiltrative appearance. (**b**) Clinical appearance 3 months following treatment with radiation therapy (total dose 25 Gy, 12 fractions)

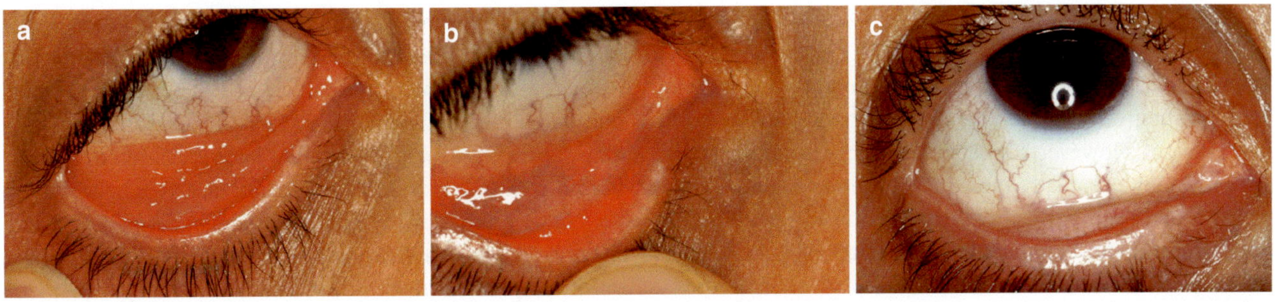

Fig. 8.13 Conjunctival lymphoma. A generally healthy 40-year-old woman with an inferior forniceal salmon patch lesion underwent an incisional biopsy that revealed a B-cell marginal zone lymphoid tissue (MALT) lymphoma. Imaging ruled out an extension of the lesion beyond the forniceal conjunctiva, and the patient was offered localized treatment with intralesional injections of rituximab 1.5 mg/0.15 cc + 0.1 cc of lidocaine on a 6 monthly injections regimen. (**a**) A pretreatment clinical picture shows the involvement of the entire inferior fornix with a pink-salmon-colored multilobulated mass. (**b**) A clinical picture taken 2 months after the completion of the treatment shows an almost complete resolution of the salmon-colored (lymphoma) tissue from the lower fornix. (**c**) Eight years later, there is no sign of recurrence, and hematological follow-up revealed no systemic spread

body (rituximab) (Fig. 8.13) [92, 93] or interferon alpha-2b (which recently is unavailable) [94]. Another common first-line treatment is with low-dose external beam radiation (20–40 Gy, usually in 2 Gy fractions) [84, 95], or brachytherapy [96, 97]. Adverse effects of external beam radiation on the ocular surface, mainly persistent dry eyes, should be considered and informed well to the patients [98]. Recently, ultra-low-dose (2 × 2 Gy = 4 Gy) radiation treatment for early-stage conjunctival MALT lymphoma was reported with good response from most patients and no ocular complications [99]. In cases of widespread lymphoma and when systemic lymphoma is diagnosed, intravenous rituximab has been used successfully with or without chemotherapy as primary treatment and in treating relapsed mucosa-associated lymphoid tissue lymphoma of the conjunctiva [80, 100–103].

8.10.4 Prognosis

Local treatment is usually effective, but semiannual systemic evaluation should be performed because of possible local recurrence and recurrence in extranodal sites. In one study, systemic lymphoma was eventually discovered in 15% of patients at 5 years and in 28% at 10 years [82].

Since most conjunctival lymphomas are low-grade, the mortality rate of conjunctival lymphoma is low. The main prognostic factor for the risk of developing systemic lymphoma is the histological subtype, with MCL and DLBCL having a markedly poorer prognosis than EMZL and FL [84]. Older age was also found to be an important prognostic factor [84, 104].

8.11 Leukemic Infiltrates

Leukemic infiltration in the eye most commonly occurs in the choroid and retina, but conjunctival infiltration is also a well-recognized complication of many types of leukemia. Conjunctival involvement in leukemia shows myriad clinical presentations that can involve one or both eyes, have focal or diffuse infiltration of the substantia propria, can occur on the bulbar or palpebral conjunctiva, and can cause microvascular changes due to hyperviscosity (leukostasis) from markedly elevated leukemic cell counts. Conjunctival lesions have also been reported as the presenting manifestation of acute leukemia in patients who were not recognized to have the disease, and in others, they signified disease relapse [105, 106]. Conjunctival leukemic involvement is consistent with good visual acuity, with no reports of vision reduction associated with the conjunctival infiltration; however, it portended a poor prognosis with a median survival of 3 months. Although clinical reports of conjunctival leukemia in the literature are relatively uncommon, autopsy studies of leukemic patients indicate that many harbor unsuspected disease and that most cases of conjunctival leukemia are probably subclinical or go unrecognized.

8.11.1 Clinical Features

Conjunctival leukemia occurs most commonly in patients with acute leukemia. Leukemic infiltrations are often firm and not tender, may appear as a pink smooth mass, and are usually associated with small areas of hemorrhage [105]. Granulocytic sarcoma (chloroma) may appear in the ocular adnexa in the course of acute myelogenous leukemia (AML) and appear as a gray-green mass in the eyelid or the forniceal or tarsal conjunctiva [107].

8.11.2 Histopathological Features

Clinicopathological studies indicate that conjunctival leukemic lesions are cellular invasions that occur at all levels of the substantia propria; they can be diffuse or patchy and are generally localized along blood vessels.

8.11.3 Treatment

The treatment includes various combinations of chemotherapy and, commonly, local radiotherapy, with good local response in most cases. However, patients who achieve a complete local response may eventually die of the systemic disease. These patients die from refractory leukemia or leukemia-related complications, most commonly from infections.

8.12 Choristoma

Choristomas are congenital lesions representing normal tissue in an abnormal location. When the lesion is composed of one type of tissue, it is considered to be a simple choristoma; when combinations of displaced tissue are involved, it is termed "complex choristoma." Epibulbar choristomas are the most common epibulbar tumors in children [108]. Among them, dermoids and dermolipomas are very common [109]. Epibulbar choristomas affect the cornea, limbus, or subconjunctival space and range in appearance from a small, flat lesion to large masses filling most of the epibulbar region. They often can cause astigmatism. Epibulbar choristomas can affect other parts of the eye and orbit and may be associated with coloboma, Goldenhar syndrome, or organoid nevus syndrome [108].

8.12.1 Dermoid

Epibulbar dermoid is a well-circumscribed firm, solitary congenital mass that involves the bulbar conjunctiva and often the corneoscleral limbus (Fig. 8.14). Rarely, more than one is found.

8.12.1.1 Clinical Features

Conjunctival dermoid is usually a solid yellow-white mass, and sometimes fine hairs protrude from the lesion. The size of epibulbar dermoids is variable, from the more common small limbal dermoid through large dermoid involving most or the entire corneal surface, to extensive dermoids that involve also the anterior chamber and the iris. The typical dermoid occurs in the inferotemporal limbus. It may be associated with Goldenhar syndrome that, in addition to the epibulbar dermoid, may include preauricular skin appendages, vertebral anomalies, eyelid coloboma, hearing loss, and mandibular hypoplasia, but also with congenital heart defects. Epibulbar dermoid, in addition to being a cosmetic blemish, can cause severe astigmatism and amblyopia, affecting the vision according to the level of corneal involvement [110].

8.12.1.2 Histopathological Features

Epibulbar dermoid is a simple choristoma that consists of dense fibrous tissue covered by stratified squamous epithelium. It usually contains dermal elements such as hair follicles, sebaceous glands, sweat glands, and sometimes adipose-connective tissue.

8.12.1.3 Treatment

When the epibulbar dermoid is very small and does not cause visual symptoms, it can be managed by observation alone. Larger dermoids can be managed by excision (lamellar keratosclerectomy) without or with conjunctival flap. In most cases, a corneal scar will remain in the excision site. Lamellar or penetrating keratoplasty may be needed in advanced cases. When amblyopia is present, early treatment is advised.

8.12.2 Dermolipoma

8.12.2.1 Clinical Features

Dermolipoma is a yellowish-tan, soft, fusiform tumor, usually localized to the temporal or supero-temporal aspect of the conjunctiva, near the lateral canthus (Fig. 8.15). Although it is congenital, it may remain asymptomatic for years until detected when it protrudes from the supero-temporal con-

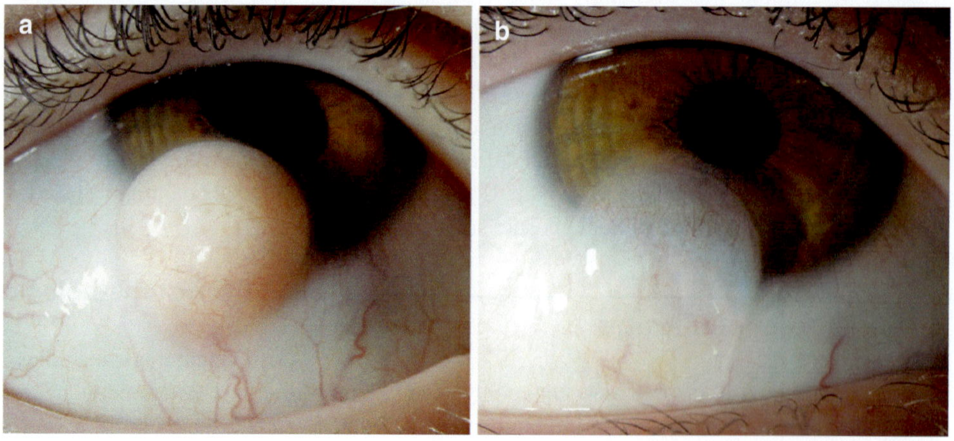

Fig. 8.14 Limbal dermoid in the lower temporal aspect of the cornea and conjunctiva. (**a**) Note hair growing from the middle of the lesion. (**b**) A residual corneal scar remains after surface excision

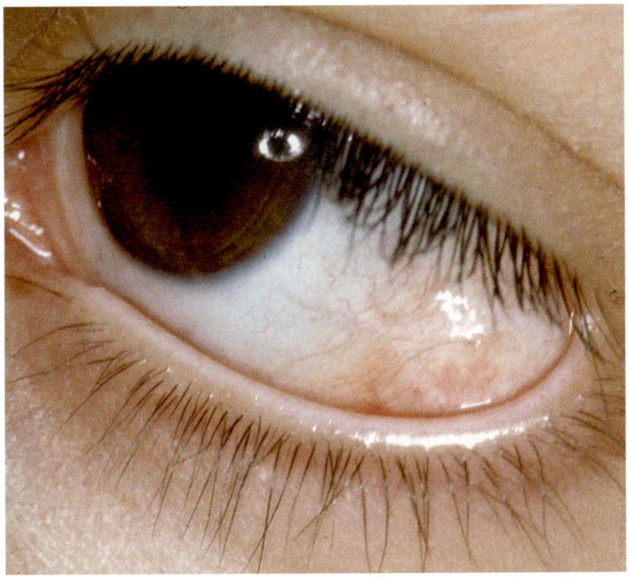

Fig. 8.15 Dermolipoma in the temporal part of the bulbar conjunctiva

junctival fornix, usually in the second and third decades. Epibulbar dermolipoma often extends between the lateral rectus and superior rectus muscles to lie close to the lacrimal gland. They also may extend posteriorly into the orbit or anteriorly toward the limbus. Dermolipoma should be differentiated from subconjunctival orbital fat prolapse [111]. Most patients have symptoms; the most common one is an increasing size of a long-standing peribulbar lump. Other symptoms include ocular irritation, episodic localized conjunctival injection, and mucoid discharge. One-third of dermolipomas have visible hair [112].

8.12.2.2 Histopathological Features

The epithelium on the surface of the dermolipoma is stratified squamous epithelium that may be partially keratinized. The stroma contains variable quantities of dense collagenous tissue and large amounts of adipose tissue, mainly in the deeper aspects of the lesion. Pilosebaceous structures are usually absent.

8.12.2.3 Treatment

The majority of dermolipomas require no treatment, but when symptomatic or cosmetically blemished, it can be managed by simple excision of the anterior portion of the lesion or by excising the entire lesion, including the orbital part through the conjunctival fornix. When the conjunctiva over the dermolipoma is adherent to the lesion and has to be excised, a rotational conjunctival flap and free conjunctival autograft have been applied to cover the conjunctival defect [113, 114].

8.12.3 Osseous Choristoma

8.12.3.1 Clinical Features

Epibulbar osseous choristoma is a rare solitary congenital lesion that most frequently presents as an isolated epibulbar lesion in the supero-temporal quadrant but may occur in other locations on the surface of the globe or in association with other choristomatous lesions such as dermolipoma [115–117]. Bilateral lesions have been reported. The lesion may be freely movable or adherent to the bulbar conjunctiva and the sclera. Not uncommonly, the lesion may involve the sheath of an extraocular muscle.

8.12.3.2 Histopathological Features

The lesion is composed of mature, compact bone surrounded by connective tissue in which additional choristomatous elements occasionally may be found.

8.12.3.3 Treatment

Epibulbar osseous choristoma typically remains undetectable until palpated by the patient, who feels the hard lesion. The diagnosis can be confirmed by ultrasonography or computed tomography that illustrates the calcifications. The tumor is generally managed by periodic observation, but if causing ocular inflammation, foreign body sensation and tearing, or is cosmetically unappealing, it may be treated by surgical excision. When lesions adhere to the sclera, superficial sclerectomy may be warranted. Imaging of the globe with the tumor may aid in the avoidance of iatrogenic globe perforation during surgical excision [115, 116].

8.12.4 Lacrimal Gland Choristoma (Ectopic Lacrimal Gland)

8.12.4.1 Clinical Features

Epibulbar lacrimal gland choristoma is a simple choristomatous congenital lesion that presents as an asymptomatic pink stromal mass, typically in the supero-temporal or temporal parts of the conjunctiva, but it has also been described in the limbal area [118, 119].

8.12.4.2 Histopathological Features

Lacrimal gland tissue, similar to the normal lacrimal gland, is seen in the conjunctival stroma. Epibulbar complex choristoma may contain lacrimal gland tissue together with other tissue elements [120, 121].

8.12.4.3 Treatment

Excision of the lesion usually suffices.

8.12.5 Complex Choristoma

Complex choristoma is a congenital, unilateral lesion that contains tissue derived from two germ layers—ectoderm and mesoderm.

8.12.5.1 Clinical Features

Epibulbar complex choristoma has a variable clinical appearance and ranges from a localized lesion to a lesion that covers much of the epibulbar surface. A large pedunculated mass protruding through the eyelid aperture has been reported [122] (Fig. 8.16a). The choristoma may invade the cornea. The consistency and color depend on the types of tissue present in the choristoma; for example, dermal elements containing adipose-connective tissue appear yellowish, while lacrimal tissue appears pink. A cases series of epibulbar choristomas containing cartilage, smooth muscle bundles, and fibrous connective tissue covered by pterygia was reported [123].

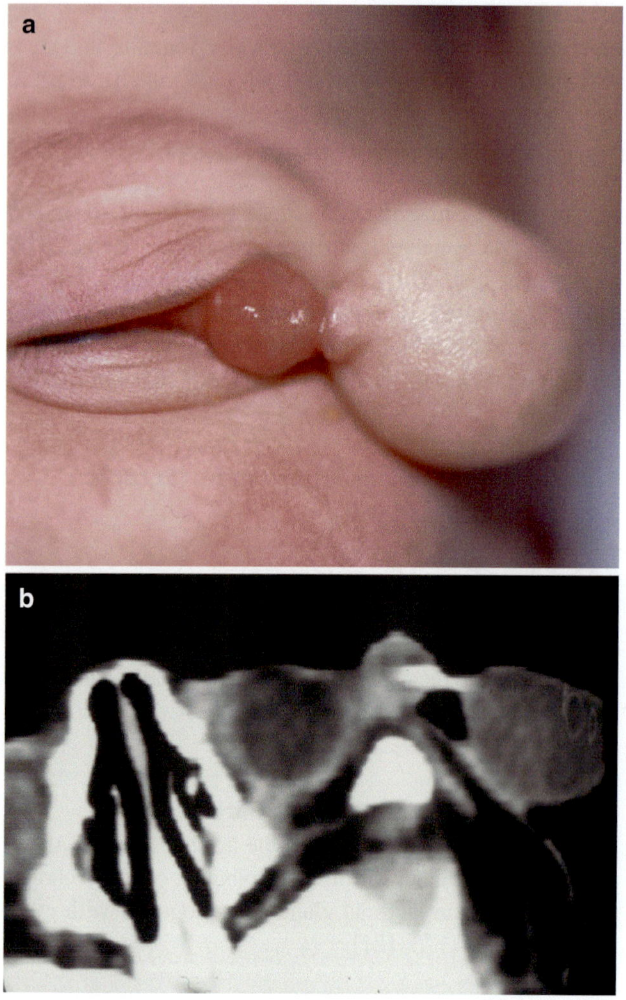

Fig. 8.16 Epibulbar complex choristoma. (**a**) The clinical appearance in a 5-day-old child who was also diagnosed with linear nevus sebaceous. A large pedunculated mass protrudes temporally through the left eyelid aperture. (**b**) CT scan shows calcifications (bone) in the tumor base and a cyst-like structure in the polypoid mass

8.12.5.2 Histopathological Features

Complex choristoma may include a variable combination of ectopic tissue such as dermal tissue containing adipose tissue, collagen and pilosebaceous structures, lacrimal gland, smooth muscle, cartilage, bone, nerves, and blood vessels. It may appear cystic (Fig. 8.16b). Epibulbar complex choristoma may be associated with organoid nevus syndrome, of which the most frequent cutaneous feature is the sebaceous nevus of Jadassohn [122].

8.12.5.3 Treatment

The management of epibulbar complex choristoma depends on the extent of the lesion and the symptoms it causes. Asymptomatic small lesions can be observed, while large symptomatic lesions should be excised. Reconstruction of the ocular surface is sometimes needed. In very advanced cases, enucleation may be needed.

8.13 Metastatic and Secondary Tumors

8.13.1 Metastatic Tumors

Metastatic tumors to the conjunctiva are rare and usually appear at an advanced stage of the systemic malignancy when there is evidence of other ocular and organ metastases [124]. Similar to sources of metastases in other ocular sites, the primary tumors are usually carcinomas, led by breast carcinoma or cutaneous melanoma.

The metastatic carcinoma appears as fleshy, yellow, or pink, vascularized stromal tumors, while metastatic cutaneous melanoma may be pigmented. The metastasis may be located in any part of the conjunctiva and is usually solitary but may be multiple. Conjunctival metastases are treated by excisional biopsy, radiotherapy, and chemotherapy. The survival time after diagnosis of conjunctival metastases is in the range of months.

8.13.2 Secondary Tumors

The conjunctiva may be secondarily involved by extraocular extension of intraocular tumors and by extension of eyelid and orbital tumors [6]. The most important tumor in this category is sebaceous gland carcinoma of the eyelid, which often exhibits pagetoid invasion into the conjunctival epithelium. Ciliary body melanoma, when extending through the sclera into the subconjunctival tissue, may simulate conjunctival melanoma. Orbital tumors, such as rhabdomyosarcoma in children, can present first in the conjunctiva.

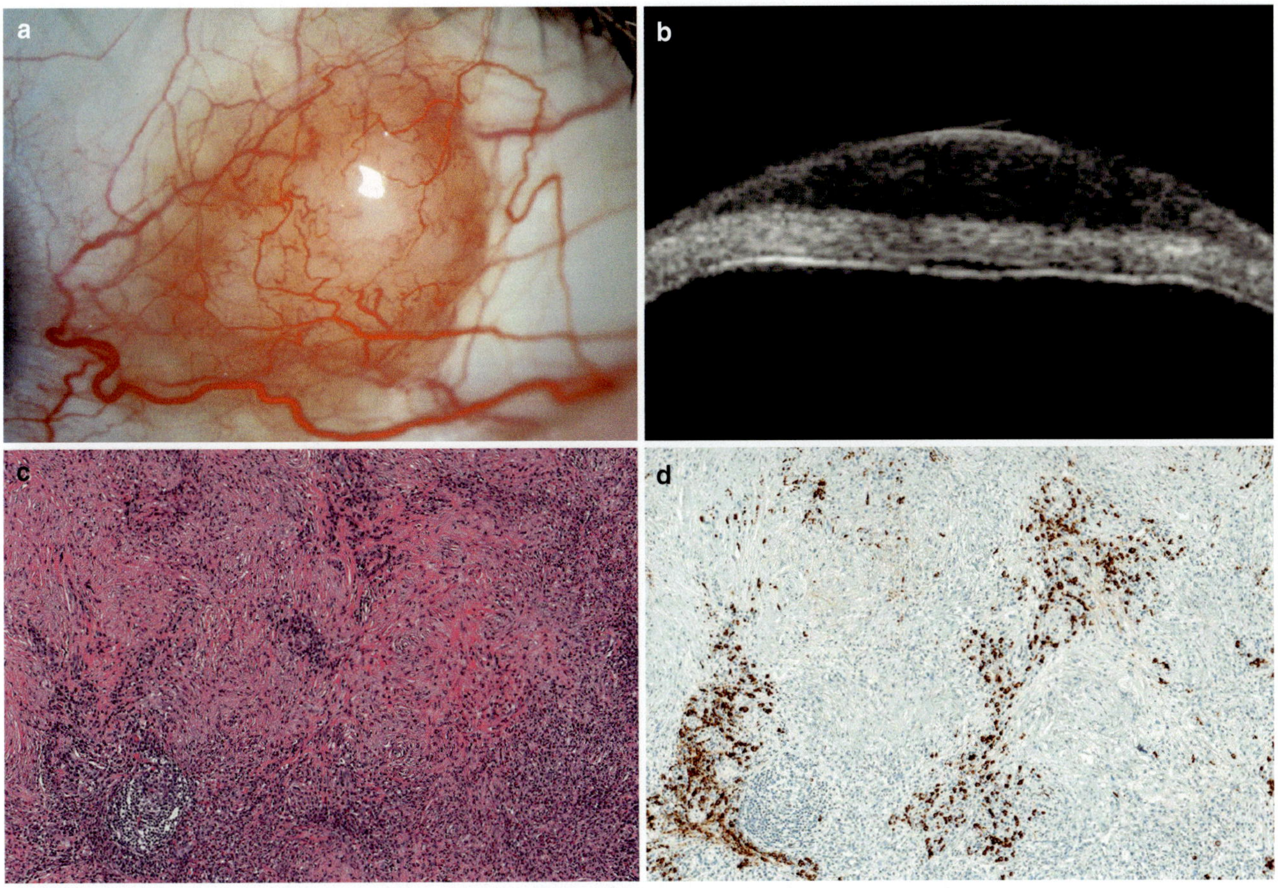

Fig. 8.17 IgG4 sclerosing disease. (**a**) Slit-lamp photos of a left eye conjunctival lesion at presentation show a temporal conjunctival bulbar lesion that is raised, tan-colored, vascular, and immobile. (**b**) Ultrasound biomicroscopy of the conjunctival lesion measuring 7.5 × 8 × 1.2 mm with low reflectivity and a shallow focal invasion into the sclera. (**c**) Histopathology demonstrates haphazard fibrosis with intermixed plasma cell-rich inflammation as well as many eosinophils and a few lymphoid follicles (hematoxylin and eosin, original magnification ×100). (**d**) Immunohistochemical stain for IgG4, in the same area as H&E. There are numerous IgG4-positive plasma cells, which, in conjunction with the H&E morphology and IgG4:IgG ratio of 64%, are diagnostic of IgG4-related disease. (Reprinted from Li et al. [127]. With permission from Wolters Kluwer Health, Inc.)

8.14 IgG4-Related Disease

Isolated conjunctival inflammation from IgG4-related disease should be on the differential diagnosis for chronic and minimally symptomatic solitary conjunctival lesions. Assessment of IgG4-RD is based on the combination of clinical history, physical exam, histopathology, laboratory results, and radiology studies [125–127] (Fig. 8.17).

8.15 Amyloidosis

Amyloid deposits in ocular adnexal structures (conjunctiva, eyelid, lacrimal gland and sac, extraocular muscles, levator palpebrae muscle, and orbit) is a rare entity. Varied presentations, vague symptoms, and rare incidences result in delayed or missed diagnoses (Fig. 8.18) [128–132]. Immunohistochemistry (IHC) [133] and, more recently, mass spectrometry (MS) allow for amyloid protein subtype analysis [134]. MS offers increased accuracy in protein subtype identification and may also allow for the identification of new protein subtypes [135]. A recent study, with a comprehensive review of the literature concluded that amyloidosis-AL is the most common form of amyloid deposit in ocular adnexal structures [136]. Hence, workup to exclude systemic involvement or associated underlying lymphoproliferative disorder is warranted.

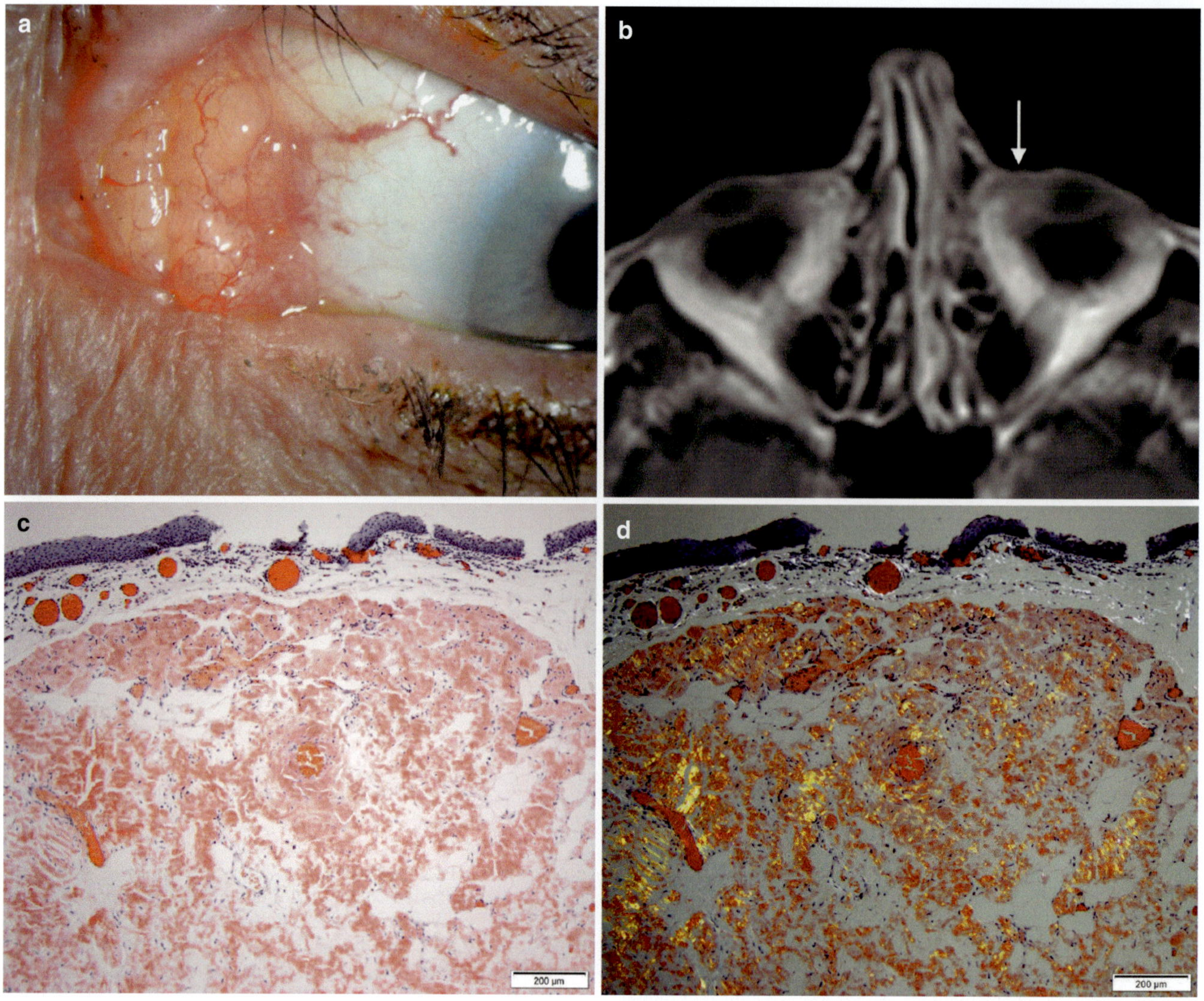

Fig. 8.18 A 63-year-old white woman with a history of sarcoidosis was noted to have an incidental left-sided conjunctival orbital mass. (**a**) The mass was yellowish in color, multinodular, and firm in consistency. Ocular motility was full, and proptosis was absent. (**b**) MRI confirmed an enhancing mass that was localized to the anterior orbit (arrow). (**c**) Congo red stained histopathology section of conjunctival mucosa shows a lobular accumulation of amorphous congophilic material in the deep stroma (Congo red), which exhibits apple-green birefringence with polarized light (**d**) compatible with amyloid deposits. (Reprinted from Blandford et al. [136]. With permission from Elsevier)

References

1. Shields JA, Mashayekhi A, Kligman BE, et al. Vascular tumors of the conjunctiva in 140 cases. Ophthalmology. 2011;118:1747–53.
2. Ferry AP. Pyogenic granulomas of the eye and ocular adnexa: a study of 100 cases. Trans Am Ophthalmol Soc. 1989;87:327–43.
3. Cameron JA, Mahmood MA. Pyogenic granulomas of the cornea. Ophthalmology. 1995;102:1681–7.
4. Millsop JW, Trinh N, Winterfield L, Berrios R, Hutchens KA, Tung R. Resolution of recalcitrant pyogenic granuloma with laser, corticosteroid, and timolol therapy. Dermatol Online J. 2014;20(3)
5. Oke I, Alkharashi M, Petersen RA, Ashenberg A, Shah AS. Treatment of ocular pyogenic granuloma with topical timolol. JAMA Ophthalmol. 2017;135:383–5.
6. Shields CL, Shields JA. Tumors of the conjunctiva and cornea. Surv Ophthalmol. 2004;49:3–24.
7. Chang TC, Estes R. Beta blocker treatment of infantile conjunctival hemangiomas—observations from 2 cases. J AAPOS. 2014;18:80–2.
8. Kiratli H, Uzun S, Tarlan B, et al. Recurrent subconjunctival hemorrhage due to cavernous hemangioma of the conjunctiva. Can J Ophthalmol. 2012;47:318–20.
9. Shields JA, Kligman BE, Mashayekhi A, et al. Acquired sessile hemangioma of the conjunctiva: a report of 10 cases. Am J Ophthalmol. 2011;152:55–9.
10. Das D, Raj SJS, Bajaj M. Acquired sessile conjunctival capillary haemangioma in an adult managed with topical timolol. BMJ Case Rep. 2020;13:e237547.
11. Grossniklaus HE, Green WR, Wolff SM, Iliff NT. Hemangiopericytoma of the conjunctiva. Two cases. Ophthalmology. 1986;93:265–7.
12. Edwards W, Craven C, Turner JR, et al. Isolated hemangiopericytoma of the conjunctiva. Am J Ophthalmol Case Rep. 2022;25:101308.
13. Kurumety UR, Lustbader JM. Kaposi's sarcoma of the bulbar conjunctiva as an initial clinical manifestation of acquired immunodeficiency syndrome. Arch Ophthalmol. 1995;113:978.

14. Rossetto JD, Molles S, Gracittelli CPG. Extensive bulbar conjunctival Kaposi's sarcoma as initial symptom of human immunodeficiency virus. Arq Bras Oftalmol. 2019;82:429–31.
15. Ghabrial R, Quivey JM, Dunn JP Jr, Char DH. Radiation therapy of acquired immunodeficiency syndrome-related Kaposi's sarcoma of the eyelids and conjunctiva. Arch Ophthalmol. 1992;110:1423–6.
16. Eduardo-Sánchez YW, Fernández-Agrafojo D. Human immunodeficiency virus-associated giant conjunctival Kaposi's sarcoma: complete remission with antiretroviral therapy and systemic chemotherapy. Arch Soc Esp Oftalmol. 2018;93:310–2.
17. Hummer J, Gass JD, Huang AJ. Conjunctival Kaposi's sarcoma treated with interferon alpha-2a. Am J Ophthalmol. 1993;116:502–3.
18. Yang J, Yin XF, Li YP, Zhou SY. Case report of ocular Kaposi's sarcoma. BMC Ophthalmol. 2017;17:143.
19. Tourlaki A, Maronese CA, Brambilla L. Successful treatment of conjunctival classic Kaposi's sarcoma with topical timolol. Ital Dermatol Venerol. 2021;156:629–30.
20. Welch J, Srinivasan S, Lyall D, et al. Conjunctival lymphangiectasia: a report of 11 cases and review of literature. Surv Ophthalmol. 2012;57:136–48.
21. Awdry P. Lymphangiectasia haemorrhagica conjunctivae. Br J Ophthalmol. 1969;53:274–8.
22. Fraunfelder FW. Liquid nitrogen cryotherapy for conjunctival lymphangiectasia: a case series. Trans Am Ophthalmol Soc. 2009;107:229–32.
23. Goshe JM, Platt S, Yeaney G, Singh AD. Surgical drainage of lymphangiectasia haemorrhagica conjunctivae. Cornea. 2017;36:116–8.
24. Han KE, Choi CY, Seo KY. Removal of lymphangiectasis using high-frequency radio wave electrosurgery. Cornea. 2013;32(4):547–9.
25. Tan JC, Mann S, Coroneo MT. Successful treatment of conjunctival lymphangiectasia with subconjunctival injection of bevacizumab. Cornea. 2016;35:1375–7.
26. Dave TV, Walvekar P. Two-year outcomes of transcutaneous non-image guided bleomycin sclerotherapy in conjunctival lymphatic malformations: a protocol-based management in 16 eyes. Ophthalmic Plast Reconstr Surg. 2023;39:64–71.
27. Spector JA, Zide BM. Carbon dioxide laser ablation for treatment of lymphangioma of the conjunctiva. Plast Reconstr Surg. 2006;117:609–12.
28. Behrendt S, Bernsmeier H, Randzio G. Fractionated beta-irradiation of a conjunctival lymphangioma. Ophthalmologica. 1991;203:161–3.
29. Foster JA, Czyz CN, Stacey A, Everman KR, Cahill KV. Percutaneous drainage and ablation as first line therapy for macrocystic and microcystic orbital lymphatic malformations. Ophthalmic Plast Reconstr Surg. 2012;28:119–25.
30. Barnacle AM, Theodorou M, Maling SJ, Abou-Rayyah Y. Sclerotherapy treatment of orbital lymphatic malformations: a large single-centre experience. Br J Ophthalmol. 2016;100:204–8.
31. Gandhi NG, Lin LK, O'Hara M. Sildenafil for pediatric orbital lymphangioma. JAMA Ophthalmol. 2013;131:1228–30.
32. Jakobiec FA, Sacks E, Lisman RL, Krebs W. Epibulbar fibroma of the conjunctival substantia propria. Arch Ophthalmol. 1988;106:661–4.
33. Delgado-Partida P, Rodriguez-Trujillo F. Fibrosarcoma (malignant fibroxanthoma) involving conjunctiva and ciliary body. Am J Ophthalmol. 1972;74:479–85.
34. Pe'er J, Maly A, Deckel Y, Frenkel S. Solitary fibrous tumor of the conjunctiva. Arch Ophthalmol. 2007;125:423–6.
35. Kim HJ, Shields CL, Eagle RC Jr, et al. Fibrous histiocytoma of the conjunctiva. Am J Ophthalmol. 2006;142:1036–43.
36. Suimon Y, Kase S, Mitsuhashi T, Ishida S. Undifferntiated pleomorphic sarcoma of the conjunctiva: a case report and review of the literature. Cancer Diagn Progn. 2022;2:232–9.
37. Ali-Ridha A, Brownstein S, O'Connor M, et al. Benign solitary fibrous histiocytoma of xanthomatous subtype of perilimbal conjunctiva and adjacent sclera in a youth. Ocul Oncol Pathol. 2018;6:341–4.
38. Pe'er J, Levinger S, Chirambo M, et al. Malignant fibrous histiocytoma of the skin and the conjunctiva in xeroderma pigmentosum. Arch Pathol Lab Med. 1991;115:910–4.
39. Singh T, Ichhpujani P. Conjunctival and corneal fibrous histiocytoma: brief review. Semin Ophthalmol. 2021;36:569–72.
40. Pe'er J, Levinger S, Ilsar M, Climenhaga H, Okon E. Malignant fibrous histiocytoma of the conjunctiva. Br J Ophthalmol. 1990;74:624–8.
41. McClintic J, Plesec T, Billings S, Singh AD. Nodular fasciitis involving the cornea: a case report and review of the literature. Cornea. 2015;34:1168–9.
42. Ferry AP, Sherman SE. Nodular fasciitis of the conjunctiva apparently originating in the fascia bulbi (Tenon's capsule). Am J Ophthalmol. 1974;78:514–7.
43. Massop DJ, Frederick PA, Li HJ, Lin A. Epibulbar nodular fasciitis. Case Rep Ophthalmol. 2016;7:262–7.
44. Kalina PH, Bartley GB, Campbell RJ, Buettner H. Isolated neurofibromas of the conjunctiva. Am J Ophthalmol. 1991;111:694–8.
45. Tanaka TS, Elner VM, Demirci H. Solitary epibulbar neurofibroma in older adult patients. Cornea. 2015;34:475–8.
46. Charles NC, Fox DM, Avendano JA, Marroquin LS, Appleman W. Conjunctival neurilemoma. Report of 3 cases. Arch Ophthalmol. 1997;115:547–9.
47. Ferry AP. Granular cell tumor (myoblastoma) of the palpebral conjunctiva causing pseudoepitheliomatous hyperplasia of the conjunctival epithelium. Am J Ophthalmol. 1981;91:234–8.
48. Marback EF, Studart E, Fonseca LE, Marback RL. Granular cell tumor located in the bulbar conjunctival space. Ocul Oncol Pathol. 2018;4:90–2.
49. See TRO, Stalhammar G, Grossniklaus H. Neurothekeoma of the eye, conjunctiva, and periorbital adnexa: A report of two cases and brief review. Surv Ophthalmol. 2019;64:852–7.
50. Fernandez NT, Saenz SG, Crespo CV, et al. Cellular neurothekeoma of the bulbar conjunctiva. A case report. Arch Soc Esp Oftalmol. 2000;75:43–6.
51. Kase S, Ishijima K, Ishida S, Rao NA. Merkel cell carcinoma of the conjunctiva. Ophthalmology. 2010;117:637.
52. Tran MN, Ratnayake G, Wong D, McGrath LM. Conjunctival Merkel cell carcinoma: case report and review of the literature. Digit J Ophthalmol. 2022;28:64–8.
53. Amber K, McLeod MP, Nouri K. The Merkel cell polyomavirus and its involvement in Merkel cell carcinoma. Dermatologic Surg. 2013;39:232–8.
54. Giller RH, Folberg R, Keech RV, Piette WW, Sato Y. Xanthoma disseminatum. An unusual histiocytosis syndrome. Am J Pediatr Hematol Oncol. 1988;10:252–7.
55. Shieh C, Daluvoy MB, Ellington KS, Proia AD. Atypical fibroxanthoma of the bulbar conjunctiva. Cornea. 2015;34:1620–2.
56. Chaudhry IA, Al-Jishi Z, Shamsi FA, Riley F. Juvenile xanthogranuloma of the corneoscleral limbus: case report and review of the literature. Surv Ophthalmol. 2004;49:608–14.
57. Kobayashi A, Shirao Y, Takata Y, Wajima R, Nonomura A, Huang AJ. Adult-onset limbal juvenile xanthogranuloma. Arch Ophthalmol. 2002;120:96–7.
58. Lee KM, Wee WR, Lee JH, Kim MK. Juvenile xanthogranuloma presenting as infiltrative conjunctival mass in an adult. Cornea. 2012;31:447–9.

59. Allaire GS, Hidayat AA, Zimmerman LE, Minardi L. Reticulohistiocytoma of the limbus and cornea. A clinicopathologic study of two cases. Ophthalmology. 1990;97:1018–22.
60. Pe'er J, Hidayat AA. Myxomas of the conjunctiva. Am J Ophthalmol. 1986;102:80–6.
61. Ríos Y, Valles-Valles D, Hernández-Ayuso I, Rodríguez-Martínez HA, Medina-Cruz A, Salcedo-Casillas G, Rodríguez-Reyes AA. Primary conjunctival myxoma: case series and review of the literature. Histopathology. 2017;71:635–40.
62. Alvarado-Villacorta R, Torres Zavala NM, Loayza LM, Rodriguez-Reyes AA. Conjunctival myxoma: a systematic review of a rare tumor. Surv Ophthalmol. 2022;67:729–40.
63. Milman T, Salomao DR, Ida CM, et al. Conjunctival myxoid lesions: clinical-pathologic multiparametric analysis, including molecular genetics (an American Ophthalmological Society thesis). Am J Ophthalmol. 2019;205:115–31.
64. Qin XY, Jin ZH, Wang YP, Zhang ZD. Conjunctival myxoid stromal tumour: a distinctive clinicopathological and immunohistochemical study. Br J Ophthalmol. 2019;103:1259–65.
65. Cameron JD, Wick MR. Embryonal rhabdomyosarcoma of the conjunctiva. A clinicopathologic and immunohistochemical study. Arch Ophthalmol. 1986;104:1203–4.
66. Polito E, Pichierri P, Loffredo A, Lasorella G. A case of primary botryoid conjunctival rhabdomyosarcoma. Graefes Arch Clin Exp Ophthalmol. 2006;244:517–9.
67. Gallego S, Zanetti I, Orbach D, et al. Fusion status in patients with lymph node-positive (N1) alveolar rhabdomyosarcoma is a powerful predictor of prognosis: experience of the European Paediatric Soft Tissue Sarcoma Study Group (EpSSG). Cancer. 2018;124:3201–9.
68. Chauhan S, Sen S, Irshad K, Kashyap S, Pushker N, Meel R, Sharma MC. Receptor tyrosine kinase gene expression profiling of orbital rhabdomyosarcoma unveils MET as a potential biomarker and therapeutic target. Hum Cell. 2024;37:297–309.
69. White VA, Damji KF, Richards JS, Rootman J. Leiomyosarcoma of the conjunctiva. Ophthalmology. 1991;98:1560–4.
70. Kenawy N, Coupland SE, Austin M, et al. Conjunctival leiomyosarcoma. Clin Experiment Ophthalmol. 2012;40:328–30.
71. Nair AG, Kaliki S, Kamal S, et al. Conjunctival leiomyosarcoma: a report of two cases. Orbit. 2015;34:274–8.
72. De Groot V, Verhelst E, Hogendoorn PCW, de Keizer RJW. Conjuctival leiomyosracoma, a rare neoplasm always originating at the limbus? Report of a new case and review of 11 published cases. Ocul Oncol Pathol. 2019;5:333–9.
73. Gameiro Filho AS, Pires Castello Branco AM, Oezati Rigueiro M, et al. Conjunctival leiomyosracoma. Am J Ophthalmol Case Rep. 2022;26:101580.
74. Lascaratos G, Gupta M, Bridges L, et al. Myofibroma of the conjunctiva invading the cornea in infancy. J Pediatr Ophthalmol Strabismus. 2010;487:47. Online:e1–3
75. Platt SM, Schoenfield L, Basti S. Recurrent conjunctival myofibrosarcoma managed with triple application of episcleral brachytherapy. Cornea. 2017;36:628–30.
76. Bryant J. Pleomorphic lipoma of the bulbar conjunctiva. Ann Ophthalmol. 1987;19:148–9.
77. Li E, Silbert J, Sinard J. Pleomorphic lipoma of the bulbar conjunctiva. BMJ Case Rep. 2018;11:e226548.
78. Miyashita K, Abe Y, Osamura Y. Case of conjunctival liposarcoma. Jpn J Ophthalmol. 1991;35:207–10.
79. Giuri S, Raica M, Munteanu M. Myxoid/round cell conjunctival liposarcoma. A case report. Romanian J Morphol Embryol. 2013;54:655–8.
80. McGrath LA, Ryan DA, Warrier SK, et al. Conjunctival lymphoma. Eye. 2023;37:837–48.
81. Coupland SE, Krause L, Deleecluse HJ, et al. Lymphoproliferative lesions of the ocular adnexa. Analysis of 112 cases. Ophthalmology. 1998;105:1430–41.
82. Coupland SE, Hellmich M, Auw-Haedrich C, Lee WR, Stein H. Prognostic value of cell-cycle markers in ocular adnexal lymphoma: an assessment of 230 cases. Graefes Arch Clin Exp Ophthalmol. 2004;242:130–45.
83. Shields CL, Shields JA, Carvalho C, Rundle P, Smith AF. Conjunctival lymphoid tumors: clinical analysis of 117 cases and relationship to systemic lymphoma. Ophthalmology. 2001;108:979–84.
84. Kirkegaard MM, Rasmussen PK, Coupland SE, et al. Conjunctival lymphoma—an international multicenter retrospective study. JAMA Ophthalmol. 2016;134:406–14.
85. Beykin G, Pe'er J, Amir G, Frenkel S. Paediatric and adolescent elevated conjunctival lesions in the plical area: lymphoma or reactive lymphoid hyperplasia? Br J Ophthalmol. 2014;98:645–50.
86. Ferreri AJ, Dolcetti R, Dognini GP, et al. Chlamydophila psittaci is viable and infectious in the conjunctiva and peripheral blood of patients with ocular adnexal lymphoma; results of a single-center prospective case–control study. Int J Cancer. 2008;125:1089–93.
87. Lee SB, Yang JW, Kim CS. The association between conjunctival MALT lymphoma and Helicobacter pylori. Br J Ophthalmol. 2008;92:534–6.
88. Carugi A, Onnis A, Antonicelli G, et al. Geographic variation and environmental conditions as cofactors in Chlamydia psittaci association with ocular adnexal lymphomas: a comparison between Italian and African samples. Hematol Oncol. 2010;28:20–6.
89. Kirkegaard MM, Coupland SE, Prause JU, Heegaard S. Malignant lymphoma of the conjunctiva. Surv Ophthalmol. 2015;60:444–58.
90. Masoomian B, Lally SE, Shields JA, Shields CL. Ophthalmic manifestations of Rosai-Dorfman disease in five patients. J Curr Ophthalmol. 2020;32:238–43.
91. Ben Artsi E, Barkley MR, Khong JJ, et al. Multiple myeloma manifesting as an ocular salmon patch—a case report. Orbit. 2020;39:379–82.
92. Ferreri AJ, Govi S, Colucci A, et al. Intralesional rituximab: a new therapeutic approach for patients with conjunctival lymphomas. Ophthalmology. 2011;118:24–8.
93. Ferreri AJM, Sassone M, Miserocchi E, et al. Treatment of MALT lymphoma of the conjunctiva with intralesional rituximab supplemented with autologous serum. Blood Adv. 2020;4:1013–9.
94. Blasi MA, Tiberti AC, Valente P, et al. Intralesional interferon-α for conjunctival mucosa-associated lymphoid tissue lymphoma: long-term results. Ophthalmology. 2012;119:494–500.
95. Platt S, Al Zahrani Y, Singh N, et al. Extranodal marginal zone lymphoma of ocular adnexa: outcomes following radiation therapy. Ocul Oncol Pathol. 2017;3(3):181–7.
96. Regueiro CA, Valcarcel FJ, Romero J, et al. Treatment of conjunctival lymphomas by beta-ray brachytherapy using a strongium-90-yttrium-90 applicator. Clin Oncol (R Coll Radiol). 2002;14:459–63.
97. Sarria GR, Cabrera CM, Sarria GJ, et al. Single-fraction low-energy electronic brachytherapy for conjunctival lymphoma. J Contemp Brachyther. 2020;12:267–72.
98. Kim SE, Yang HJ, Yang SW. Effects of radiation therapy on the Meibomian glands and dry eye in patients with ocular adnexal mucosa-associated lymphoid tissue lymphoma. BMC Ophthalmol. 2020;20:24.
99. Lee MJ, Lee MY, Choe JY, et al. Ultra-low-dose radiation treatment for early stage ocular adnexal MALT lymphoma. Eur J Ophthalmol. 2022;32:3092–6.
100. Nuckel H, Meller D, Steuhl KP, Duhrsen U. Anti-CD20 monoclonal antibody therapy in relapsed MALT lymphoma of the conjunctiva. Eur J Haematol. 2004;73:258–62.

101. Kim SY, Yang SW, Lee WS, et al. Frontline treatment with chemoimmunotherapy for limited-stage ocular adnexal MALT lymphoma with adverse factors: a phase II study. Oncotarget. 2017;8:68583–90.
102. Castillejo Becerra CM, Dalvin LA, Jevremovic D, et al. Clinical characteristics and outcomes of ocular adnexal mantle cell lymphoma. Orbit. 2022;41:97–104.
103. Frenkel S, Gaitonde SS, Azar N, Wood MG, Schmidt ML. Conjunctival marginal zone b-cell lymphoma in a 13-year-old child. J Pediatr Ophthalmol Strabismus. 2011;48 Online:e1–4. Epub 2010 May 21
104. Nam SW, Woo KI, Kim YD. Characteristics of primary extranodal marginal zone B-cell lymphoma in Korea: conjunctiva versus other ocular adnexa. Br J Ophthalmol. 2018;102:502–8.
105. Lee SS, Robinson MR, Morris JC, Mirtsching BC, Shen D, Chan CC. Conjunctival involvement with T-cell polymorphocytic leukemia: report of a case and review of the literature. Surv Ophthalmol. 2004;49:525–36.
106. Mozaheb Z, Khooei A. Bilateral conjunctival infiltration as an extramedullary relapse of AML. Case Rep Hematol. 2018;2018:9590469.
107. Aggarwal E, Mulay K, Honavar SG. Orbital extra-medullary granulocytic sarcoma: clinicopathologic correlation with immunohistochemical features. Surv Ophthalmol. 2014;59:232–5.
108. Mansour AM, Barber JC, Reinecke RD, Wang FM. Ocular choristomas. Surv Ophthalmol. 1989;33:339–58.
109. Huang JJ, Li B, Liang QF, Xu XL, Gao F, Zhang ZB. The clinical and histopathological analysis of 2 053 cases of conjunctival neoplasms. Zhonghua Yan Ke Za Zhi. 2016;52:738–44.
110. Zhong J, Deng Y, Zhang P, et al. New grading system for limbal dermoid: a retrospective analysis of 261 cases over a 10-year period. Cornea. 2018;37:66–71.
111. Kim E, Kim HJ, Kim YD, et al. Subconjunctival fat prolapse and dermolipoma of the orbit: differentiation on CT and MR imaging. AJNR Am J Neuroradiol. 2011;32:465–7.
112. Vahdani K, Rose GE. The presentation and surgical treatment of peribulbar dermolipoma. Ophthalmic Plast Reconstr Surg. 2021;37:226–9.
113. Sa HS, Kim HK, Shin JH, Woo KI, Kim YD. Dermolipoma surgery with rotational conjunctival flaps. Acta Ophthalmol. 2012;90:86–90.
114. Choi YJ, Kim IH, Choi JH, Lee MJ, Kim N, Choung HK, et al. Early results of surgical management of conjunctival dermolipoma: partial excision and free conjunctival autograft. Br J Ophthalmol. 2015;99:1031–6.
115. Gayre GS, Proia AD, Dutton JJ. Epibulbar osseous choristoma: case report and review of the literature. Ophthalmic Surg Lasers. 2002;33:410–5.
116. Vachette M, Moulin A, Zografos L, Schalenbourg A. Epibulbar osseous choristoma: a clinicopathological case series and review of the literature. Klin Monatsbl Augenheilkd. 2012;229:420–3.
117. Herdiana TR, Takahashi Y, Valencia MRP, et al. Epibulbar osseous choristoma within a dermolipoma: case report and literature review. Orbit. 2019;38:407–11.
118. Pfaffenbach DD, Green WR. Ectopic lacrimal gland. Int Ophthalmol Clin. 1971;11:149–59.
119. Tuncer S, Araz B, Peksayar G, Buyukbabani N. Solitary lacrimal gland choristoma of the limbal conjunctiva. Ophthalmic Surg Lasers Imaging. 2010;41 Online:e1–2.
120. Pokorny KS, Hyman BM, Jakobiec FA, Perry HD, Caputo AR, Iwamoto T. Epibulbar choristomas containing lacrimal tissue. Clinical distinction from dermoids and histologic evidence of an origin from the palpebral lobe. Ophthalmology. 1987;94:1249–57.
121. Grob SR, Jakobiec FA, Stagner AM, Colby KA. Diffuse epibulbar complex lacrimal-cartilaginous choristoma: diagnostic clues and management. Cornea. 2015;34:1321–3.
122. Pe'er J, Ilsar M. Epibulbar complex choristoma associated with nevus sebaceous. Arch Ophthalmol. 1995;113:1301–4.
123. Zhang Z, Yang Z, Pan Q, Qin X, Deng Y, Cao Y. Epibulbar complex cartilaginous choristoma: a distinctive clinicopathological case series and literature review. Medicine (Baltimore). 2018;97:e9902.
124. Kiratli H, Shields CL, Shields JA, DePotter P. Metastatic tumours to the conjunctiva: report of 10 cases. Br J Ophthalmol. 1996;80:5–8.
125. Goto H, et al. Diagnostic criteria for IgG4-related ophthalmic disease. Jpn J Ophthalmol. 2015;59(1):1–7.
126. Aziz H, Villa-Forte A, Plesec T, Singh A. Isolated conjunctival inflammation suggestive of IgG4-related disease. Ocul Oncol Pathol. 2015;2:51–3.
127. Li A, Plesec TP, Mileti L, Singh AD. Isolated conjunctival inflammation as manifestation of IgG4 related disease. Cornea. 2018;37:1182.
128. Mora-Horna ER, Rojas-Padilla R, Lopez VG, et al. Ocular adnexal and orbital amyloidosis: a case series and literature review. Int Ophthalmol. 2016;36:281–98.
129. Aryasit O, Preechawai P, Kayasut K. Clinical presentation, treatment, and prognosis of periocular and orbital amyloidosis in a university-based referral center. Clin Ophthalmol. 2013;7:801–5.
130. Demirci H, Shields CL, Eagle RC Jr, Shields JA. Conjunctival amyloidosis: report of six cases and review of the literature. Surv Ophthalmol. 2006;51:419–33.
131. Leibovitch I, Selva D, Goldberg RA, et al. Periocular and orbital amyloidosis: clinical characteristics, management, and outcome. Ophthalmology. 2006;113:1657–64.
132. Suesskind D, Ziemssen F, Rohrbach JM. Conjunctival amyloidosis—clinical and histopathologic features. Graefes Arch Clin Exp Ophthalmol. 2015;253:1377–83.
133. Collins AB, Smith RN, Stone JR. Classification of amyloid deposits in diagnostic cardiac specimens by immunofluorescence. Cardiovasc Pathol. 2009;18:205–16.
134. Vrana JA, Gamez JD, Madden BJ, et al. Classification of amyloidosis by laser microdissection and mass spectrometry-based proteomic analysis in clinical biopsy specimens. Blood. 2009;114:4957–9.
135. Gilbertson JA, Theis JD, Vrana JA, et al. A comparison of immunohistochemistry and mass spectrometry for determining the amyloid fibril protein from formalin-fixed biopsy tissue. J Clin Pathol. 2015;68:314–7.
136. Blandford AD, Yordi S, Kapoor S, et al. Ocular adnexal amyloidosis: a mass spectrometric analysis. Am J Ophthalmol. 2018;193:28–32.

9 Conjunctival and Adnexal Lymphoma

Mary E. Aronow, Brian T. Hill, and Arun D. Singh

9.1 Introduction

Conjunctival and adnexal lymphoma encompasses a complex group of lymphoproliferative neoplasms that involve the eyelid, conjunctiva, lacrimal apparatus, extraocular muscles, and orbit. Involvement can be unilateral or bilateral, limited to a single site, multifocal, or overlapping multiple adnexal structures. Furthermore, disease can be localized to the ocular adnexal region, or it can affect regional, central, and peripheral lymph nodes, as well as distant, extranodal sites. The spectrum of lymphoma subtypes that comprise conjunctival and adnexal lymphoma is heterogeneous and ranges from low-grade extramarginal zone lymphoma (EMZL) to high-grade diffuse large B-cell lymphoma (DLBCL). Treatment selection and overall survival are dependent upon the lymphoma subtype. While aggressive forms exist, the majority of conjunctival and adnexal lymphoma are low-grade and generally follow an indolent clinical course. While disease-related morbidity is relatively common, the overall 10-year disease-specific mortality rate is estimated to be as low as 5–10%. This chapter covers historical aspects of conjunctival and adnexal lymphoma as well as recent advances that have yielded improvement in the diagnosis, staging, and treatment of this complex disease.

M. E. Aronow
Early Clinical Development-Ophthalmology, Genentech, a Member of the Roche Group, South San Francisco, CA, USA

B. T. Hill
Hematology and Medical Oncology, Taussig Cancer Center, Cleveland Clinic, Cleveland, OH, USA

A. D. Singh (✉)
Department of Ophthalmic Oncology, Cole Eye Institute, Cleveland Clinic, Cleveland, OH, USA
e-mail: SINGHA@ccf.org

9.2 Epidemiological Aspects

Conjunctival and adnexal lymphoma accounts for approximately 8% of all cases of extranodal non-Hodgkin's lymphoma (NHL). Conjunctival and adnexal lymphoma is rare, with an estimated incidence of 0.2 per 100,000 persons [1]. Most clinical series have demonstrated a slight female predominance (60% of cases) [2, 3]. Using database from the North American Association of Central Cancer Registries for ocular and orbital lymphomas between 1995 and 2018, standardized incidence rate (ASIR) of 2.6 persons per million was reported with the highest incidence among Asia-Pacific Islanders. The incidence has increased significantly from 1995 to 2003 (average percent change, APC = 2.1%) but has declined thereafter until 2018 (APC = −0.7%) [4]. However, incidence is increasing in the Danish population for unknown reasons [5] Overall, there is a higher prevalence of OAL in Asia than in Western countries [6]. OAL is uncommon in children [6, 7].

Of all ophthalmic neoplasms, conjunctival and adnexal lymphoma accounts for 6–8% of orbital and 10–15% of adnexal tumors [8, 9]. Localized, ocular-only disease is present at diagnosis in 60–80% of individuals, while the remainder have evidence of systemic involvement at the time of ophthalmic presentation. Bilateral involvement is observed in 10–15% of cases of ocular-only lymphoma, and is frequently asymmetric [10]. Among affected adnexal sites, the frequency of involvement is as follows: orbit/lacrimal gland 46–74%, conjunctiva 20–33%, and eyelid 5–20% [11]. In some cases, the distinction of involvement between sites is difficult to determine; therefore, the reported frequency of overlapping sites may be underreported.

9.3 Etiology and Pathogenesis: B-Cell Biology and Lymphomagenesis

Lymphoma is a malignant lymphoid tumor arising as clonal proliferation of either B-lymphocytes or T-lymphocytes, or less commonly natural killer (NK) cells [12]. Lymphoma

© The Author(s), under exclusive license to Springer Nature Switzerland AG 2024
J. Pe'er et al. (eds.), *Clinical Ophthalmic Oncology*, https://doi.org/10.1007/978-3-031-72443-5_9

Table 9.1 Immunophenotypic expression of OAL

Type	Precursor cell	CD3	CD5	CD10	CD20	CD23	CD43	CD79a	Bcl-2	Bcl-6	Cyclin D1	MUM1
EMZL	Memory B cell	–	–	–	+	–	+	+	+	–	–	–
FL	Centrocyte	–	–	+	+	±	–	+	+	+	–	–
MCL	Mantle cell	–	+	–	+	–		+	+	–	+	–
LPL	Memory B cell	–	–	–	+	–		+	+	–	–	+/–
DLBCL	Centroblast	–	–	+/–	+	+/–		+	+/–	+/–	–	+/–

EMZL extranodal marginal zone lymphoma, *FL* follicular lymphoma, *MCL* mantle cell lymphoma, *LPL* lymphoplasmacytic lymphoma, *DLBCL* diffuse large B-cell lymphoma

arises from germinal centers (follicular lymphoma), the mantle zone (mantle cell lymphoma), or memory B-cells (EMZL). Each lymphoma subtype demonstrates a unique immunophenotypic expression profile (Table 9.1). During normal lymphocyte maturation, errors may occur in which an antigen–receptor–gene region is juxtaposed to an oncogene region, resulting in dysregulation of the oncogenic region. Less often, a novel oncogenic protein is formed by fusion of two other genes. Chromosomal translocations underlying these alterations are well described in as many as 90% of systemic lymphoma [13]. Limited data suggests that such translocations are less common in OAL [14, 15].

The infection/inflammation/mutation (IMM) model of lymphomagenesis refers to the theory that lymphoma develops because of errors in the normal lymphocyte response to infection and/or inflammation. The evidence basis for this includes known associations between lymphoma and specific infections and autoimmune disorders. A classic example is the relationship between gastric (EMZL) of mucosal-associated lymphoid tissue (MALT) and chronic *H. pylori* infection. Conjunctival and adnexal lymphoma surgical biopsy specimens have demonstrated the presence of DNA from both *C. psittaci* and *H. pylori* [16, 17]. While infectious agents have been implicated in lymphoma etiology, this association varies widely depending upon geographical regions worldwide as well as by subpopulations within specific geographical areas [16]. These observations have important implications related to therapy selection. In some regions, antibiotics have been shown to be efficacious for conjunctival and adnexal lymphoma, while in other parts of the world antimicrobials have been minimally effective in the treatment of this disease [18].

9.4 Classification

Conjunctival and adnexal lymphoma encompasses the malignant end of the spectrum of ocular adnexal lymphoproliferative disorders. Reactive lymphoid hyperplasia (RLH), in contrast, represents the benign end of the spectrum of lymphoproliferative disorders. With advances in molecular diagnosis, the vast majority of RLH have more recently been reclassified as low-grade malignant lymphoma. OAL is a localized form of lymphoma that has been integrated into the schema of lymphoproliferative diseases described in two major classification systems: the Revised European American Lymphoma classification [18] and more recently the 2016 edition of the World Health Organization (WHO) Classification of Tumors of Hematopoietic and Lymphoid Tissue [19].

Conjunctival and adnexal lymphoma can be divided by the type and site(s) of tissue involvement. The vast majority of conjunctival and adnexal lymphoma are of the non-Hodgkin's B-cell type. Despite the multitude of systemic lymphoma subtypes, most conjunctival and adnexal lymphoma belong to one of five subtypes: EMZL (or MALT lymphoma), follicular lymphoma (FL), DLBCL, mantle cell lymphoma (MCL), and lymphoplasmacytic lymphoma (LPL) (Table 9.2) [20]. Most conjunctival and adnexal lymphoma, approximately 75%, are of the EMZL/MALT subtype [21]. Conjunctival and adnexal lymphoma is termed solitary if limited to the ocular adnexa, secondary when contiguous sites are involved, and systemic if remote involvement is present. Conjunctival and adnexal lymphoma is solitary in 60–80% of cases at presentation [22, 23].

Table 9.2 Distribution of various types of OAL

Author	Year	Patients	EMZL (%)	FL (%)	MCL (%)	LPL (%)	DLBC (%)	Plasmacytoma (%)	T cell (%)
Nakata	1999	44	77	–	4	2	14	–	–
Jenkins	2000	192	54	11	2	24	8	–	<1
Stafford	2001	48	60	–	–	–	4	–	–
MtKelvie	2001	70	63	17	3	–	11	–	1
Mannami	2001	43	86	–	2	–	12	–	–
Bhatia	2001	47	17	53	–	–	26	–	–
Coupland	2003	230	59	12	3	4	13	4	3
Fung	2003	98	57	18	4		7	–	–
Sharara	2003	17	47	12	18	6	18	–	–
Cho	2003	57	98	–	2	–	–	–	–
Sullivan	2005	69	35	22	1	4	7	3	6
Rosado	2006	62	89	–	–	–	<1	–	–
Ferry	2007	353	52	23	5	1	8	–	<1
Oh	2007	128	75	–	3	1	5	1	4
Yun	2007	69	87	–	–	–	–	3	–
Hatef	2007	43	44	21	1	–	21	–	<1
Rootman	2011	122	60	12	1	4	4	–	–
Watkins	2011	57	28	2	5	–	4	4	5
Zanni	2012	41	63	10	5	5	17	–	–
Parikh	2015	79	75	25	–	–	–	–	
Woolf	2015	81	88	6	–	–	–	–	1
Konig	2016	52	52	14	–	–	–	–	–
Olsen	2018	797	57	11	8	–	15	–	–
Hsu	2021	112	68	8	–	–	10	–	–
Kirkegaard	2022	263	68	16	7	2	5	2	–
Fernandez	2022	133	70	16	4	–	4	–	–
Total		3307	17–98	2–53	1–18	1–24	1–26	1–4	1–6

EMZL extranodal marginal zone lymphoma, *FL* follicular lymphoma, *MCL* mantle cell lymphoma, *LPL* lymphoplasmacytic lymphoma, *DLBCL* diffuse large B-cell lymphoma

9.5 Clinical Features

9.5.1 Symptoms

Subjective complaints in conjunctival and adnexal lymphoma are broad and may include a visible mass, exophthalmos, pain, pressure, tearing, or diplopia. If the lacrimal gland is involved, dry eye symptoms can occur. Many patients are asymptomatic at the time of diagnosis.

9.5.2 Signs

Conjunctival and adnexal lymphoma have site-specific presentations that affect diagnosis (Fig. 9.1). In the conjunctiva, lesions are characteristically a salmon-pink color (73%) followed by a follicular appearance (15%) and a nodular or subconjunctival mass (7%) [24].

Clinical appearance does not allow for the distinction of benign from malignant lymphoproliferative disease.

In the orbit, lacrimal gland, and eyelid, conjunctival and adnexal lymphoma often present as a mass. If palpable, these masses are typically firm. Mobility is variable depending upon attachment to other structures. Diplopia may occur depending upon the size and timeframe over which the mass develops. Exophthalmos and decreased retropulsion of the globe may be the only clinical signs. Secondary ptosis can also occur. Rare manifestations include isolated lateral rectus muscle infiltration [25].

Orbital lymphoma when visualized at the time of biopsy appears as a whitish pink mass reflecting its leukocytic and vascular characteristics. Involvement of the nasolacrimal drainage system can result in epiphora. Compression or invasion of the optic nerve can lead to neuropathy and vision loss.

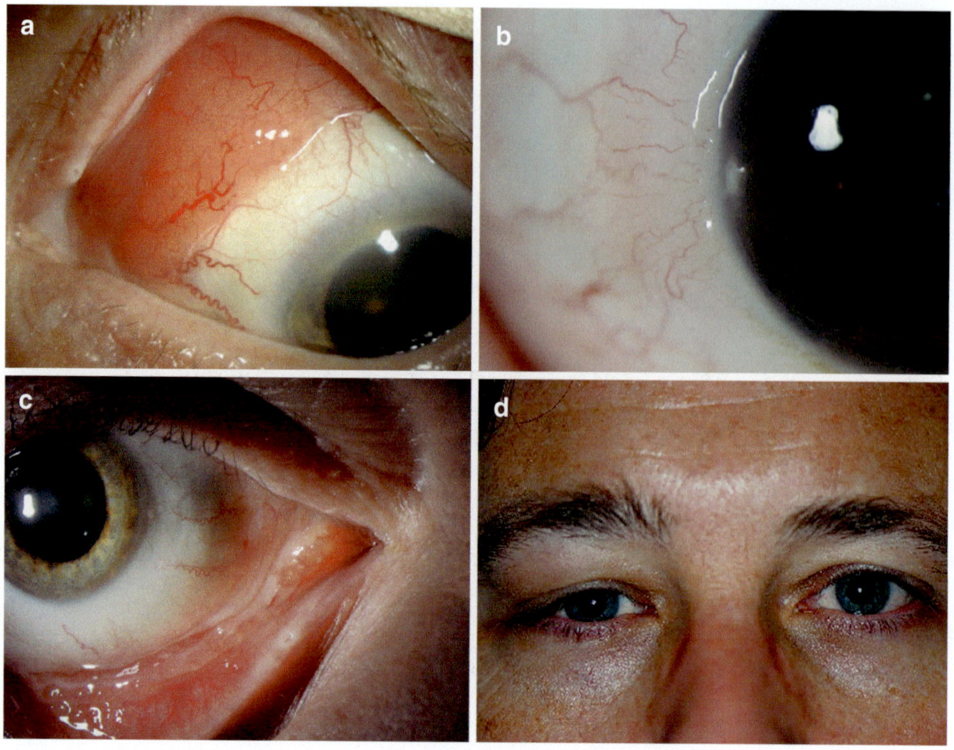

Fig. 9.1 Conjunctival adnexal lymphoma. Spectrum of clinical features. Typical salmon patch appearance (**a**), subtle bulbar conjunctival infiltration with small cell lymphoma (**b**), inferior forniceal infiltration with mantle cell lymphoma (**c**), and orbital fulness due to follicular lymphoma of the lacrimal gland (**d**)

9.6 Diagnostic Evaluation

Evaluation of conjunctival and adnexal lymphoma involves characterization of the lesion and staging. Biopsy should ideally be obtained by open methods (incisional or excisional biopsy, rather than fine-needle aspiration biopsy) to allow for sufficient tissue for multiple special studies: histopathology, lymphocyte immunophenotypical analysis, and molecular genetics studies to identify gene rearrangements indicative of clonality and/or translocations.

While there is variability in biopsy technique, several general principles apply. If lymphoma is suspected, specimens should be sent fresh and kept moist. Wrapping tissue in gauze soaked in saline is preferable to immersing samples in saline (tissue should not be left to dry or immersed in a fixative). When sending fresh samples, it is advisable to communicate with the pathology team ahead of time and deliver samples from the operating room within 60 min of collection. Samples should be obtained with as minimal trauma as possible, being careful not to induce crush artifact. Cautery should be used sparingly and preferably after an adequately sized biopsy has been obtained. Specimens should be oriented and labeled with the site and exact location in order to facilitate the pathologist in their analysis. It is also helpful to provide the pathologist with a brief patient history as well as any relevant prior biopsy reports.

9.7 Local Imaging Studies

Imaging studies play an important role in conjunctival and adnexal lymphoma but are performed at different times depending upon presentation.

High-resolution anterior segment optical coherence tomography (HR-OCT) appears promising in differentiating from closely simulating entities such as conjunctival amyloidosis. In lymphoma, HR-OCT images typically show homogenous, dark subepithelial lesions with smooth borders, containing monomorphic dot-like infiltrates amyloidosis appears as heterogeneous, dark lesions with irregular borders, often containing hyperreflective linear infiltrates (Fig. 9.2) [26].

With conjunctival disease, the lesion is frequently biopsied first, and imaging of the orbit follows to assess for the possibility of occult ipsilateral or contralateral orbital involvement. For orbital and eyelid disease, the orbit is usually imaged up front to optimize the biopsy approach. Contrast-enhanced CT and MRI of the orbits will show enhancing lesions that can be discrete or diffuse (Fig. 9.3). Lymphoid lesions typically mold to structures such as the globe or bony orbit. Larger lesions are FDG avid on PET scan. Neuroimaging will reveal occult orbital involvement in up to 50% of clinically unsuspected cases [27]. Paranasal sinus involvement is not uncommon.

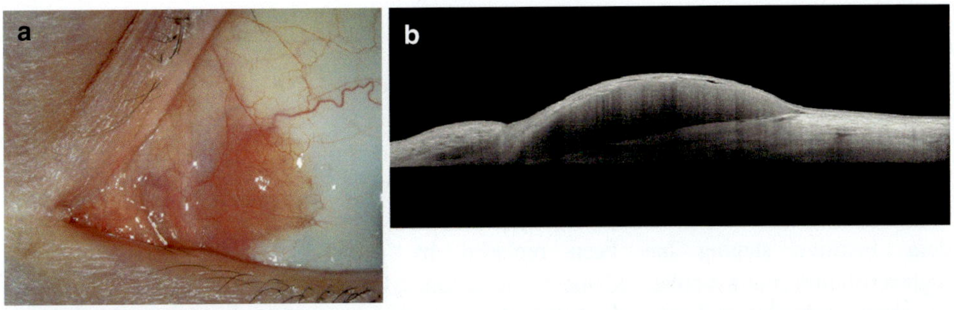

Fig. 9.2 Conjunctival adnexal lymphoma. Clinical appearance (**a**). Anterior segment optical coherence tomography showing homogeneous, dark subepithelial lesions with smooth borders, containing monomorphic dot-like infiltrates

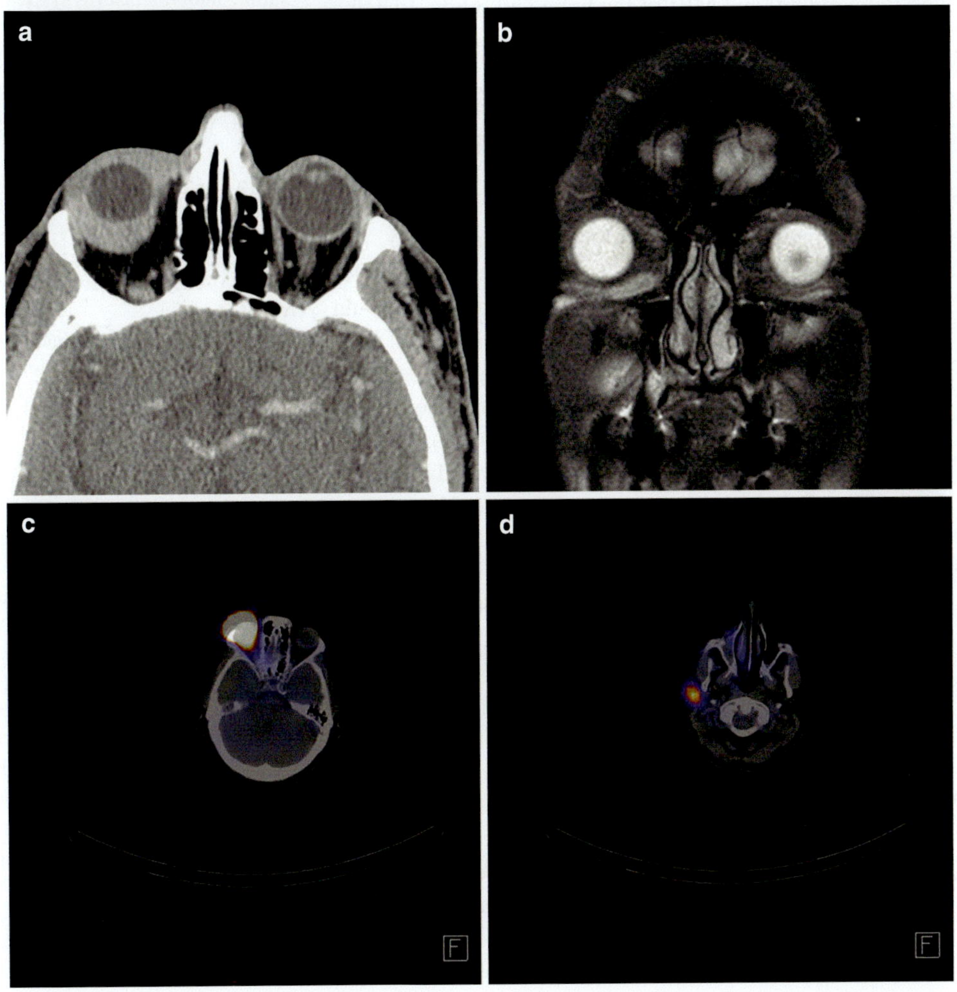

Fig. 9.3 Conjunctival adnexal lymphoma. Imaging studies. Axial CT, showing superior orbital mass molding to the orbital wall (**a**). Coronal MRI scan (T2-weighted image) demonstrating inferior orbital involvement (**b**). PET positivity of the orbital lymphoma (**c**). Also note uptake in the cervical lymph node (**d**)

It is important to emphasize the relatively high rate of overlap that occurs between conjunctival and adnexal lymphoma and uveal lymphoma [28, 29]. Dilated fundus examination and ancillary imaging studies such as B-scan ultrasonography and angiography are useful for characterizing disease extent and laterality. This is particularly important in cases with subtle extra-scleral extension (ESE) or occult involvement of the fellow eye. B-scan ultrasonography is a sensitive modality for detecting ESE. The pattern of ESE may be crescentic thickening, a discrete mass (often adjacent to the optic nerve), or diffuse choroidal thickening. Fluorescein (FA) and indocyanine green angiography (ICG) are useful in suspected cases of uveal involvement. ICG demonstrates a characteristic pattern of focal hypo-filling corresponding to clinically observed choroidal infiltrates. These foci may represent regions of choroidal non-perfusion secondary to space-occupying choroidal infiltration by lymphoma cells. ICG is superior to FA in visualizing the choroidal circulation and is therefore preferred for confirming the diagnosis and extent of disease burden [30]. When performed, FA may show early hyperfluorescence, hypofluorescent spots corresponding clinically observed choroidal infiltrates, choroidal folds, or a normal angiogram.

9.8 Staging Procedures

Conjunctival and adnexal lymphoma can occur in the setting of systemic lymphoma; therefore, when the disease presents at an ocular site, initial staging is performed. This includes a thorough physical examination, ideally performed by a medical oncologist with expertise in lymphoproliferative disorders. Invasive staging has been replaced by using high-resolution contrast-enhanced imaging techniques: CT of the chest, abdomen, and pelvis (or full-body positron emission tomography) and MRI of the brain and orbits. Imaging of the neck is performed if cervical nodes are palpated or suspected to be enlarged. Laboratory evaluation includes complete blood count (CBC), hepatic enzymes, and serum lactate dehydrogenase (LDH). Although part of the formal staging process for systemic lymphoma, bone marrow aspiration and biopsy may have low yield in OAL in the absence of cytopenia or radiographic evidence of systemic disease.

An understanding of the staging process is important for multidisciplinary management of OAL. Historically, the Ann Arbor system was used in most centers. In this system, lymphoma types were divided into low-grade or high-grade based on their expected clinical behavior. Low-grade (indolent) lymphoma (EMZL, FL, LPL) was divided into two stages, while high-grade lymphoma (DLBCL, MZL) was divided into three stages (Table 9.3). The Ann Arbor staging system has several deficiencies for characterizing conjunctival and adnexal lymphoma, particularly as it results in a disproportionate staging distribution. Two-thirds of primary OAL present as a localized mass, which are classified as stage IE [2, 10, 23, 31]. Overall rates for initial staging are 60–80% for IE, 4–25% for IIE, and 16–18% for stages III and IV combined [32, 33]. Studies using criteria of extra-orbital disease showed stages III and IV rates of 22–36% at diagnosis [22, 23]. The disproportionate number of cases staged as IE precludes the ability to differentiate the majority of conjunctival and adnexal lymphoma from one another in terms of disease extent within the ocular adnexal structures. This in turn can have important prognostic implications.

In recent years, the tumor–node–metastasis (TNM) -based staging system for primary conjunctival and adnexal lymphoma has been developed under the guidance of the American Joint Committee on Cancer (AJCC) [34] and has now been adopted by most centers. This system addresses many of the deficiencies of the Ann Arbor system and more precisely defines disease extent. The T-staging describes the extent of disease within the ocular adnexal region. Specifically, T1, T2, and T3 correspond to the involvement of the conjunctiva, orbit, and eyelids, respectively. T4 designation indicates the OAL involvement of structures adjacent to the ocular adnexal region, including bone and brain. Currently in its eighth edition, the TNM-based staging system continued to be refined with each successive edition. Ultimately the goal is to facilitate future studies aimed at identifying clinical and histopathological features of OAL of prognostic significance and to assess treatment outcomes. TNM staging continues to evolve and to be evaluated with regard to its prognostic significance for OAL [35].

Table 9.3 Staging of OAL by Ann Arbor and tumor-node-metastasis systems

Ann Arbor system	
Indolent lymphomas: EMZL, FL, LPL	
Stage I	Localized disease (Ann Arbor [AA] I, IE and II, IIE)
Stage II	Disseminated disease (Ann Arbor [AA] III and IV)
Aggressive lymphomas: DLBCL, MCL	
Stage I	Localized or extranodal disease (Ann Arbor [AA] I or IE)
Stage II	Two or more nodal sites; three or more extranodal sites
Stage III	Stage II with additional poor prognostic features
Tumor-node-metastasis system[a]	
T classification	
TX	Lymphoma extent not specified
T0	No evidence of lymphoma
T1	Conjunctival lymphoma alone
T2	Orbital lymphoma with or without conjunctival involvement
T3	Preseptal eyelid lymphoma with or without conjunctival/orbital disease
T4	Orbital and extra-orbital lymphoma with invasion of adjacent structures (bone, sinus, brain)
N classification	
NX	Lymph node involvement not assessed
N0	No evidence of lymph node involvement
N1	Involvement of lymph node regions superior to the mediastinum
N1a	Involvement of a single lymph node region superior to the mediastinum
N1b	Involvement of two or more lymph node regions superior to the mediastinum
N2	Involvement of lymph node regions of the mediastinum
N3	Diffuse or disseminated involvement of peripheral and central lymph node regions
M classification	
M0	No evidence of involvement of other extra nodal sites
M1a	Noncontiguous involvement of tissue or organs (parotids, liver, spleen, kidney, breast)
M1b	Lymphomatous involvement of the bone marrow
M1c	Both M1a and M1b involvement

EMZL extranodal marginal zone lymphoma, *FL* follicular lymphoma, *MCL* mantle cell lymphoma, *LPL* lymphoplasmacytic lymphoma, *DLBCL*, diffuse large B-cell lymphoma, *E* extranodal disease

[a]Modified from the American Joint Committee on Cancer (AJCC) eighth edition TNM-based staging manual for OAL

9.9 Differential Diagnosis

The differential diagnosis for conjunctival and adnexal lymphoma is extensive. It includes inflammatory lesions (Fig. 9.4), reactive lymphoid hyperplasia lesions (Fig. 9.5), epithelial tumors, lightly melanocytic tumors, and infectious lesions.

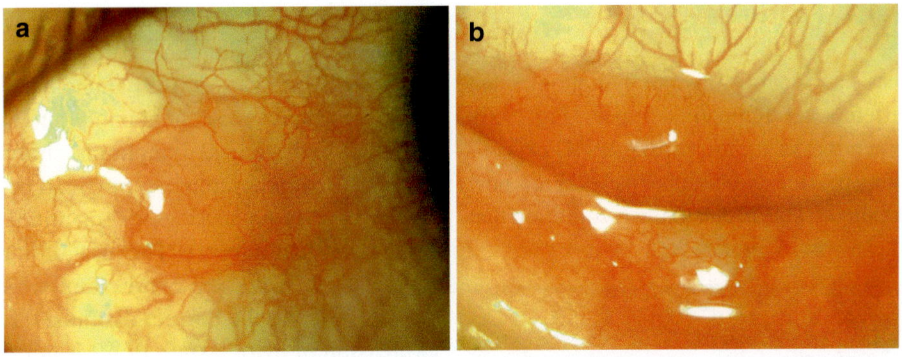

Fig. 9.4 Conjunctival adnexal lymphoma. Simulating condition. Bulbar (**a**) and forniceal (**b**) idiopathic inflammatory conjunctival granuloma

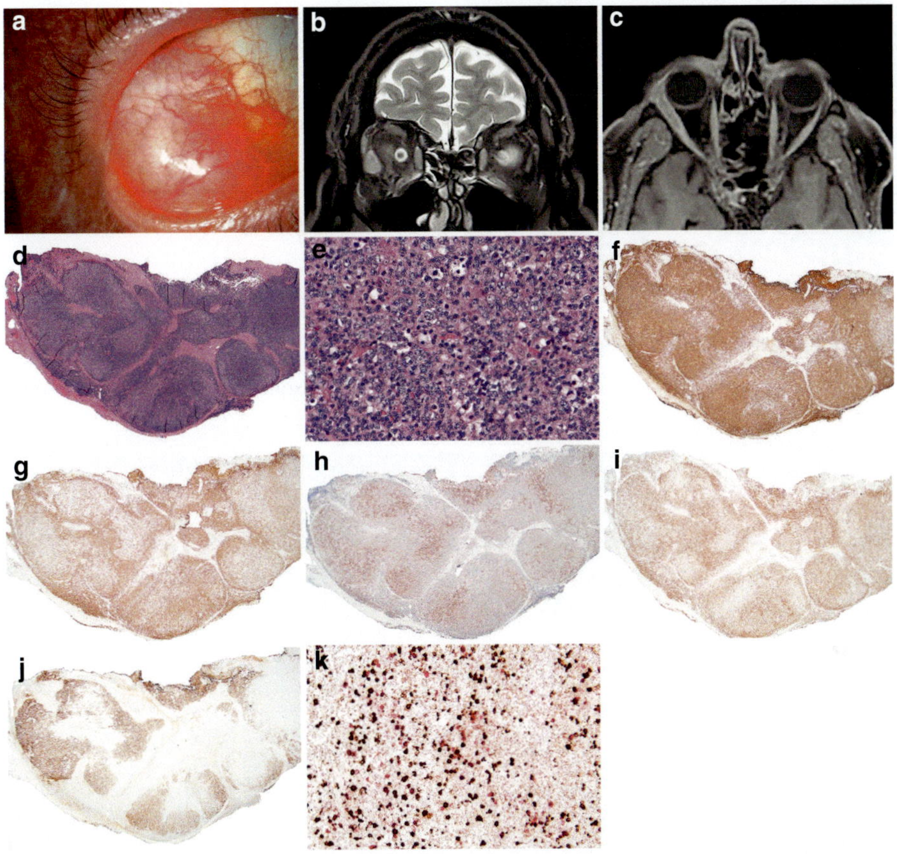

Fig. 9.5 Clinical presentation and histopathological features of reactive lymphoid hyperplasia. A 63-year-old man presented for evaluation of a conjunctival lesion of the right eye that was noticed a month ago. A firm, nodular, nonmobile lesion attached to sclera at temporal and inferotemporal quadrant was noted with engorged feeder vessels. (**a**) 0.4 mm of proptosis was measured without limitation of ocular motility. Orbital MRI revealed a homogeneously enhancing expansile lesion of the anterior right lateral rectus muscle (**b**) involving the tendinous insertion. Excisional biopsy not achievable due to posterior extension into the lateral rectus muscle (C0); therefore, subtotal excision was performed using lid swing technique. Representative H&E section demonstrates several variably sized and shaped secondary follicles (**a**, 2× magnification). Close-up of a germinal center composed of a mixture of centroblasts, centrocytes, tingible-body macrophages, and scattered histiocytes and follicular dendritic cells (**b**, 40×). CD20 marks B-cells (**c**) while CD3 (**d**) marks interfollicular T-cells (2×). BCL6 (**e**, 2×) highlights the germinal center B-cells, while BCL2 (**f**, 2×) highlights background T-cells and non-germinal center B-cells. CD21 shows intact follicular dendritic cell meshworks associated with the follicles (**g**, 2×). Dual ultrasensitive chromogenic in situ hybridization (CISH) for kappa and lambda light chain-encoding mRNA demonstrates polytypic B-cells and polytypic plasma cells within a representative germinal center (**h**, 20×). Additionally, concurrent flow cytometric analysis performed on this conjunctival lesion revealed no monoclonal B-cells or aberrant T-cells, and PCR studies for B-cell clonality (BIOMED 2) detected no clonal rearrangements in the immunoglobulin heavy chain or kappa light chain gene loci. (Courtesy of Anna Beata Owczarczyk, MD, PhD. Hematopathologist, Robert J. Tomsich Pathology and Laboratory Medicine, Cleveland Clinic, Cleveland, OH, USA)

9.10 Pathological Features

Pathological analysis can identify obvious lymphomas but cannot reliably differentiate lymphoma types (Fig. 9.6). Recent data has shown that using the current WHO classification, 76% of lesions previously classified as RLH are now reclassified as lymphomas. This is due to the recognition that a small number of malignant lymphocytes, whose presence is indicative of lymphoma, can be overshadowed by surrounding normal or reactive lymphoid cells.

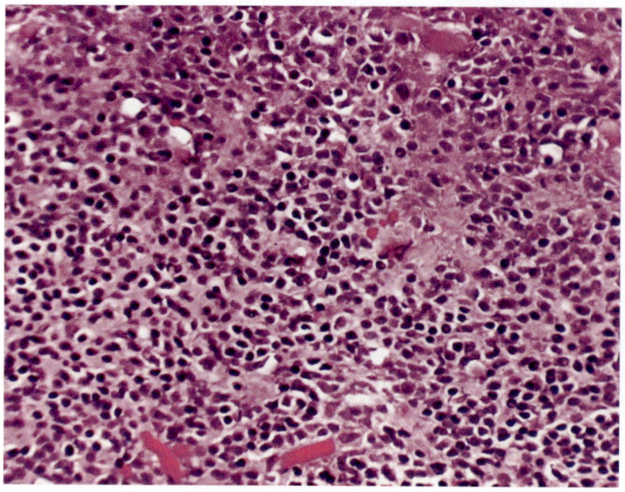

Fig. 9.6 Conjunctival adnexal lymphoma. Photomicrograph of monomorphic lymphocytes typical of EMZL (H&E, original magnification ×100)

The common immunophenotypic expressions of conjunctival and adnexal lymphoma subtypes are shown in Table 19.1. Immunophenotyping can be carried out qualitatively on tissue sections or quantitatively on dispersed cells (flow cytometry). The use of intact tissue allows localization of marker expression, which can be critical for establishing the correct diagnosis. For example, overexpression of cytoplasmic Bcl-2 is not seen in normal follicular structures and is consistent with follicular lymphoma (Fig. 9.7) [36]. Immunohistochemistry may not detect critically important cells when the sampling effect limits their presence. Flow cytometry, in contrast, does not give anatomic information but can accurately assign the immunophenotype of involved cells in very small samples.

9.11 T-Cell Lymphoma

In rare cases, conjunctival and adnexal lymphoma can be of T-cell origin. In a review of 353 individuals with OAL, only a single case (0.3%) was of T-cell lineage [10]. The most common presenting symptoms of T-cell lymphoma of the

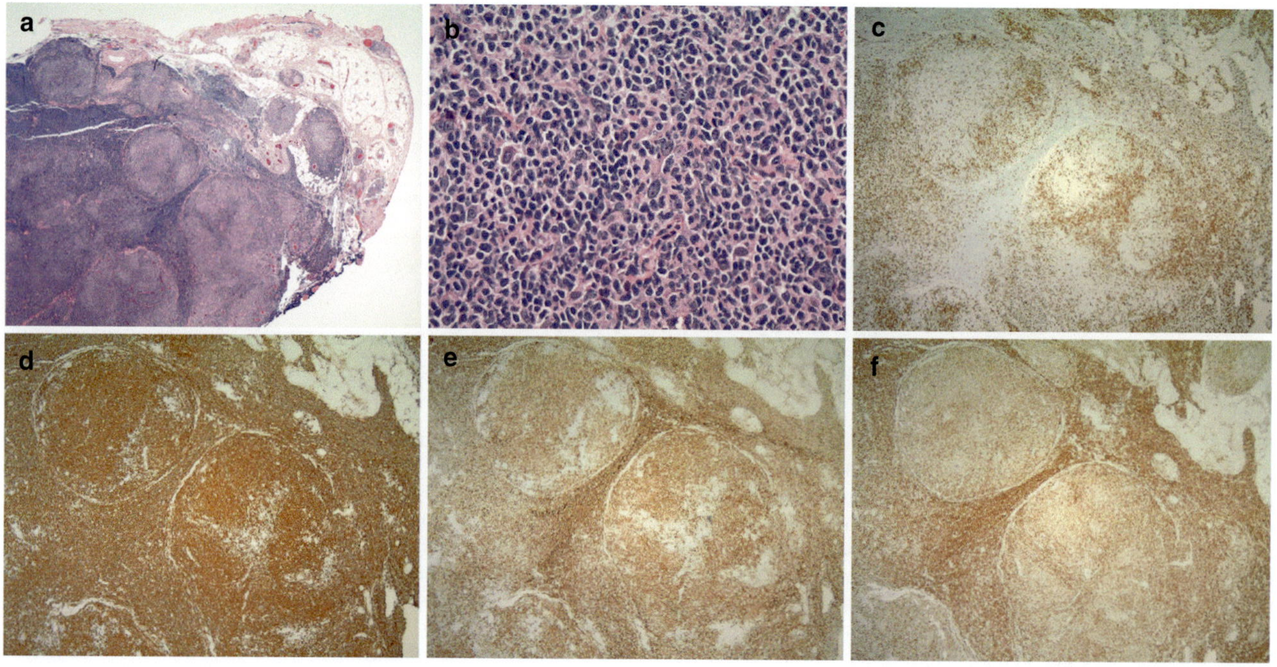

Fig. 9.7 Conjunctival adnexal lymphoma. Immunohistochemical characterization of follicular lymphoma (WHO 4th revised edition/ICC grade 1–2, low grade). Histological sections demonstrate fragments of soft tissue with an atypical nodular lymphoid infiltrate largely effacing the underlying tissue architecture (**a**). The lymphoid cells are predominantly small to medium in size with angulated nuclei (**b**). Immunohistochemical stains were performed to clarify the morphologic findings. CD3 and CD5 highlight interspersed T-cells (**c**). CD20 and PAX5 highlight most cells in the atypical lymphoid infiltrate with a predominantly nodular pattern (**d**). They show extensive coexpression of CD10 (**e**) and are positive for dim Bcl-2 (**f**) and BCL6. CD21 shows expanded interspersed dendritic meshworks. Cyclin D1 was negative in the lymphoid cells

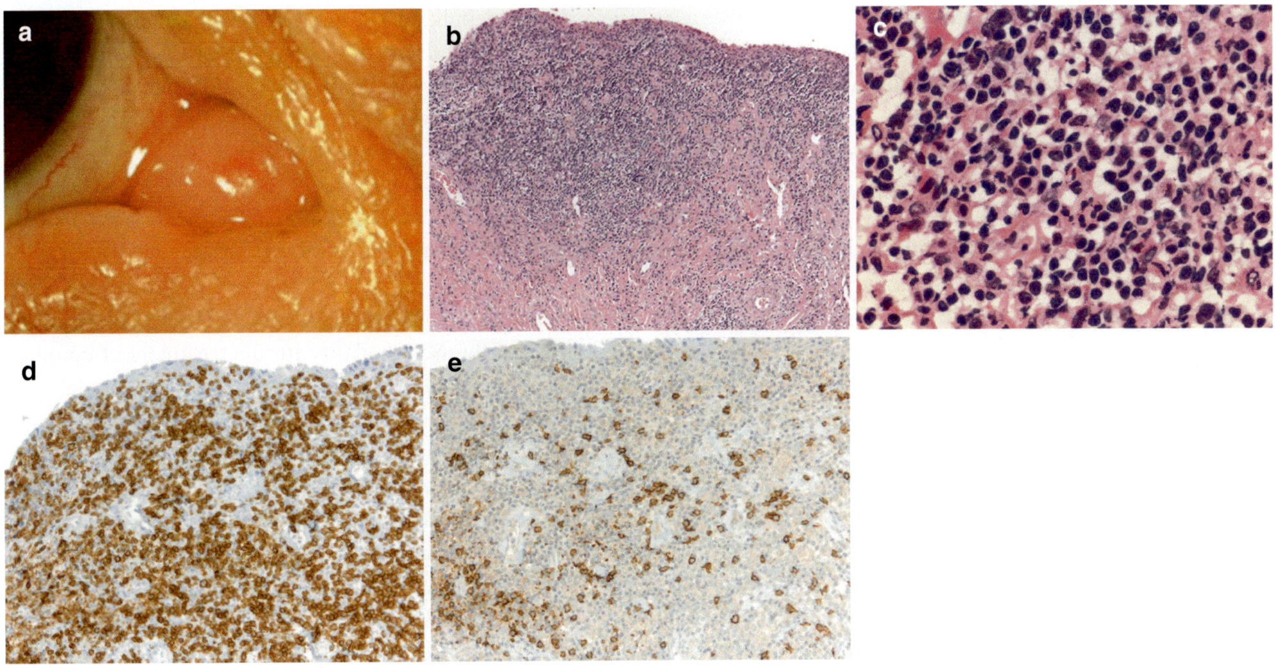

Fig. 9.8 Ocular adnexal lymphoma. T-cell lymphoma of the caruncle in a patient with slowly progressive mycosis fungoides (**a**). Histology shows conjunctival mucosa with a diffuse population of small mononuclear cells (**b**, H&E 100×). High power shows atypical cells with scant cytoplasm, irregular clefted nuclei, and prominent nucleoli (**c**; H&E 600×). Immunohistochemistry shows that most of the cells are CD3-positive T lymphocytes (**d**, CD3 IHC 200×) with only a few B-cells (**e**; CD20 IHC 200×). The T-cells also expressed CD4, CD5, partial CD2, and had loss of CD7 (not shown). T-cell receptor gene rearrangement studies confirmed the presence of a monoclonal T-cell population. (Courtesy Gabrielle A. Yeaney, MD, Division of Ocular Pathology, Diagnostics Institute, Cleveland Clinic, Cleveland, OH, USA)

ocular adnexa were ulcerated eyelid skin lesions (40%) followed by eyelid swelling (13.3%) and lacrimal passageways obstruction (13%) [37].

As with B-cell neoplasms, a heterogeneous group of T-cell lymphomas can involve the ocular adnexal structures (Fig. 9.8). Most T-cell lymphomas affecting the ocular adnexal structures are aggressive and carry a poor prognosis. Advanced stage at diagnosis leads to almost certain death from the disease despite aggressive local and systemic treatment [37].

Most non-B-cell lymphomas are an extension of the malignant stage of mycosis fungoides or a secondary manifestation of systemic T-cell lymphoma. In a series of seven individuals with OAL of T-cell origin, three cases were peripheral T-cell lymphomas (PTCL) demonstrating positivity for CD3, CD8, and βF1 and negativity for CD56. Two cases were positive for CD3 and CD30 while negative for CD56 and were classified as anaplastic large-cell lymphomas of T-cell type (T-ALCL) [38]. The remaining two cases were positive for CD3 and CD56 and negative for βF1. These two cases were positive for Epstein–Barr virus (EBV) by in situ hybridization, consistent with T-cell/natural killer (NK)-cell lymphoma of nasal type (also referred to as lethal midline granuloma) [38].

9.12 Treatment

There is no current consensus regarding optimal treatment algorithms for conjunctival and adnexal lymphoma. Treatment remains an area of controversy, progress, and change. Currently, conjunctival and adnexal lymphoma treatment choice depends on whether the disease is localized or systemic. Local disease can be effectively managed with radiotherapy alone. Systemic disease is frequently treated in a manner like other indolent lymphomas, typically using rituximab or other immunotherapies alone, or in combination with cytotoxic chemotherapy. With the recognition that the vast majority of conjunctival and adnexal lymphoma are of the low-grade EMZL/MALT type and that there may be an infectious basis for this subgroup of conjunctival and adnexal lymphoma, there is a possibility of deferring cytotoxic modalities. A second controversy is whether to treat BRL and indolent conjunctival and adnexal lymphoma. In recent years, there has been a paradigm shift in the management of indolent systemic lymphoma. Rather than upfront treatment and systemic imaging surveillance repeated at regular intervals, many patients are now being monitored with a "watch and wait" approach. In the absence of symptoms, treatment for indolent systemic lymphoma can in many cases be deferred. It may be reasonable then to apply this strategy to asymptomatic cases of RLH and low-grade conjunctival and adnexal lymphoma. A survey of treatment modalities follows.

9.13 Observation

Watchful waiting (WW) in asymptomatic patients may be considered in exceptional cases (elderly, monocular comorbidities, patient preference) [39].

9.14 Antimicrobial Treatment

A recent development in conjunctival and adnexal lymphoma management is based on the IMM model of lymphomagenesis. There is increasing evidence of the role of chronic infection in conjunctival and adnexal lymphoma. Both *C. psittaci* and *H. pylori* have been implicated [16, 17]. Follow-up data from *C. psittaci* detection studies have suggested a therapeutic effect following antibiotic therapy with doxycycline, presumably by eradication of the infection that underlies lymphomagenesis. Other studies have shown an effect in small numbers of patients using anti-*H. pylori* triple therapy [40]. Overall, antibiotic treatment regimens have shown variable results by study group and geographical location.

In a retrospective case series of 67 patients with conjunctival EMZL who received doxycycline as their primary treatment and were followed up for at least 5 years, only 25 patients (37%) achieved a complete response, with a partial response in an additional 8 patients (12%). Almost 50% showed stable or progressive disease [41]. Larger studies are needed to clarify the role of antibiotics in the treatment of conjunctival and adnexal lymphoma.

9.15 Surgery

Surgery has been reported to be successful in managing certain cases of highly localized OAL and has been recommended for stage I MALT systemic lymphoma in some sites. Its applicability remains dubious for most conjunctival and adnexal lymphoma due to the diffuse nature and frequent juxtaposition of conjunctival and adnexal lymphoma to sensitive ocular tissues. Surgery should therefore be reserved for localized, isolated lesions of the conjunctiva [32].

9.16 Cryotherapy

Cryotherapeutic ablation of conjunctival and adnexal lymphoma has limited use in the management of conjunctival and adnexal lymphoma [42]. It has resulted in variable success due to debulking the tumor without complete elimination of malignant tissue. It may have application in a limited number of patients with conjunctival and adnexal lymphoma who are unable to receive other treatment modalities, accepting higher chances of recurrence [43].

9.17 Radiation

Historically, external beam radiation (EBRT) has been the most frequently used modality for the treatment of conjunctival and adnexal lymphoma. Analysis of this modality is confounded by small patient numbers in most series, the use of early and inaccurate classification schemes, short follow-up times, and apparent lack of ophthalmic follow-up. Complications were detected at a rate of up to 50% higher when close ophthalmic follow-up was performed.

Both electron and photon irradiation have been successfully employed in OAL (Fig. 9.9) [21]. Dosage is based on the tumor grade or type [22, 23]. Typical doses are 24–30 Gy for low-grade OAL and 30–40 Gy for high-grade conjunctival and adnexal lymphoma [44]. In a recent review of 77 eyes with OAL treated with radiation alone (mean follow-up of 38 months), highly fractionated EBRT with a mean dose of 25 Gy was found to be effective, providing high local control and low risk of visually significant complications (Fig. 9.10) [46]. Overall RT responses are excellent [47].

Radiation complications are minor [48]. The long-term RT toxicities included dry eye (16%) and cataract (13%) (Fig. 9.11) [49]. These findings are consistent with results from a phase III randomized trial[46] and guidelines from the International Lymphoma Radiation Oncology Group recommendations for extranodal lymphoma of all sites [50]. Methods such as lens-sparing electron irradiation technique can be used to reduce cataract formation [51].

Burden of multiple treatment sessions (12 fractions) can be minimized by using ultra-low-dose radiotherapy (ULDRT) (2 × 2 Gy) for symptomatic control of low-grade lymphomas [52]. In a small case series (seven treated patients), five (71%) patients had complete response and two patients had partial response with minimal toxicity over the median follow-up time of 22 months [53]. Similar favorable results have been reported in studies with larger number of patients (17 patients) [54] or with longer follow-up (median 44 months, range 30–54 months) [55].

A phase II multicenter single-arm trial to evaluate the efficacy and safety of low-dose radiotherapy of 12 Gy in four fractions of 3 Gy in indolent lymphoma (follicular lymphoma grade (marginal zone lymphoma, chronic lymphocytic leukemia/small lymphocytic lymphoma) is underway (NCT05543070) [56].

Limited favorable experience of treating EMZL of the fornix (three patients) with a focused single dose of 14 Gy kilovoltage

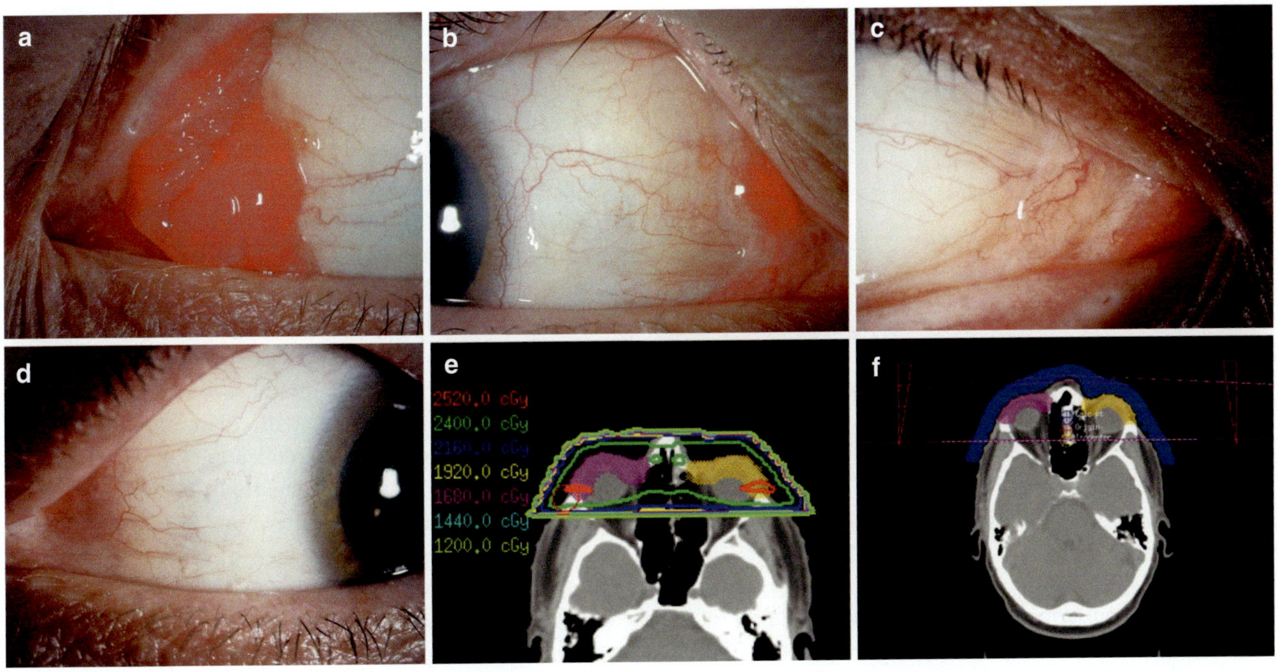

Fig. 9.9 Conjunctival adnexal lymphoma (EMZL) OU. Response to radiation therapy. Before (**a**, right eye; **b**, left eye) and 3 months (**c**, right eye; **d**, left eye) after 24 Gy (**e**) fractionated radiation therapy delivered using opposed lateral fields (**f**). Note total regression of the infiltration. Three years later, the patient underwent cataract surgery for radiation-induced cataracts

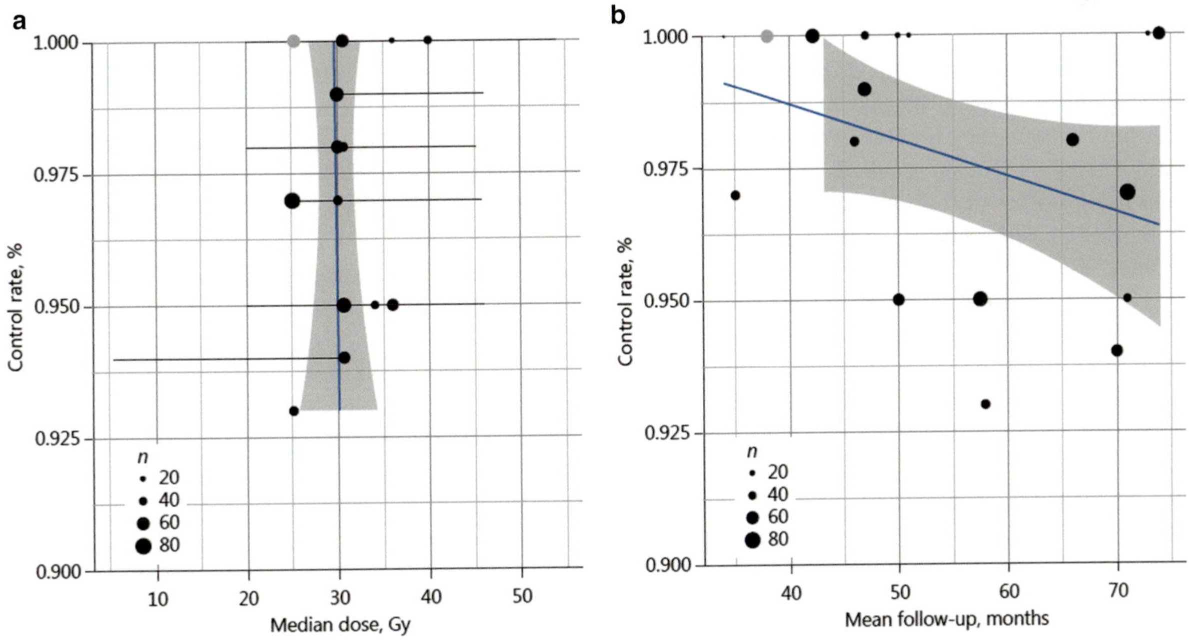

Fig. 9.10 Conjunctival adnexal lymphoma. Radiation therapy. Published studies. Association between median dose and control rate. The x-axis shows the radiation dose in Gy. Points represent the median dose reported in a study, and the whiskers represent the range of radiation dose in the study. The size of the point corresponds to the number of subjects in the study. The y-axis is the reported local control rate of the study (**a**). Association between mean follow-up duration (months) and control rate. The x-axis represents the reported follow-up time of the study, and the y-axis is the reported control rate. The size of the point represents the number of subjects in the study. The blue line represents the line of best fit weighted by the number of subjects in the study. The gray areas represent the standard error associated with the line of best fit (**b**). (Reproduced with permission from Platt et al. [45])

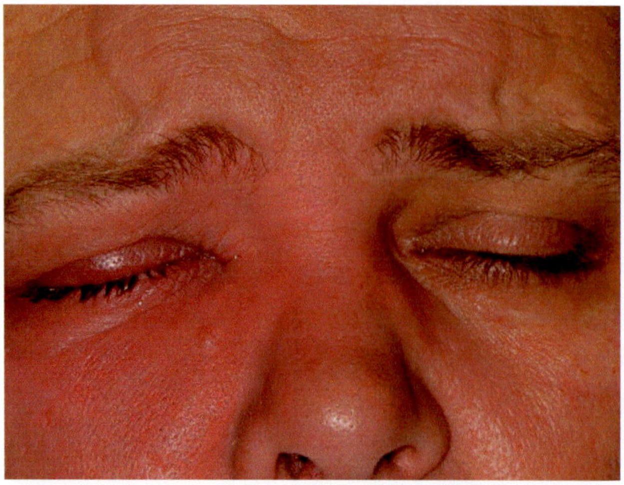

Fig. 9.11 Conjunctival adnexal lymphoma. Post-treatment radiation dermatitis

brachytherapy (prescribed to the maximum thickness of the lesion) needs to assessed in larger number of patients [57].

9.18 Chemotherapy

Since conjunctival and adnexal lymphoma frequently presents as localized disease (stage IE), chemotherapy is rarely used except for aggressive DLBCL. The review of chemotherapy used in lymphoma is beyond the scope of this chapter. Standard chemotherapy for OAL when it is part of more advanced disease is that of standard systemic lymphoma regimens using single-agent rituximab alone or in combination with cyclophosphamide, doxorubicin, vincristine, and prednisone (CHOP), the alkylating agent chlorambucil, and, more recently, bendamustine, which has dual properties of an alkylating agent and a purine analogue. While some have used systemic corticosteroids for tumor suppression of OAL, steroids generally offer ineffective long-term control.

9.19 Immunotherapy

Interferon (IFN-alpha) has been used rarely for conjunctival and adnexal lymphoma despite its long-standing use in systemic lymphoma. One report of five cases showed 80% initial complete response with short-term follow-up [58]. One patient with stage IIA disease died of systemic lymphoma at 1 year. More data regarding local and systemic efficacy are needed prior to acceptance of this modality.

Antilymphocyte antibodies are a recent form of lymphoma treatment. The most commonly used is rituximab, an anti-CD-20 monoclonal antibody, which leads to the destruction of B-cells using mechanisms of complement and antibody-mediated destruction as well as induction of apoptosis. These antibodies are effective when used alone but also significantly increase the remission rates when used in combination with chemotherapy. Local control rates of conjunctival and adnexal lymphoma to rituximab may be less than that reported with radiation therapy [59]. Single-agent rituximab used for bilateral ocular or with systemic presence of EMZL used in 11 patients showed progression in 7 (64%), all in the ocular adnexa and none at systemic sites (Fig. 9.12) [59]. In a systematic review, efficacy of systemic rituximab in a systematic review was in CR in 21 patients (63%), PR in 11 patients (33%), and SD in 1 patient (3%) after 20.5 months of follow-up [61].

Patients with indolent conjunctival lymphomas may be suitable candidates for intralesional therapies [62]. While standardly administered as an intravenous infusion, intralesional injection of rituximab (50 mg/1 ml) for low-grade conjunctival and adnexal lymphoma has shown promise in early studies [52, 63]. Rituximab injected subconjunctivally (50 mg in 5 ml) surrounding the tumor monthly in 12 eyes led to complete response in 11 eyes (73%) and partial in 4 eyes (27%). Similar results have been reported in a prospective phase 2 trial of 20 patients, wherein 11 (55%) patients achieved tumor regression, 8 had stable disease (40%), and 1 (5%) had progressive disease [64]. In a systematic review (38 cases), CR was observed in 28 patients (75%), PR in 7 patients (19%), SD in 1 patient (2%), and progressive disease in 2 patients (4%) over 20.4 months of follow-up [61]. As this treatment can be done in the office setting with good tolerance and few systemic side effects, it may be a suitable alternative in selected cases [62]. However, the role of subcutaneous rituximab for conjunctival and adnexal lymphoma has yet to be established.

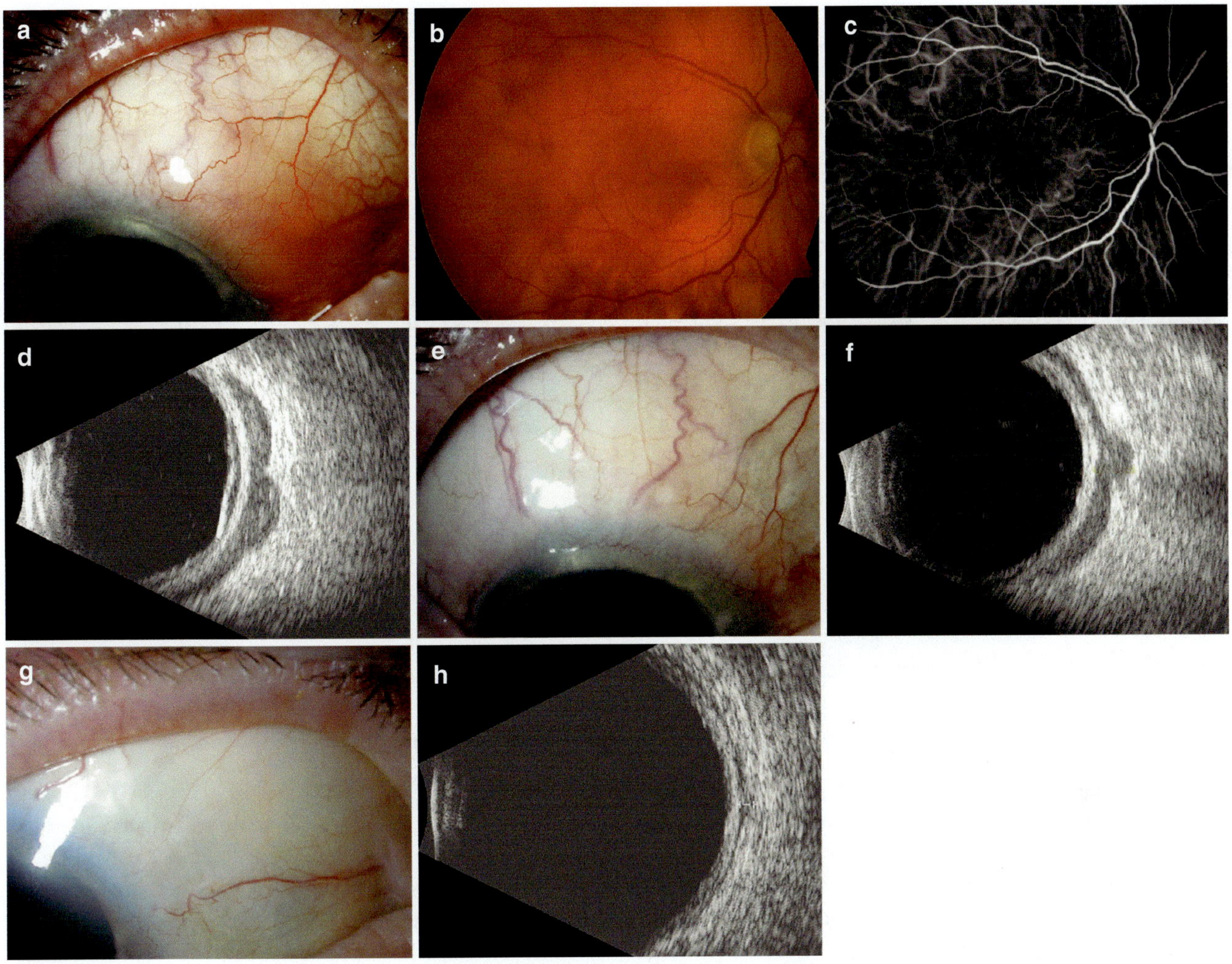

Fig. 9.12 Conjunctival adnexal lymphoma. Response to rituximab. A 68-year-old otherwise healthy man with a history of refractory, unilateral open-angle glaucoma in his right eye was referred for evaluation before a glaucoma filtering procedure. External examination of the right eye demonstrates episcleral venous dilation in the right eye associated with faintly demarcated, slightly raised, pink subconjunctival infiltrates restricted to the superior nasal quadrant with subtle inferior perilimbal extension (**a**). Fundus photography: fundus photographs demonstrate flat, yellow, choroidal infiltrates in both eyes, which extend into the periphery as discrete lesions (**b**). Indocyanine green angiography: indocyanine angiography confirms the presence of infiltrative lesions in the choroid as demonstrated by persistent hypofluorescence in both eyes (**c**). B-scan ultrasonography: representative selections illustrate the presence of hyperechoic choroidal lesions with orbital extension in both eyes, more prominent in the right than in the left (**d**). Given his bilateral eye involvement, he was started on rituximab infusion at a dose of 750 mg weekly for 4 weeks as an upfront systemic therapy causing limited response (**e**, **f**) necessitating radiation therapy consisting of 25 Gy in 14 fractions to both eyes. At 5-year follow-up, the patient was in complete remission (**g**, **h**). Visual acuity is 20/40 right eye and 20/20 left eye with symmetric IOP off medical therapy. (Reproduced with permission from: Sears et al. [60])

9.20 Prognosis

Prognosis is evaluated in three ways: local control, progression to systemic involvement, and death from lymphoma. The AJCC/TNM tumor stage eighth edition classification has prognostic value for relapse and survival among patients with OAL [65]. While certain anatomic sites, such as orbital involvement, are presently assigned a higher TNM stage and have traditionally been associated with a poorer prognosis (in comparison to conjunctival lymphoma), the lymphoma subtype is the most significant indicator of prognosis (Fig. 9.13) [66].

The disease-specific mortality increased through T-categories from T1 to T3 disease in ocular adnexal EMZL but not for other subtypes of OAL (FL, DLBCL, or MCL) [67].

Validation of newer staging protocols will provide future evidence in this regard. Excellent local control has been reported using external beam radiation. Among conjunctival and adnexal lymphoma, EMZL has a quantitatively better prognosis than other tumor types with regard to the spread of tumor and lymphoma-related death. EMZL and FL patients had a markedly better prognosis (10-year disease-specific survival of 92% and 71%, respectively) than DLBCL and

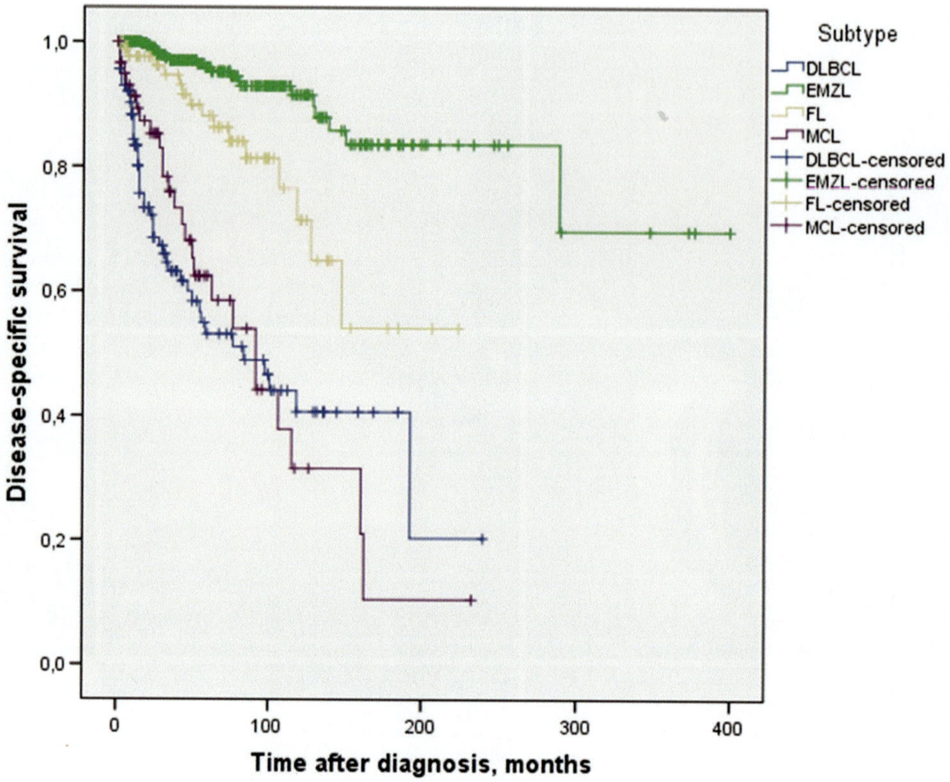

Fig. 9.13 Conjunctival adnexal lymphoma. Disease-specific survival by lymphoma subtype. The low-grade lymphoma subtypes extranodal marginal zone B-cell lymphoma (green) and follicular lymphoma (yellow) have a more favorable disease-specific survival than the high-grade lymphoma subtypes diffuse large B-cell lymphoma (blue) and mantle cell lymphoma (purple). (Reproduced with permission from Olsen et al. [66])

MCL patients (10-year disease-specific survival of 41% and 32%, respectively) [66].

Extra-orbital spread can occur in over 45% of EMZL cases after a mean follow-up of 63 months, suggesting that long-term follow-up is needed [22, 23, 32]. A recent large single-center report with long-term outcomes from patients with primary low-grade OAL found that age < 60 years was associated with improved progression-free survival and that while individuals with indolent disease may survive decades without treatment, up to 4% of OAL can transform to more aggressive variants [68].

A total of 689 patients were followed up for 42 months (median). The median age was 62 years (range, 8–100 years), and the majority were in Ann Arbor stage IE (90%, 485/541 patients) and American Joint Committee on Cancer stage T2 (61%, 340/557 patients) at the time of diagnosis. The orbit (66%, 452/689 patients) and the conjunctiva (37%, 255/689 patients) were the most frequently involved anatomical structures. The 5-year, 10-year, and 20-year disease-specific survival (DSS) rates were 96%, 91%, and 90%, respectively [69].

9.21 Future Research

Our evolving ability to characterize conjunctival and adnexal lymphoma on a molecular level will increase the potential for developing newer and less toxic therapies. Recent advances in next-generation sequencing have allowed for more comprehensive genomic profiling of OAL. In one series of 36 samples, 53% harbored a potentially actionable mutation [70]. In another recent series of 69 OAL tumors, whole-exome sequencing identified candidate driver genes clustered in the B-cell receptor (BCR), NF-κB, NOTCH, and NFAT signaling pathways [71]. With the introduction of targeted pathway therapeutics such as BTK inhibitors and immunotherapeutics including bispecific antibiotics, there are now an increasing number of treatment options for patients with conjunctival and adnexal lymphoma.

References

1. Cohen VM, Sweetenham J, Singh AD. Ocular adnexal lymphoma. What is the evidence for an infectious aetiology? Br J Ophthalmol. 2008;92(4):446–8.
2. Hatef E, Roberts D, McLaughlin P, Pro B, Esmaeli B. Prevalence and nature of systemic involvement and stage at initial examination in patients with orbital and ocular adnexal lymphoma. Arch Ophthalmol. 2007;125(12):1663–7.
3. Bayraktar S, Bayraktar UD, Stefanovic A, Lossos IS. Primary ocular adnexal mucosa-associated lymphoid tissue lymphoma (MALT): single institution experience in a large cohort of patients. Br J Haematol. 2011;152(1):72–80.
4. Alfaar AS, Yousef YA, Matthew WW, Hassanain O, Kakkassery V, Moustafa M, et al. Declining incidence and improving survival of ocular and orbital lymphomas in the US between 1995 and 2018. Sci Rep. 2024;14(1):7886.

5. Holm F, Mikkelsen LH, Kamper P, Rasmussen PK, Larsen TS, Sjo LD, et al. Ocular adnexal lymphoma in Denmark: a nationwide study of 387 cases from 1980 to 2017. Br J Ophthalmol. 2021;105(7):914–20.
6. Alnaim AF, Alhawsawi A, AlSomali A, Jannadi R, Alsolami SM, Alotaibi HA. Conjunctival pediatric-type follicular lymphoma in a young male: a case report and literature review. Cureus. 2022;14(2):e22023.
7. Moustafa GA, Topham AK, Aronow ME, Vavvas DG. Paediatric ocular adnexal lymphoma: a population-based analysis. BMJ Open Ophthalmol. 2020;5(1):e000483.
8. Shields JA, Bakewell B, Augsburger JJ, Flanagan JC. Classification and incidence of space-occupying lesions of the orbit. A survey of 645 biopsies. Arch Ophthalmol. 1984;102(11):1606–11.
9. Spraul CW, Grossniklaus HE. Analysis of 24,444 surgical specimens accessioned over 55 years in an ophthalmic pathology laboratory. Int Ophthalmol. 1997;21(5):283–304.
10. Ferry JA, Fung CY, Zukerberg L, Lucarelli MJ, Hasserjian RP, Preffer FI, et al. Lymphoma of the ocular adnexa: a study of 353 cases. Am J Surg Pathol. 2007;31(2):170–84.
11. Knowles DM, Jakobiec FA, McNally L, Burke JS. Lymphoid hyperplasia and malignant lymphoma occurring in the ocular adnexa (orbit, conjunctiva, and eyelids): a prospective multiparametric analysis of 108 cases during 1977 to 1987. Hum Pathol. 1990;21(9):959–73.
12. McGrath LA, Ryan DA, Warrier SK, Coupland SE, Glasson WJ. Conjunctival lymphoma. Eye (Lond). 2023;37(5):837–48.
13. Ye H, Liu H, Attygalle A, Wotherspoon AC, Nicholson AG, Charlotte F, et al. Variable frequencies of t(11;18)(q21;q21) in MALT lymphomas of different sites: significant association with CagA strains of H pylori in gastric MALT lymphoma. Blood. 2003;102(3):1012–8.
14. Takada S, Yoshino T, Taniwaki M, Nakamura N, Nakamine H, Oshima K, et al. Involvement of the chromosomal translocation t(11;18) in some mucosa-associated lymphoid tissue lymphomas and diffuse large B-cell lymphomas of the ocular adnexa: evidence from multiplex reverse transcriptase-polymerase chain reaction and fluorescence in situ hybridization on using formalin-fixed, paraffin-embedded specimens. Mod Pathol. 2003;16(5):445–52.
15. Kirkegaard MK. Ocular adnexal lymphoma: subtype-specific clinical and genetic features. Acta Ophthalmol. 2022;100(Suppl 270):3–37.
16. Ferreri AJ, Guidoboni M, Ponzoni M, De Conciliis C, Dell'Oro S, Fleischhauer K, et al. Evidence for an association between Chlamydia psittaci and ocular adnexal lymphomas. J Natl Cancer Inst. 2004;96(8):586–94.
17. Chan CC, Smith JA, Shen DF, Ursea R, LeHoang P, Grossniklaus HE. Helicobacter pylori (H. pylori) molecular signature in conjunctival mucosa-associated lymphoid tissue (MALT) lymphoma. Histol Histopathol. 2004;19(4):1219–26.
18. Harris NL, Jaffe ES, Stein H, Banks PM, Chan JK, Cleary ML, et al. A revised European-American classification of lymphoid neoplasms: a proposal from the International Lymphoma Study Group. Blood. 1994;84(5):1361–92.
19. Swerdlow S, Campo E, Harris NL, Jaffe ES, Pileri SA, Stein H, et al. Cancer TIAFRO. WHO classification of tumours of haematopoietic and lymphoid tissue (IARC WHO classification of tumours). 4th ed. World Health Organization; 2008.
20. Aronow ME. Ocular adnexal lymphoma: evidence-based treatment approach. Int Ophthalmol Clin. 2015;55(1):97–109.
21. Yen MT, Bilyk JR, Wladis EJ, Bradley EA, Mawn LA. Treatments for ocular adnexal lymphoma: a report by the American Academy of Ophthalmology. Ophthalmology. 2018;125(1):127–36.
22. Fung CY, Tarbell NJ, Lucarelli MJ, Goldberg SI, Linggood RM, Harris NL, et al. Ocular adnexal lymphoma: clinical behavior of distinct World Health Organization classification subtypes. Int J Radiat Oncol Biol Phys. 2003;57(5):1382–91.
23. Jenkins C, Rose GE, Bunce C, Wright JE, Cree IA, Plowman N, et al. Histological features of ocular adnexal lymphoma (REAL classification) and their association with patient morbidity and survival. Br J Ophthalmol. 2000;84(8):907–13.
24. Jung SK, Paik JS, Park GS, Cho SG, Yang SW. Refractory follicular conjunctival lesions: overlook as just inflammation or not? Br J Ophthalmol. 2019;103(11):1660–5.
25. Rafizadeh SM, Nozarian Z, Sonbolestan SA. Isolated lateral rectus muscle large B cell lymphoma: a rare case report and review of the literature. Am J Ophthalmol Case Rep. 2022;28:101736.
26. Venkateswaran N, Sripawadkul W, Karp CL. The role of imaging technologies for ocular surface tumors. Curr Opin Ophthalmol. 2021;32(4):369–78.
27. Stafford SL, Kozelsky TF, Garrity JA, Kurtin PJ, Leavitt JA, Martenson JA, et al. Orbital lymphoma: radiotherapy outcome and complications. Radiother Oncol. 2001;59(2):139–44.
28. Fuller ML, Sweetenham J, Schoenfield L, Singh AD. Uveal lymphoma: a variant of ocular adnexal lymphoma. Leuk Lymphoma. 2008;49(12):2393–7.
29. Aronow ME, Portell CA, Sweetenham JW, Singh AD. Uveal lymphoma: clinical features, diagnostic studies, treatment selection, and outcomes. Ophthalmology. 2014;121(1):334–41.
30. Saatci AO, Arikan G, Ozcan MA, Ozkal S, Kargi A, Undar B. Indocyanine green angiographic features of systemic non-Hodgkin's lymphoma and bilateral choroidal involvement. Ophthalmic Surg Lasers Imaging. 2006;37(3):236–9.
31. Rath S, Connors JM, Dolman PJ, Rootman J, Rootman DB, White VA. Comparison of American Joint Committee on Cancer TNM-based staging system (7th edition) and Ann Arbor classification for predicting outcome in ocular adnexal lymphoma. Orbit. 2014;33(1):23–8.
32. Coupland SE, Hellmich M, Auw-Haedrich C, Lee WR, Stein H. Prognostic value of cell-cycle markers in ocular adnexal lymphoma: an assessment of 230 cases. Graefes Arch Clin Exp Ophthalmol. 2004;242(2):130–45.
33. McKelvie PA, McNab A, Francis IC, Fox R, O'Day J. Ocular adnexal lymphoproliferative disease: a series of 73 cases. Clin Experiment Ophthalmol. 2001;29(6):387–93.
34. Coupland SE, White VA, Rootman J, Damato B, Finger PT. A TNM-based clinical staging system of ocular adnexal lymphomas. Arch Pathol Lab Med. 2009;133(8):1262–7.
35. Aronow ME, Portell CA, Rybicki LA, Sweetenham JW, Singh AD. Ocular adnexal lymphoma: assessment of a tumor-node-metastasis staging system. Ophthalmology. 2013;120(9):1915–9.
36. Liu H, Ye H, Dogan A, Ranaldi R, Hamoudi RA, Bearzi I, et al. T(11;18)(q21;q21) is associated with advanced mucosa-associated lymphoid tissue lymphoma that expresses nuclear BCL10. Blood. 2001;98(4):1182–7.
37. Manta AI, Wilson-Pogmore AA, Sullivan TJ. Thirty years of experience with ocular adnexal T-cell lymphoma. Ophthalmic Plast Reconstr Surg. 2023;39(3):266–74.
38. Coupland SE, Foss HD, Assaf C, Auw-Haedrich C, Anastassiou G, Anagnostopoulos I, et al. T-cell and T/natural killer-cell lymphomas involving ocular and ocular adnexal tissues: a clinicopathologic, immunohistochemical, and molecular study of seven cases. Ophthalmology. 1999;106(11):2109–20.
39. Mizuhara K, Kobayashi T, Nakao M, Takahashi R, Kaneko H, Shimura K, et al. Watchful waiting is an acceptable treatment option for asymptomatic primary ocular adnexal mucosa-associated lymphoid tissue lymphoma: a retrospective study. Cancer Med. 2023;12(3):3134–44.
40. Abramson DH, Rollins I, Coleman M. Periocular mucosa-associated lymphoid/low grade lymphomas: treatment with antibiotics. Am J Ophthalmol. 2005;140(4):729–30.

41. Choi SH, Yang MK, Kim TM, Choi HJ. Feasibility of oral doxycycline as first-line therapy for conjunctival mucosa-associated lymphoid tissue lymphoma. Eye. 2024;38(1):282–28.
42. Lee J, Oh D, Choi BO, Eom KY, Lee JH, Kim JH, et al. Patterns of care for orbital marginal zone B-cell lymphoma of mucosa-associated lymphoid tissue in Korea throughout 2016: results from a multicenter cross-sectional cohort study (KROG 16-19). Asia Pac J Clin Oncol. 2019;15(6):358–63.
43. Fernandez CA, Henry RK, Shields CL, Bilyk JR, Lally SE, Eagle RC, et al. Ocular adnexal lymphoma: a single-institution retrospective study. Saudi J Ophthalmol. 2021;35(3):230–8.
44. Uno T, Isobe K, Shikama N, Nishikawa A, Oguchi M, Ueno N, et al. Radiotherapy for extranodal, marginal zone, B-cell lymphoma of mucosa-associated lymphoid tissue originating in the ocular adnexa: a multiinstitutional, retrospective review of 50 patients. Cancer. 2003;98(4):865–71.
45. Platt S, Al Zahrani Y, Singh N, et al. Extranodal marginal zone lymphoma of ocular adnexa: outcomes following radiation therapy. Ocul Oncol Pathol. 2017;3(3):181–7.
46. Lowry L, Smith P, Qian W, Falk S, Benstead K, Illidge T, et al. Reduced dose radiotherapy for local control in non-Hodgkin lymphoma: a randomised phase III trial. Radiother Oncol. 2011;100(1):86–92.
47. Saul EE, Alderuccio JP, Reis IM, Zhao W, Iyer SG, Rodriguez G, et al. Long-term outcomes of patients with conjunctival extranodal marginal zone lymphoma. Am J Hematol. 2023;98(1):148–58.
48. Eze C, Friedrich I, Hadi I, Schmidt-Hegemann NS, Hartoyo SN, Trauth R, et al. Primary radiation therapy in stage I/II indolent orbital lymphoma—a comprehensive retrospective recurrence and toxicity analysis. Eur J Haematol. 2022;109(1):21–30.
49. Pereira-Da Silva MV, Di Nicola ML, Altomare F, Xu W, Tsang R, Laperriere N, et al. Radiation therapy for primary orbital and ocular adnexal lymphoma. Clin Transl Radiat Oncol. 2023;38:15–20.
50. Yahalom J, Illidge T, Specht L, Hoppe RT, Li YX, Tsang R, et al. Modern radiation therapy for extranodal lymphomas: field and dose guidelines from the International Lymphoma Radiation Oncology Group. Int J Radiat Oncol Biol Phys. 2015;92(1):11–31.
51. Hoffmann C, Ringbaek T, Eckstein A, Deya W, Santiago A, Heintz M, et al. Long-term follow-up of patients with conjunctival lymphoma after individualized lens-sparing electron radiotherapy: results from a longitudinal study. Cancers (Basel). 2023;15(22)
52. Fasola CE, Jones JC, Huang DD, Le QT, Hoppe RT, Donaldson SS. Low-dose radiation therapy (2 Gy x 2) in the treatment of orbital lymphoma. Int J Radiat Oncol Biol Phys. 2013;86(5):930–5.
53. de Castro B, Peixeiro RP, Mariz JM, Oliveira A. Ultra-low dose radiotherapy in the management of low-grade orbital lymphomas. Rep Pract Oncol Radiother. 2022;27(3):467–73.
54. Park J, Yea JW, Oh SA, Kim MK, Son JH, Park JW. Prospective study of 4 Gy Radiotherapy for Orbital Mucosa-Associated Lymphoid Tissue Lymphoma (FORMAL). Cancers (Basel). 2022;14(17)
55. Lee MJ, Lee MY, Choe J-Y, Choi SH, Kim HJ. Ultra-low-dose radiation treatment for early-stage ocular adnexal MALT lymphoma. Eur J Ophthalmol. 2022;32(5):3092–6.
56. Gao LR, Wang X, Xia C, Song YW, Wang L, Li X, et al. Multicenter phase II study of moderate low-dose radiotherapy in indolent non-Hodgkin lymphoma: CLCG-iNHL-01 protocol. Future Oncol. 2024;20(2):71–81.
57. Sarria GR, Cabrera CM, Sarria GJ, Buitrago M, Fuentes P, Serpa S, et al. Single-fraction low-energy electronic brachytherapy for conjunctival lymphoma. J Contemp Brachytherapy. 2020;12(3):267–72.
58. Blasi MA, Gherlinzoni F, Calvisi G, Sasso P, Tani M, Cellini M, et al. Local chemotherapy with interferon-alpha for conjunctival mucosa-associated lymphoid tissue lymphoma: a preliminary report. Ophthalmology. 2001;108(3):559–62.
59. Portell CA, Aronow ME, Rybicki LA, Macklis R, Singh AD, Sweetenham JW. Clinical characteristics of 95 patients with ocular adnexal and uveal lymphoma: treatment outcomes in extranodal marginal zone subtype. Clin Lymphoma Myeloma Leuk. 2014;14(3):203–10.
60. Sears NC, Singh A, Singh AD. Ocular adnexal lymphoma presenting as refractory unilateral open-angle glaucoma. J Glaucoma. 2016;25:e741–e4.
61. Serbest Ceylanoglu K, Guneri Beser B, Singalavanija T, Juntipwong S, Worden FP, Demirci H. Targeted therapy and immunotherapy for advanced malignant conjunctival tumors: systematic review. Ophthalmic Plast Reconstr Surg. 2024;40(1):18–29.
62. Demirci H, Ozgonul C, Diniz Grisolia AB, Elner VM. Intralesional rituximab injection for low-grade conjunctival lymphoma management. Ophthalmology. 2020;127(9):1270–3.
63. Davies A, Merli F, Mihaljevic B, Mercadal S, Siritanaratkul N, Solal-Celigny P, et al. Efficacy and safety of subcutaneous rituximab versus intravenous rituximab for first-line treatment of follicular lymphoma (SABRINA): a randomised, open-label, phase 3 trial. Lancet Haematol. 2017;4(6):e272–e82.
64. Ferreri AJM, Sassone M, Miserocchi E, Govi S, Cecchetti C, Corti ME, et al. Treatment of MALT lymphoma of the conjunctiva with intralesional rituximab supplemented with autologous serum. Blood Adv. 2020;4(6):1013–9.
65. Kwon M, Lee JS, Lee C, Yoon DH, Sa HS. Prognostic factors for relapse and survival among patients with ocular adnexal lymphoma: validation of the eighth edition of the American Joint Committee on Cancer (AJCC) TNM classification. Br J Ophthalmol. 2021;105(2):279–84.
66. Olsen TG, Holm F, Mikkelsen LH, Rasmussen PK, Coupland SE, Esmaeli B, et al. Orbital lymphoma-an international multicenter retrospective study. Am J Ophthalmol. 2019;199:44–57.
67. Vest SD, Coupland SE, Esmaeli B, Finger PT, Graue GF, Grossniklaus HE, et al. Specific location of ocular adnexal lymphoma and mortality: an international multicentre retrospective study. Br J Ophthalmol. 2023;107(9):1231–8.
68. Desai A, Joag MG, Lekakis L, Chapman JR, Vega F, Tibshirani R, et al. Long-term course of patients with primary ocular adnexal MALT lymphoma: a large single-institution cohort study. Blood. 2017;129(3):324–32.
69. Hindso TG, Esmaeli B, Holm F, Mikkelsen LH, Rasmussen PK, Coupland SE, et al. International multicentre retrospective cohort study of ocular adnexal marginal zone B-cell lymphoma. Br J Ophthalmol. 2020;104(3):357–62.
70. Cani AK, Soliman M, Hovelson DH, Liu CJ, McDaniel AS, Haller MJ, et al. Comprehensive genomic profiling of orbital and ocular adnexal lymphomas identifies frequent alterations in MYD88 and chromatin modifiers: new routes to targeted therapies. Mod Pathol. 2016;29(7):685–97.
71. Magistri M, Happ LE, Ramdial J, Lu X, Stathias V, Kunkalla K, et al. The genetic landscape of ocular adnexa MALT lymphoma reveals frequent aberrations in NFAT and MEF2B signaling pathways. Cancer Res Commun. 2021;1(1):1–16.

10 Caruncle Tumors

Hans E. Grossniklaus, Daniel R. Capiz-Correa, and Jill R. Wells

10.1 Caruncle Tumors

The caruncle (diminutive of the Latin word Caro = flesh) is a fleshy structure located at the inner canthus at the lacrimal lake. It has a tail that blends to the skin of the medial canthal angle and a round to ovoid head medial to the plica semilunaris. The distance from the common canaliculus is about 0.85 mm [1–3]. The caruncle develops from the nasal aspect of the lower lid fold and is sequestered from the lower lid by the growth of the lower canaliculus. It has an irregular surface, measuring about 5 mm vertically, 3 mm transversely, and 1.5 mm in thickness, containing conjunctival and skin elements. The caruncle has a nonkeratinized stratified squamous epithelium with goblet cells. The stroma contains fibroblasts and melanocytes interspersed with collagen, adipose tissue, sebaceous glands associated with hair follicles, striated muscle fibers (Horner's muscle), inflammatory cells, and, in some individuals, sweat glands and accessory lacrimal tissue. Its blood supply is from the medial palpebral artery. The lymphatics drain to the submaxillary lymph nodes and are innervated by the infratrochlear nerve. The function of the caruncle is not well understood, but it may participate in lacrimal drainage through contractions of Horner's muscle [1–4].

Because the caruncle is a transitional zone structure, it can give rise to tumors found in the skin, conjunctiva, and lacrimal gland. Few caruncle lesion series have been published since the first report by Von Graefe in 1858 [4–11]. Lesions of the caruncle are rare, and because of their multiple components, clinical diagnosis and management can be difficult. Caruncle lesions correspond to 0.3–1.1% of all specimens submitted to an ophthalmic pathology laboratory [4–9]. Inconsistency between clinical and histopathological diagnoses as high as 50% has been reported [5–9]. In a report by Ostergaard of 574 caruncle lesions, 96% of lesions were classified as benign, with the benign nature of these tumors being recognized in only 29% prior to histopathological study [9].

In the series reported by Ostergaard, tumors were classified as benign in 96% of lesions, premalignant in 1.7%, and malignant in 2.4%. The most affected age group was from 20 to 29 years (71%). Nevus and papilloma were the most common benign neoplasms, occurring in 43% and 22% of cases, respectively. Less common lesions included inclusion cysts (6.1%), sebaceous gland hyperplasia (5.4%), and chronic inflammatory lesions (4.4%). Rare lesions included oncocytoma in 16 cases, primary basal cell carcinoma in 3 cases of secondary basal cell carcinoma, lymphoma in 4 cases and sebaceous gland carcinoma [2], melanoma [2], and Kaposi's sarcoma [2]. Vascular tumors were also found, corresponding to nine hemangiomas, seven pyogenic granulomas, and four lymphangiomas. Ectopic lacrimal gland was found in seven cases (Table 10.1) [9].

H. E. Grossniklaus (✉) · J. R. Wells
Department of Ophthalmology, Emory University School of Medicine/Emory Eye Center, Atlanta, GA, USA
e-mail: ophtheg@emory.edu; jwells4@emory.edu

D. R. Capiz-Correa
Department of Orbit and Oculoplastic, Fundacion Hospital Nuestra Senora de la Luz, I.A.P., Mexico City, Mexico

© The Author(s), under exclusive license to Springer Nature Switzerland AG 2024
J. Pe'er et al. (eds.), *Clinical Ophthalmic Oncology*, https://doi.org/10.1007/978-3-031-72443-5_10

Table 10.1 Pathological diagnoses of lesions of the caruncle

Category	*n*	%
Benign	550	96
Degeneration		
Elastoid degeneration	2	0.3
Amyloid deposits	1	0.2
Inflammation		
Chronic inflammation	25	4.4
Chalazion	4	0.7
Foreign body	3	0.5
Abscess	1	0.2
Folliculitis	1	0.2
Neoplasia		
Cystic		
Inclusion cyst	35	6.1
Ductal cyst	9	1.6
Epithelial		
Papilloma	127	22.1
Sebaceous gland hyperplasia	31	5.4
Oncocytoma	16	2.8
Ectopic lacrimal gland	7	1.2
Sebaceous gland adenoma	3	0.5
Hidrocystoma	1	0.2
Lymphoid		
Reactive lymphoid hyperplasia	2	0.3
Mesenchymal		
Leiomyoma	1	0.2
Melanocytic		
Nevus	248	43.2
Primary acquired melanosis	5	0.9
Vascular		
Hemangioma	9	1.6
Lymphangioma	4	0.7
Pyogenic granuloma	7	1.2
Miscellaneous		
Normal tissue	5	0.9
Dermoid tumor	1	0.2
Fribrolipoma	1	0.2
Xanthoma	1	0.2
Premalignant	10	1.7
Neoplasia		
Papilloma with dysplasia	4	0.7
Dysplasia	2	0.3
Melanocytic		
Primary acquired melanosis with atypia	4	0.7
Malignant	14	2.4
Neoplasia		
Epithelial		
Basal cell carcinoma (primary)	1	0.2
Basal cell carcinoma (secondary)	3	0.5
Sebaceous gland carcinoma	2	0.3
Lymphoid		
Lymphoma	4	0.7
Melanocytic		
Melanoma	2	0.3
Vascular		
Kaposi's sarcoma	2	0.3
Total	574	100.0

Modified from Ostergaard et al. [9]. With permission from Wiley

10.2 Epithelial Lesions

10.2.1 Squamous Papilloma

Papillomas are benign epithelial tumors of the conjunctiva with a cauliflower-like appearance, most of which are exophytic, and can be sessile or pedunculated, and they are more common in adults between 20 and 39 years of age and children. They can be solitary or multiple [4, 5, 11, 13]. They are intimately related to human papilloma virus especially serotypes 6 and 11 [4, 5, 8, 9, 12, 13]. Histologically, they are composed of multiple fronds or fingerlike projections of conjunctival epithelium, which enclose cores of vascularized connective tissue [8, 13]. After removal, recurrence rates range from 6% to 27% [8]. Topical alpha-interferon can be used in case of recurrence or multiple lesions (Fig. 10.1).

10.2.2 Sebaceous Hyperplasia

Sebaceous hyperplasia can present as a slow-growing, painless, yellow, "greasy," granular, nodular lesion, which is associated with overlying telangiectatic vessels of unknown etiology, although some reports present cases experiencing pain [4, 14]. Histologically, they are formed of hyperplastic glandular lobules situated around a single duct where the sebaceous cells maintain their normal maturation with a single, outer, dark, germinal layer changing abruptly to clear vacuolated cells in the inner layers. Excisional biopsy is recommended if malignancy is suspected to improve cosmesis or lesion debulking (Fig. 10.2).

10.2.3 Oncocytoma

Oncocytomas constitute 5.1% of caruncle lesions [15]. In the ocular region, they are most commonly found in the caruncle, but can arise from the conjunctiva, eyelid, lacrimal gland, and lacrimal sac. Clinically, they are slow-growing nodules, red, orange-tan, or red-blue in color, sometimes with a lobulated, fleshy, or cystic appearance, found in patients over 50 years of age (range, 51–89), with slightly higher prevalence in women. They develop from oncocytic metaplasia of the lacrimal or salivary acinar cells, or from conjunctiva adjacent to the caruncle. Histologically, they are composed of polygonal epithelial cells with round, central to paracentral, nuclei and abundant, finely granular, eosinophilic cytoplasm containing abundant mitochondria. Lymphocytes can be present but are scanty, and lymphoid follicles are rare (Fig. 10.3).

Fig. 10.1 Squamous papilloma. (**a**) Pedunculated and sessile papilloma arising from the caruncle (clinical photograph). (**b**) Acanthotic epithelium arranged in a papillomatous configuration overlaying central vascular cores (H&E stain, 10×)

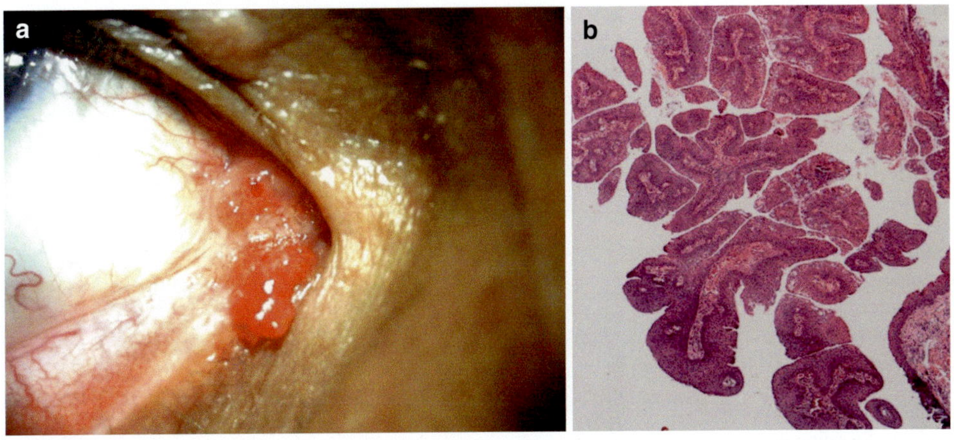

Fig. 10.2 Sebaceous hyperplasia: lobules of enlarged subepithelial sebaceous glands, with normal maturation (H&E stain, 25×)

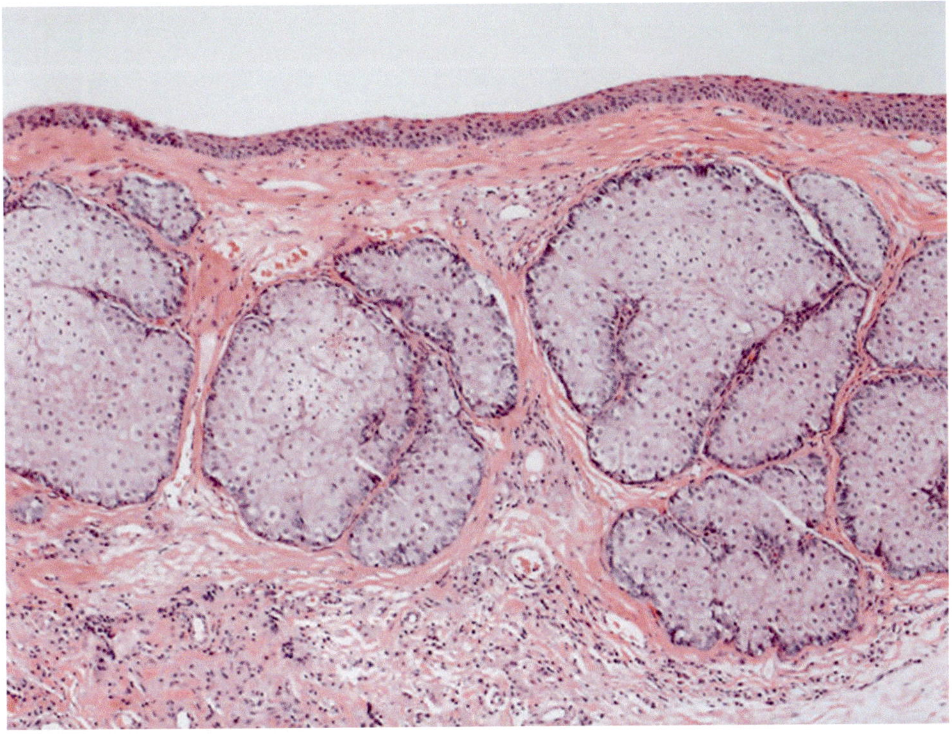

Fig. 10.3 Oncocytoma. (**a**) Dark subepithelial nodule (clinical photograph). (**b**) Oncocytes forming glands. These cells have small, displaced nuclei with abundant eosinophilic cytoplasm (H&E stain, 100×)

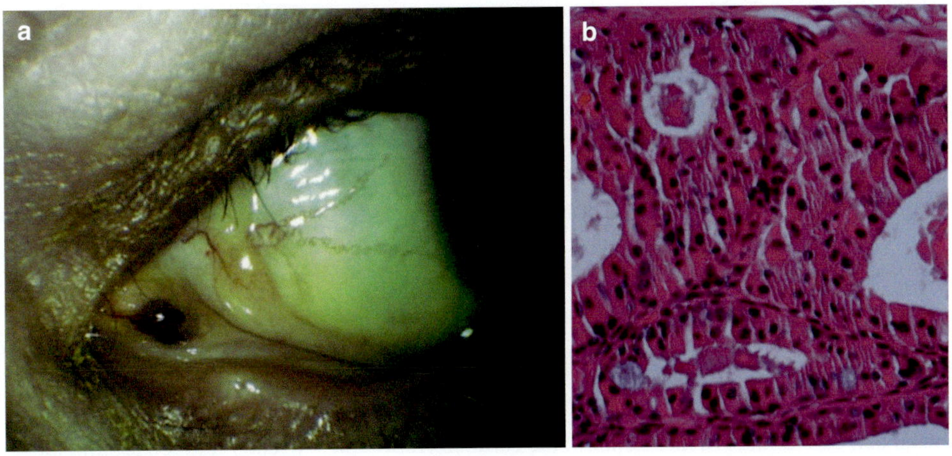

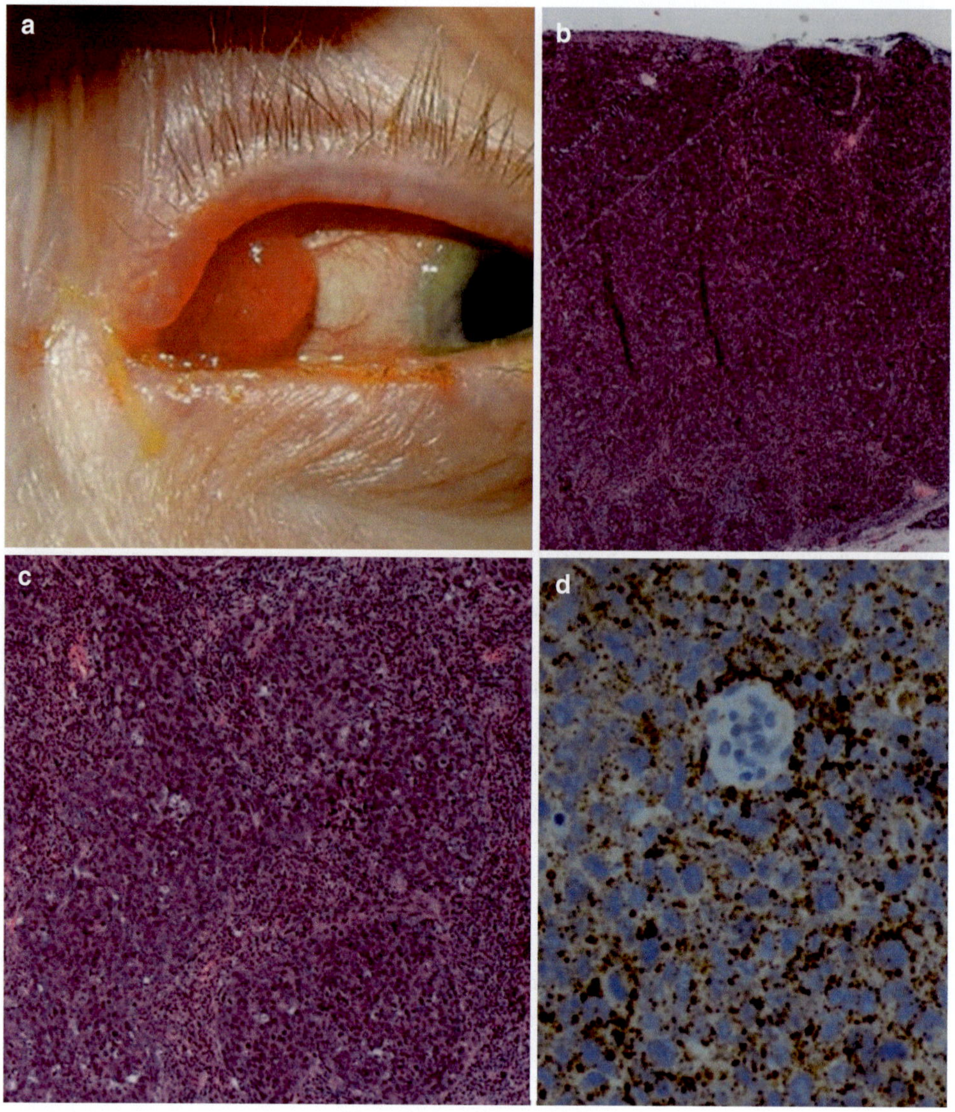

Fig. 10.4 Sebaceous carcinoma. (**a**) Fleshy nodule arising from the caruncle (clinical photograph). (**b**) Tumor composed of lobules of hyperplastic sebaceous glands (H&E stain, 10×). (**c**) Higher magnification showing cells with sebaceous differentiation, pleomorphic amphophilic nuclei with prominent nucleoli, lobules of tumor surrounded by chronic inflammatory cells (H&E stain, 40×). (**d**) Sebaceous differentiation, with positive staining for adipophilin (adipophilin immunostain, 100×)

10.2.4 Sebaceous Carcinoma

More than 95% of sebaceous carcinomas originate in the eyelids, usually from the Meibomian glands of the tarsus and less often from the Zeiss glands, with only about 2–5% developing in the caruncle [16, 17]. Clinically, they can be misdiagnosed as sebaceous gland hyperplasia. Histologically, this tumor is composed of lobules of sebaceous gland with pleomorphic vacuolated cells and mitotic activity. The standard local treatment is complete surgical removal with negative margins and map biopsies to rule out pagetoid spread and regional and distant metastasis. Follow-up is recommended (Fig. 10.4).

10.2.5 Basal Cell Carcinoma

Basal cell carcinoma is a rare tumor of the caruncle, although some studies report the incidence as being similar to that of melanoma [4, 7, 9]. Because of its close proximity to the medial canthus, it is not rare to find caruncular involvement from a basal cell carcinoma arising in the skin of the medial canthus. Clinically, most lesions are vascularized and nodular, more common in men, between the range of 24 and 82 years [18]. Basal cell carcinoma can arise from basal cells of the epithelium or infundibular cells of the hair follicles or from pluripotent stem cells. They should be treated by complete excision whenever possible.

10.3 Pigmented Lesions

10.3.1 Nevus

Nevus is the most commonly reported lesion of the caruncle [4–6, 8, 9, 15]. In a report by Shields, caruncular nevus accounted for 15% of all conjunctival nevi [19]. They are usually noticed around the age of puberty and are regarded as hamartomas. They are mildly elevated, brown, pigmented lesions with a cystic component, but they can be amelanotic. Feeder and intrinsic vessels can be seen in up to one of three

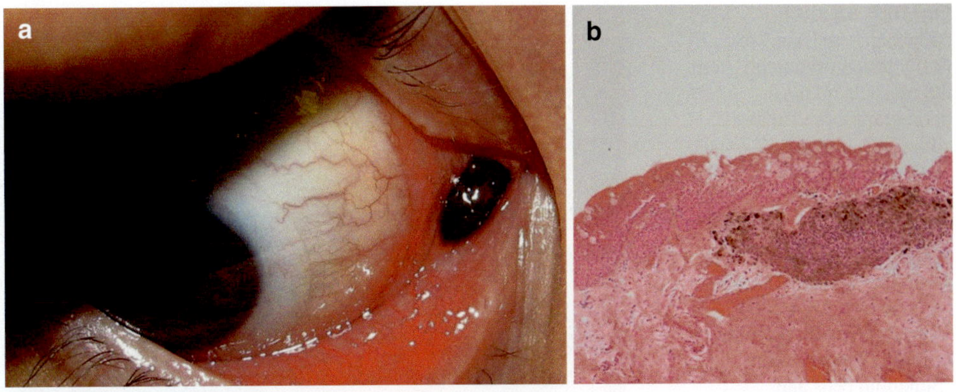

Fig. 10.5 Caruncle nevus. (**a**) Dark pigmented lesion with well-demarcated margin; note the absence of cysts (clinical photograph). (**b**) Subepithelial nest of nevus cells, some with melanin pigment in their cytoplasm (H&E stain, 25×)

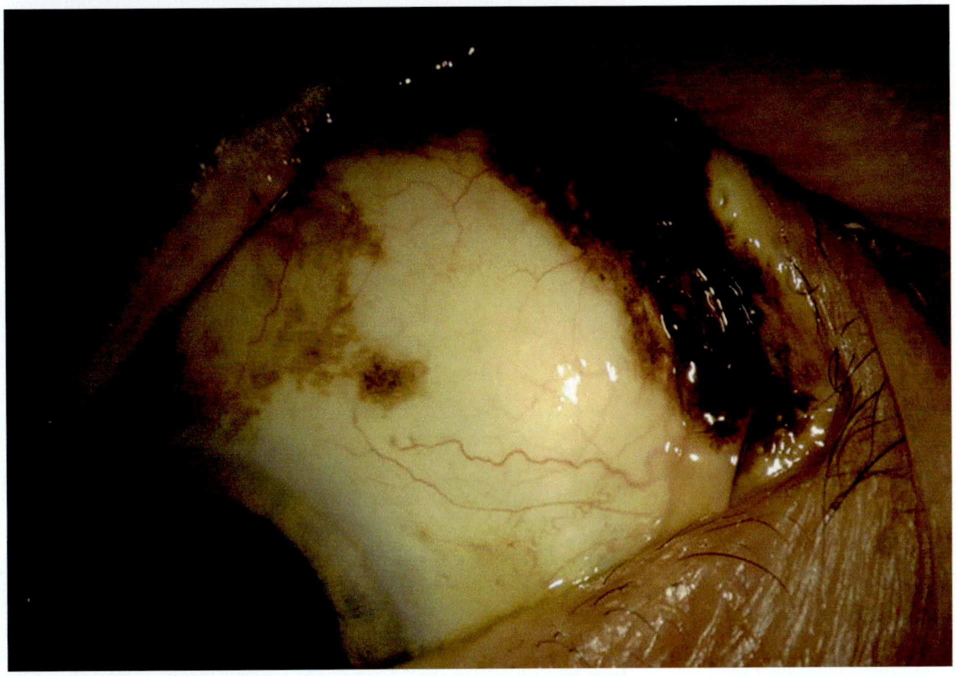

Fig. 10.6 Caruncle PAM with associated conjunctival melanoma. Extensive areas of PAM extending to the bulbar and tarsal conjunctiva, and the caruncle. Melanoma arising from PAM affecting the superior fornix (clinical photograph)

cases. Nevi are usually asymptomatic, but occasionally the patient can report a foreign body sensation. Surgical removal is mainly done for cosmetic reasons or if there is a clinical suspicion of malignancy. Histologically, nevi are composed of nest of nevus cells. Most are compound nevi, but some can have a subepithelial or junctional component (Fig. 10.5).

10.3.2 Melanoma

Melanoma has been reported to be the most prevalent malignant lesion of the caruncle. Melanoma involving the caruncle has a relatively poor prognosis (together with melanomas in the palpebral conjunctiva, plica semilunaris, and fornix) compared to epibulbar conjunctival lesions. One feature to distinguish melanoma from nevus is the absence of intralesional cysts on slit-lamp examination. Treatment for conjunctival melanoma includes surgical removal with clear margins plus cryotherapy and/or radiotherapy, with topical chemotherapy for diffuse disease and exenteration if there is orbital invasion. Melanoma can arise from primary acquired melanosis in up to 40% of cases, from nevi in 30% or de novo in 30% of cases [5] (Figs. 10.6 and 10.7).

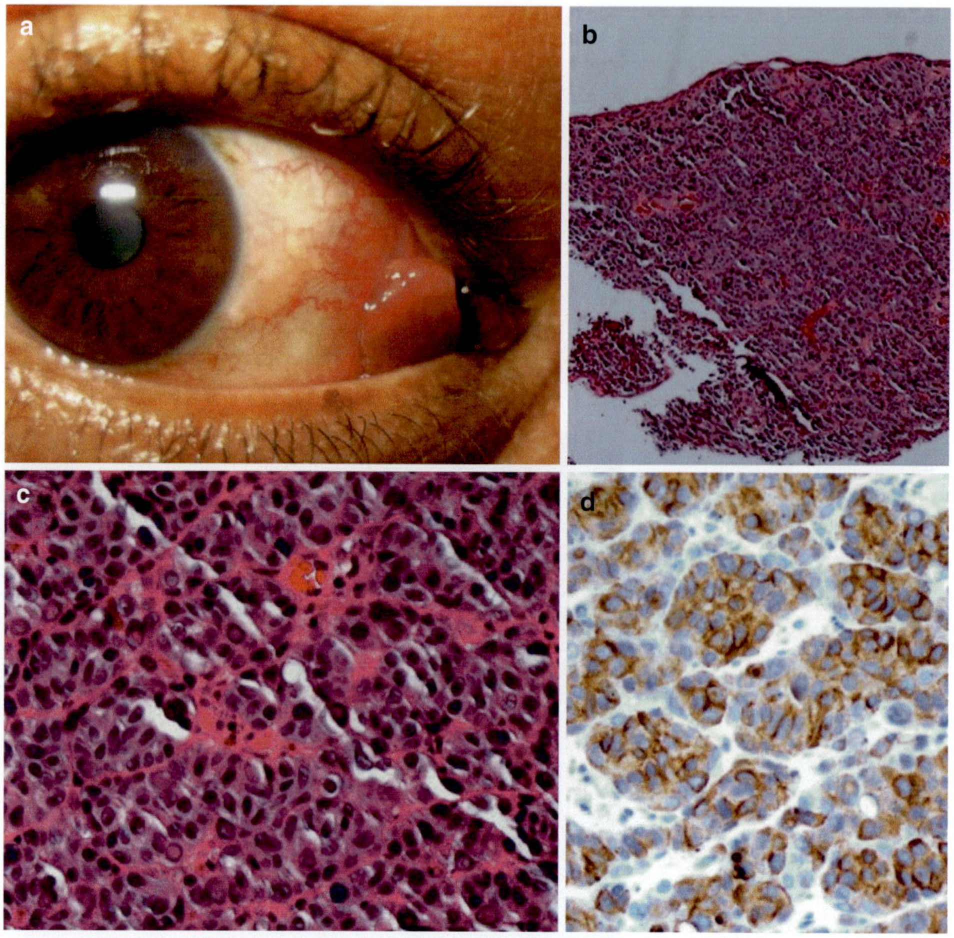

Fig. 10.7 Caruncle melanoma. (**a**) Exophytic, fleshy lesion originating from the caruncle (clinical photograph). (**b**) Tumor composed of sheets of spindle and epithelioid cells with a moderate amount of eosinophilic cytoplasm (H&E stain, 25×). (**c**) Higher magnification showing cells with spindle-shaped and round nuclei with prominent nucleoli. There are also epithelioid cells and occasional mitotic Figs. (100×). (**d**) Caruncle melanoma: positive staining for HMB-45 immunostain in tumor cells (HMB-45 immunostain, 100×)

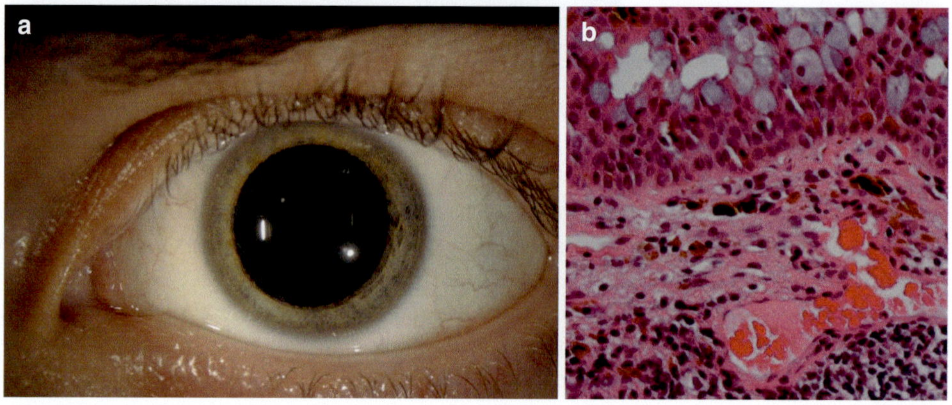

Fig. 10.8 Chronic inflammation with secondary pigmentation. (**a**) Mild redness of caruncle and plica. (**b**) Cellular infiltrate with reactive vascular channels and secondary pigmentation (H&E stain, 100×)

10.4 Inflammatory Lesions

Most inflammatory lesions of the caruncle have been reported as unspecified nongranulomatous chronic inflammation [8, 9]. Other reported inflammatory lesions include foreign body granuloma, abscess, folliculitis, actinomycosis, inflammatory pseudotumor, ocular cicatricial pemphigoid, cytomegalovirus infection, *molluscum contagiosum*, and spherocytosis (Fig. 10.8).

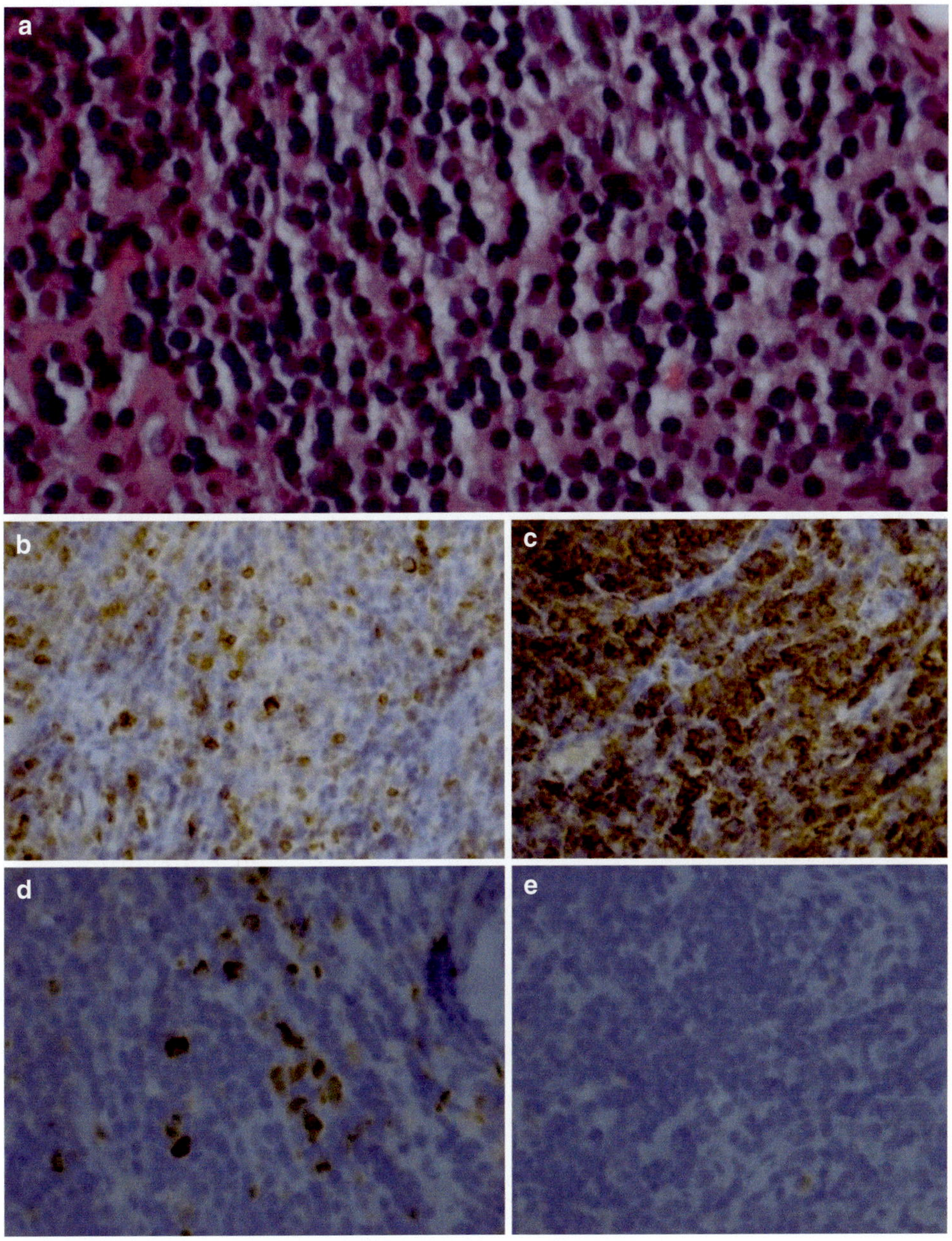

Fig. 10.9 Marginal zone B-cell (MALT type) lymphoma. (**a**) Lymphocytic infiltrate in the substantia propria, composed of small, round lymphocytes and occasional plasma cells (H&E stain, 150×). (**b**) CD3-positive staining in lymphocytes (CD3 immunostain, 100×). (**c**) CD20-positive staining in many lymphocytes (CD20 immunostain, 100×). (**d**) Kappa light chain-positive staining in scattered CD20 positive lymphocytes (Kappa light chain immunostain, 150×). (**e**) Lambda light chain-positive staining is negative (lambda light chain immunostain, 150×)

10.5 Lymphoproliferative Tumors

Reactive lymphoid hyperplasia is the most common lymphoproliferative disorder affecting the caruncle, accounting for up to 3% of all caruncular lesions [9, 10]. A few caruncular lymphomas have been reported in the different series, of which low-grade B-cell lymphoma (MALT) was the most common. The clinical presentation of a salmon-colored mass on the caruncle should raise suspicion of a lymphoproliferative disorder. Incisional biopsy is recommended (Fig. 10.9).

10.6 Vascular Tumors

10.6.1 Capillary Hemangioma

A case report on capillary hemangioma of the caruncle by Ozdal reported three patients who developed a rapidly growing mass arising in the caruncle, without history of surgery or trauma, and all three lesions were nodular, lobulated and ulcerated, and excised because malignancy was suspected [20]. Histologically, capillary hemangiomas are composed by lobules of small, thin, and irregular vessels lined by a

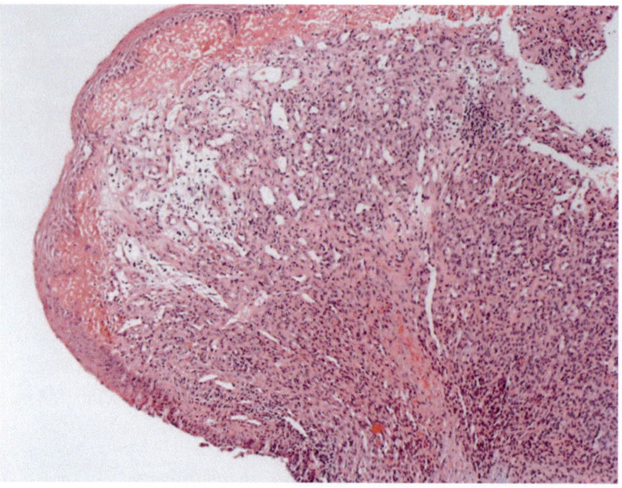

Fig. 10.10 Capillary hemangioma: small and irregular vessels lined by a single row of endothelial cells with surrounding fibrous septa (25×)

single layer of flattened, mature endothelial cells separated by thin fibrous septa (Fig. 10.10).

References

1. Spencer W. Ophthalmic pathology: an atlas and textbook, vol. 1. 4th ed. Saunders: Philadelphia; 1996.
2. Kathuria SS, Howarth D, Hurwitz JJ, Oestreicher J. An anatomic and histologic study of the caruncle. Ophthalmic Plast Reconstr Surg. 1999;15(6):407–11.
3. Mori M. The structure of the caruncula lacrimalis of Japanese. Okajimas Folia Anat Jpn. 1965;41(5):277–83.
4. Kaeser PF, Uffer S, Zografos L, Hamédani M. Tumors of the caruncle: a clinicopathologic correlation. Am J Ophthalmol. 2006;142(3):448–55.
5. Luthra CL, Doxanas MT, Green WR. Lesions of the caruncle: a clinicohistopathologic study. Surv Ophthalmol. 1978;23(3):183–95.
6. Santos A, Gómez-Leal A. Lesions of the lacrimal caruncle. Clinicopathologic features. Ophthalmology. 1994;101(5):943–9.
7. Shields CL, Shields JA, White D, Augsburger JJ. Types and frequency of lesions of the caruncle. Am J Ophthalmol. 1986;102(6):771–8.
8. Levy J, Ilsar M, Deckel Y, Maly A, Pe'er J. Lesions of the caruncle: a description of 42 cases and a review of the literature. Eye (Lond). 2009;23(5):1004–18.
9. Ostergaard J, Prause J, Heegard S. Caruncular lesions in Denmark 1978–2002: a histopathological study with correlation to clinical referral diagnosis. Acta Ophthalmol Scand. 2006;84:130–6.
10. Solari HP, Ventura MP, Orellana ME, Novais GA, Cheema DP, Burnier MN Jr. Histopathological study of lesions of the caruncle: a 15-year single center review. Diagn Pathol. 2009;4:29.
11. Graefes Von A. Geschwulste der Tranenkarunkel. Arch Ophthalmol. 1854;1:289–91.
12. Sjö NC, Heegaard S, Prause JU, Buchwald C, von Lindeberg H. Human papillomavirus in conjunctival papilloma. Br J Ophthalmol. 2001;85(7):785–7.
13. Eagle R. Eye pathology and atlas and text. 2nd ed. Lippincot Willims and Wilkins/Wolters Kluwer: Philladelphia; 2011.
14. Ogawa M, Shinzawa M, Dogru M, Miyauchi J, Tanaka Y, Ogawa Y, Obata H, Tsubota K, Shimazaki J. Caruncular and pericaruncular sebaceous gland hyperplasia: a report of 2 cases and literature review. Eye Contact Lens. 2016;44(Suppl 1):S316–9.
15. Kapil JP, Proia AD, Puri PK. Lesions of the lacrimal caruncle with an emphasis on oncocytoma. Am J Dermatopathol. 2011;33(3):227–35.
16. Shields JA, Shields CL, Marr BP, Eagle RC Jr. Sebaceous carcinoma of the caruncle. Cornea. 2006;25(7):858–9.
17. Pfeiffer ML, Yin VT, Myers J, Esmaeli B. Regional nodal recurrence of sebaceous carcinoma of the caruncle 11 years after primary tumor resection. JAMA Ophthalmol. 2013;131(8):1091–2.
18. Ugurlu S, Ekin MA, Altinboga AA. Primary basal cell carcinoma of the caruncle: case report and review of the literature. Ophthalmic Plast Reconstr Surg. 2014;30(3):e62–4.
19. Shields CL, Fasiuddin AF, Mashayekhi A, Shields JA. Conjunctival nevi: clinical features and natural course in 410 consecutive patients. Arch Ophthalmol. 2004;122(2):167–75.
20. Ozdal PC, Kargi S, Göka S, Callejo SA, Hucumenoglu S, Burnier MN Jr. Capillary hemangioma of the caruncle. Can J Ophthalmol. 2004;39(5):560–2.

Conjunctival Tumors in Children

11

Jacob Pe'er and Shahar Frenkel

11.1 Introduction

The conjunctiva is a translucent vascularized mucous membrane composed of many histological elements that form the epithelium and stroma and can be the origin of many types of tumors. The entire conjunctiva is external tissue, and because of its exposure, most of the conjunctival tumors are diagnosed early.

Conjunctival lesions can be classified into epithelial tumors, melanocytic tumors, and stromal tumors. Two other classes exist: developmental (hamartomas and choristomas) and lesions of the caruncular area, which is a mixture between conjunctival and skin. Metastatic and secondary tumors are rare.

Conjunctival lesions in children are nearly always benign [1–3]. Shields et al. [3] found that 97% of conjunctival lesions in children are benign, but being a series of a tertiary referral center, this is probably an underestimation. The rare malignant conjunctival tumors in children are usually larger and appear in older age. Children with xeroderma pigmentosum are a unique group in whom malignant conjunctival tumors can appear at an early age [4].

In this chapter, we describe conjunctival lesions in children according to their tissue of origin.

11.2 Benign Epithelial Lesions

11.2.1 Squamous Papilloma

Conjunctival squamous papillomas in children are commonly associated with papillomavirus, mostly types 6, 11, and 16 [5–7]. They appear as sessile or pedunculated pink/red lesions with an irregular surface (Fig. 11.1). Usually, these are solitary lesions, but they can be bilateral and multiple and may become confluent (Table 11.1).

These lesions are often asymptomatic. However, when large and more pedunculated, they can be symptomatic and may cause foreign body sensation, mucous secretion, hemorrhagic tears, and incomplete eyelid closure.

Histologically, the squamous papilloma of childhood is composed of epithelial projections covered by non-keratinized acanthotic stratified squamous epithelium, which may have goblet cells and have a fibrovascular core in which acute and chronic inflammatory cells are often found. Papillomavirus of various types can be demonstrated by immunohistochemical and molecular techniques.

In many cases, treatment is not needed, and observation is the practice, but when needed, complete surgical excision is performed. Such papillomas can be treated also by cryotherapy with or without excision. Recurrence is common, mainly when multiple lesions are caused by papillomavirus. Such lesions may be treated by adjuvant interferon α2b (IFNa2b) [8, 9], locally or systemically, topical mitomycin C [10], or oral cimetidine [11].

11.2.2 Conjunctival Epithelial Cysts

Conjunctival cysts are common and may be congenital or acquired. The acquired ones are more common and are mostly epithelial inclusions cysts (Fig. 11.2) that can occur spontaneously or following surgical and nonsurgical trauma [12].

The conjunctival cyst is a smooth translucent lesion that contains clear or turbid fluid and sometimes can show a "pseudohypopyon"-like layer. In dark-skinned patients, the cyst can be pigmented.

Histologically, the epithelial inclusion cyst is lined by conjunctival epithelium. The lumen can be clear, or it can contain mucinous material, epithelial debris, or keratin. Ductal cysts are lined by two layers of epithelium, usually of the apocrine type, and may contain PAS-positive material (Fig. 11.3).

J. Pe'er (✉) · S. Frenkel
Ocular Oncology Service and Ophthalmic Pathology Laboratory, Department of Ophthalmology, Hadassah—Hebrew University Medical Center, Jerusalem, Israel
e-mail: peer@hadassah.org.il

© The Author(s), under exclusive license to Springer Nature Switzerland AG 2024
J. Pe'er et al. (eds.), *Clinical Ophthalmic Oncology*, https://doi.org/10.1007/978-3-031-72443-5_11

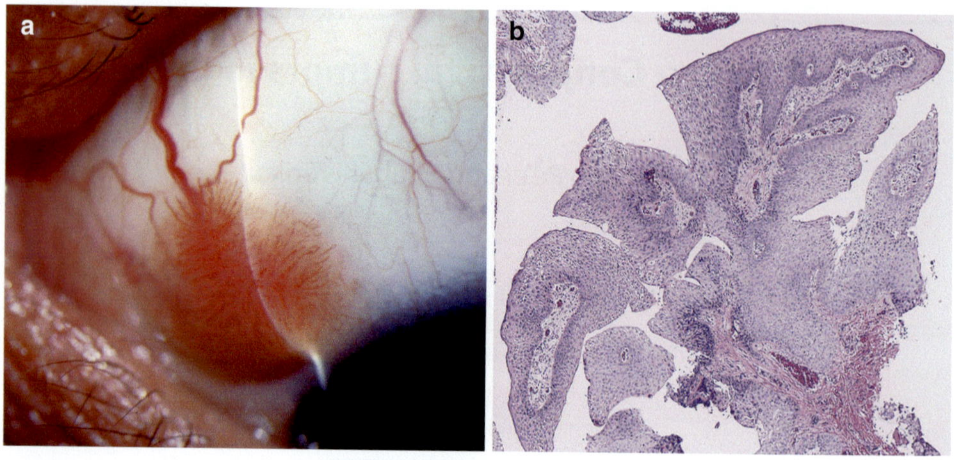

Fig. 11.1 *Solitary sessile squamous papilloma* of the bulbar conjunctiva. Clinical appearance (**a**). Histopathology shows papillomatous fronds of acanthotic nonkeratinized squamous epithelium with central fibrovascular cores (**b** hematoxylin and eosin, original magnification ×4)

Table 11.1 Conjunctival lesions in children

Epithelial lesions
Squamous papilloma
Epithelial cysts
(Squamous cell carcinoma)
Melanocytic lesions
Junctional nevus
Compound nevus
Inflamed juvenile conjunctival nevus
Complexion-related melanosis
Congenital ocular melanosis
(Malignant melanoma)
Stromal lesions
Vascular lesions
Pyogenic granuloma
Capillary hemangioma
Cavernous hemangioma
Racemose hemangioma
Varix
Lymphangioma
Lymphangiectasia
Fibrous lesions
Benign fibrous histiocytoma
Neural lesions
Neurofibroma
Neurilemoma (schwannoma)
Histiocytic lesions
Juvenile xanthogranuloma
Myogenic lesions
Rhabdomyosarcoma
Lipomatous lesions
Herniated orbital fat
Lymphoproliferative lesions
Benign reactive lymphoid hyperplasia
Lymphoma
Leukemic infiltrates (AML)
Choristomas
Dermoid
Dermolipoma
Oseous choristoma
Lacrimal gland choristoma
Complex choristoma
Caruncular lesions
of conjunctival tissue origin
of epidermic and skin appendages origin
Xeroderma pigmentosum

If asymptomatic, such cysts can be observed and be excised if enlarged and symptomatic. In many cases, over a long-term follow-up, the cyst eventually undergoes spontaneous resolution.

11.2.3 Pre-malignant and Malignant Epithelial Lesions

Conjunctival intraepithelial neoplasia and squamous cell carcinoma are very rare in children [1–3]. It happens more frequently in young patients with xeroderma pigmentosum (XP) [4]. Conjunctival tumors in XP are discussed separately.

11.3 Benign Melanocytic Lesions

Most benign melanocytic conjunctival lesions are nevi. Primary acquired melanosis (PAM), typical and atypical, is seen only in adulthood. Complexion-related melanosis is found in the more pigmented races. In congenital melanosis, the pigmentation, usually bluish, is in the sclera and not in the conjunctiva (Fig. 11.4).

11.3.1 Conjunctival Nevi

Conjunctival nevi are the most common conjunctival lesions in children and are commonly seen in the bulbar conjunctiva, plica semilunaris, and the caruncle [1–3]. Practically, they do not exist on the palpebral conjunctiva, and if they appear, they should be suspected of malignancy. They rarely encroach upon the cornea.

Nevi that appear in birth or within the first 6 months of life are considered by many experts to be congenital nevi, and those that appear more than 6 months after birth are considered to be acquired. Most acquired conjunctival nevi appear during the first two decades of life. Conjunctival nevi can be classified histologically into junctional, com-

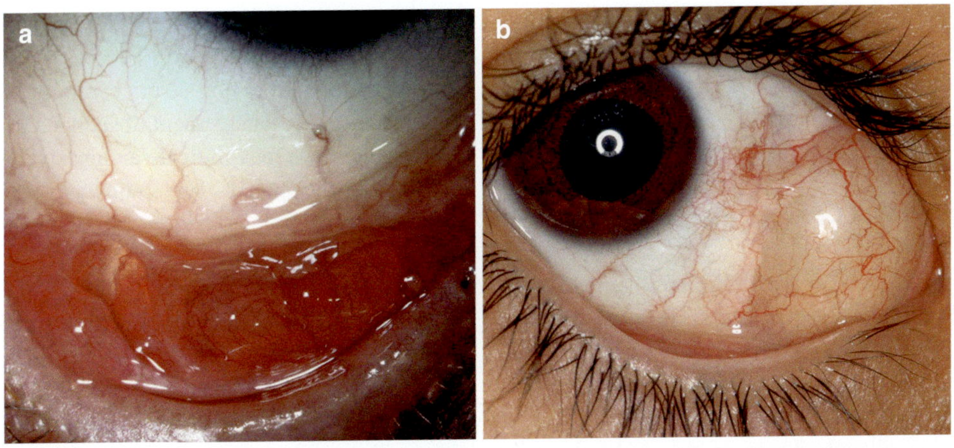

Fig. 11.2 Epithelial inclusion cyst. Multiple cysts in the inferior fornix (**a**). A large conjunctival cyst in the nasal bulbar conjunctiva that occurred after strabismus surgery (**b**)

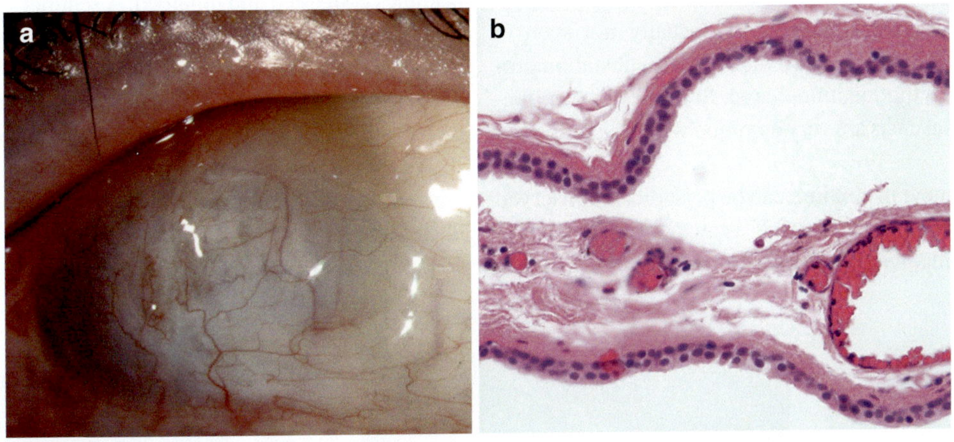

Fig. 11.3 Ductal cyst. Bluish cyst in the temporal bulbar conjunctiva. Posterior margin of the cyst cannot be visualized (**a**). The cyst lined by two cell layers, with luminal cells showing apical snouts, consistent with apocrine differentiation. The double cell lining is consistent with a ductal-type cyst, possibly from an accessory lacrimal gland. Apocrine differentiation may be metaplastic (**b**. hematoxylin and eosin stain, 40× magnification). (Reprinted with permission from Bryn Mawr Communications. Aponte EP, Schoenfield L, Stern RM, Singh AD. A ductal cyst of lacrimal origin. Adv Ocul Care. 2010:29–30)

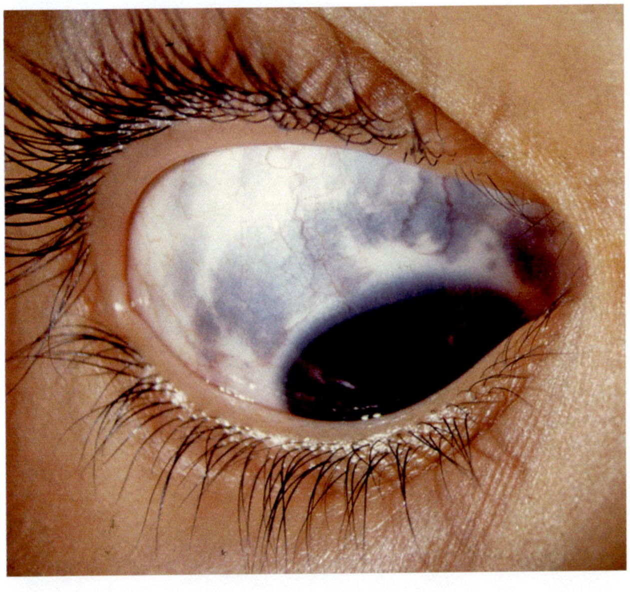

Fig. 11.4 *Congenital melanosis oculi* with gray-blue pigmentation of the sclera

pound, and subepithelial nevi; the later ones are rare in children. In childhood and adolescence, conjunctival nevi may be more pink and congested due to inflammatory infiltration. These inflamed nevi are discussed separately. The overall risk for malignant transformation during childhood is very low [1–3].

11.3.2 Conjunctival Junctional Nevus

Junctional conjunctival nevus is typically diagnosed in children or young adolescents. They may wrongly be misdiagnosed as PAM, which is usually diagnosed in adults. They are located typically in the interpalpebral bulbar, common in the juxtalimbal conjunctiva, and rarely involve the cornea.

Clinically, these are focal, flat, well-circumscribed lesions moving freely over the ocular surface. Epithelial cysts may or may not be detectable.

Histopathologically, one can find the intraepithelial proliferation of nevus cells anterior to the epithelial basement membrane, which is generally intact. The epithelium over it may be thin.

11.3.3 Conjunctival Compound Nevus

Compound conjunctival nevi are well-circumscribed, variably pigmented, slightly elevated sessile lesions, which in most cases contain cystic structures (Fig. 11.5). They may vary in size from tiny lesions to ones that occupy large parts of the bulbar conjunctiva. Nevi may become darker or lighter but usually will not change in size and color after adolescence.

Histologically, the compound nevus represents an intermediate stage between the early junctional and late subepithelial nevus stages; the latter one is usually not seen in children. Nests of nevus cells are found in the substantia propria in addition to the junctional area. Solid nests of epithelium and epithelial cysts are very common within a compound nevus.

Conjunctival nevi in children can be periodically observed with photographic comparison. If growth or recent color change is documented, local excision of the entire lesion should be considered. Sometimes, excision for cosmetic reasons is desired. If the lesion adheres to the sclera, a thin lamella of the underlying sclera can be removed. This is in contrast with the management of such occurrences in adults, where adherence may indicate an invasive malignant lesion, indicating the need for adjuvant therapy such as brachytherapy.

11.3.4 Inflamed Juvenile Conjunctival Nevus

Inflamed juvenile conjunctival nevus (IJCN) is a compound nevus that appears only in children and adolescents, most of them with symptomatic or asymptomatic allergic conjunctivitis (Fig. 11.6). Most lesions are amelanotic, and about 25% show pigmentation. It may be worrisome when it grows quickly and becomes congested and inflamed. A sentinel vessel is common [13]. More so than other types of conjunctival nevi, IJCNs have a higher tendency to change their size and color and may become more or less pigmented or more or less pink depending on the activity of the inflammatory allergic process.

Histologically, it is a compound nevus with marked chronic inflammation. Eosinophils are common. Architectural disorder is often seen but with no atypical cells [14, 15]. Increased expression of nerve growth factor (NGF),

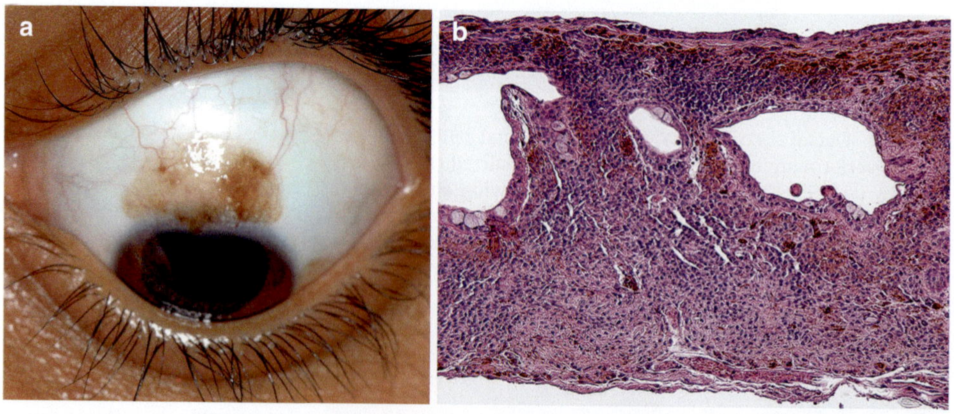

Fig. 11.5 A typical partially pigmented *compound conjunctival nevus* with cystic elements in an atypical location in the upper bulbar conjunctiva at the limbus (**a**). Histopathology of a compound nevus of the conjunctiva with cystic structures lined by conjunctival epithelium (**b**. hematoxylin and eosin, original magnification ×10)

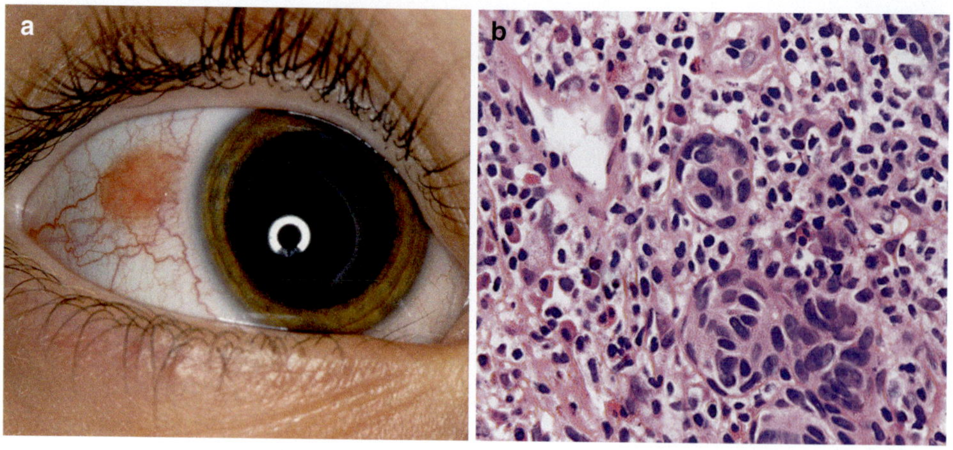

Fig. 11.6 *Amelanotic inflamed juvenile conjunctival nevus* in the temporal conjunctiva with cystic elements and dilated vessels around it. (**a**) Histopathology showing nevus nests with marked chronic inflammation around them and a remarkable number of eosinophils (**b**. hematoxylin and eosin, original magnification ×40)

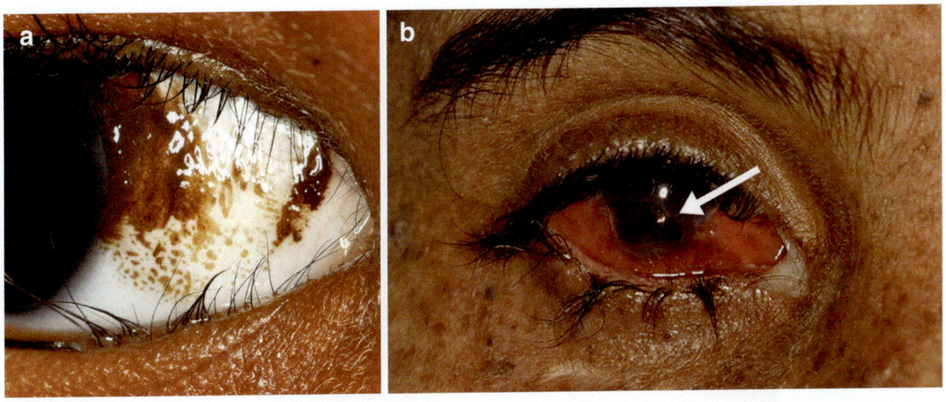

Fig. 11.7 Conjunctival melanoma. (**a**) A healthy 2-year-old girl with a dark complexion had a pigmented conjunctival lesion since birth that started growing at the age of 6 months. It took over a year to reach a specialist. By this time, the melanoma had grown over the limbus. (**b**) A 10-year-old girl with xeroderma pigmentosa (XP) was noticed to have a dark pigmented mass over her inferior limbus (arrow). The lesion could be scraped over the cornea, without involvement underneath Bowman's layer but was invasive under the conjunctival epithelium

eosinophils, and mast cells in IJCN and modulation of eosinophils properties by lesion fibroblasts partly through NGF suggest a possible association between IJCN and allergic inflammation [16].

Since these are benign lesions, observation alone is recommended. If the lesion is growing over the limbus and becomes elevated, excision should be performed. Recurrence is not common.

11.3.5 Melanoma

Conjunctival melanoma in children (Fig. 11.7a) is very rare, and only case reports and small case series have been published [17, 18]. In a review of 40 years of the medical literature [17, 18], only 28 cases were found, and only 8 of them had adequate details. Conjunctival melanoma may appear at an earlier age in patients with xeroderma pigmentosum (Fig. 11.7b). Conjunctival melanoma in children may often be misdiagnosed. Due to its rarity in children, more common diagnoses should be considered in the work-up. However, any rapidly growing, vascularized mass that changes color should also be biopsied in children. Because of its rarity in children, the knowledge of the management and prognosis of this condition is very limited.

For clinical and histopathological features and treatment options of conjunctival melanoma, see Chap. 7.

11.4 Conjunctival Stromal Lesions

The conjunctival stroma contains various tissue elements, such as vascular, fibrous, neural, lymphatic, and others. However, conjunctival stromal lesions are rare, and, in children, they are almost always benign.

11.4.1 Vascular Lesions

Vascular tumors of the conjunctiva are uncommon, and, in children, they are always benign, although they may have a functional effect. The most common conjunctival vascular lesions are pyogenic granuloma, capillary hemangioma, and lymphangioma/lymphangiectasia [1–3, 19]

11.4.1.1 Pyogenic Granuloma

The term "pyogenic granuloma" is a misnomer since it is neither pyogenic nor granulomatous but a granulation tissue. Pyogenic granuloma is a fibrovascular response to tissue insults such as surgical or nonsurgical trauma or inflammation, although may be spontaneous. It is commonly seen after strabismus surgery, chalazion surgery, and excision of conjunctival lesions and in anophthalmic sockets after enucleation. It has been reported in every part of the conjunctiva [20].

Clinically, pyogenic granuloma appears as a fleshy, elevated, red, often pedunculated vascularized mass. Histologically, it is composed of granulation tissue with marked chronic inflammation with lymphocytes, plasma cells, and neutrophils and proliferation of small, mostly capillary-sized blood vessels (Fig. 11.8).

Pyogenic granuloma often responds to topical corticosteroids when diagnosed early, but, in many cases, surgical excision is required. In a recent report, conjunctival pyogenic granuloma showed complete resolution after treatment with topical timolol 0.5% [21].

11.4.1.2 Capillary Hemangioma

Conjunctival capillary hemangioma appears during early infancy, and, like in the skin, it may grow over several months and then regress spontaneously within several years. The hemangioma is a distinct or diffuse red, elevated conjunctival lesion

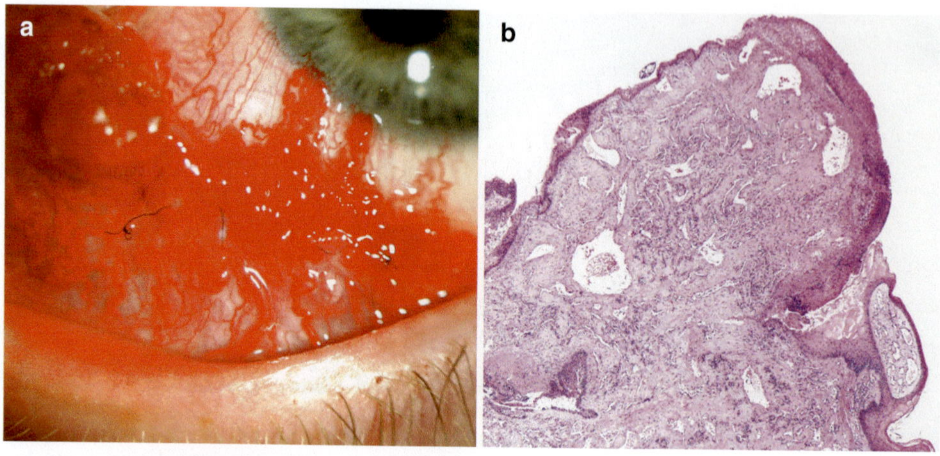

Fig. 11.8 Pyogenic granuloma (**a**) A rapidly growing recurrent conjunctival vascular growth in the infero-nasal conjunctival fornix. Note: prominent vascularity. (**b**) Polypoid lesion with a lobular pattern of capillary proliferation. The vessels are variably dilated (Original magnification ×4)

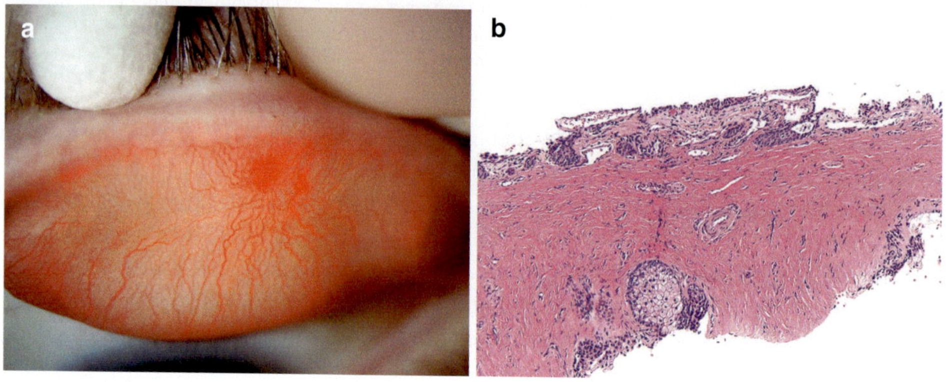

Fig. 11.9 Capillary hemangioma. (**a**) Color photograph of a circumscribed vascular conjunctival lesion overlying the upper tarsus. (**b**) On histopathology examination, the tarsal conjunctival stroma revealed numerous thin-walled capillary-type vessels, most of which contained red blood cells within their lumen (H&E ×10)

that can occur anywhere in the conjunctiva. It may be limited to the conjunctiva or in association with eyelid or orbital capillary hemangioma. Histologically, it shows numerous capillary channels and proliferation of endothelial cells [3, 19] (Fig. 11.9).

In most cases, no treatment is needed for conjunctival capillary hemangioma, and the child should only be observed. When the lesion is large and potentially amblyogenic, it should be treated. Local or systemic corticosteroids or surgical excision can be employed [3]. The experience in treating conjunctival capillary hemangioma by beta-blockers is still limited [22].

11.4.1.3 Cavernous Hemangioma

Cavernous hemangioma can appear clinically as a red or blue multiloculated lesion in the conjunctival stroma of children and adolescents. The lesion is usually isolated but may be associated with syndromes [19]. It may cause recurrent subconjunctival hemorrhage [23] (Fig. 11.10).

Histologically, it is composed of large blood-filled spaces lined by endothelial cells and separated by fibrous septa. It can be treated by surgical excision.

11.4.1.4 Varix and Racemose Hemangioma

These are rare vascular malformations of dilated blood channels in the conjunctival stroma [19].

A varix is a mass of venous channels that may be a single channel or complex venous channels; many of them are anterior extensions of the orbital varix. The color ranges from blue-red to black. These lesions are usually

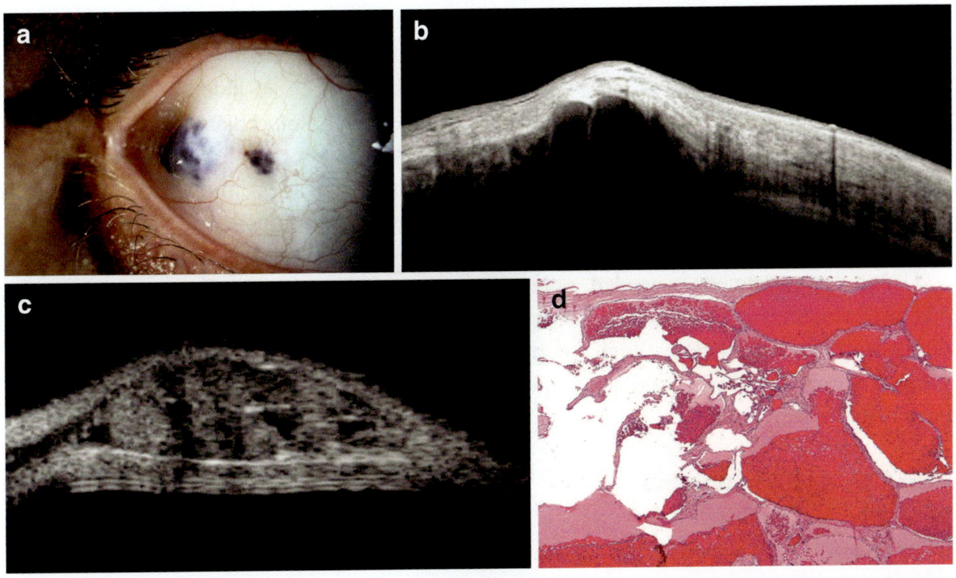

Fig. 11.10 Cavernous hemangioma. (**a**) A clustered "grape-like" lesions involving the temporal conjunctiva was observed on slit-lamp examination. (**b**) On OCT, there were clear spaces located in the subepithelial layer of the conjunctiva. (**c**) Ultrasonography showed two well-defined lesions with many low reflective intrinsic cystic-like pockets. (**d**) Large, well-circumscribed vascular proliferation of thin-walled veins that completely replaced the conjunctival stroma (H&E ×4). Most of the lumina were engorged with blood

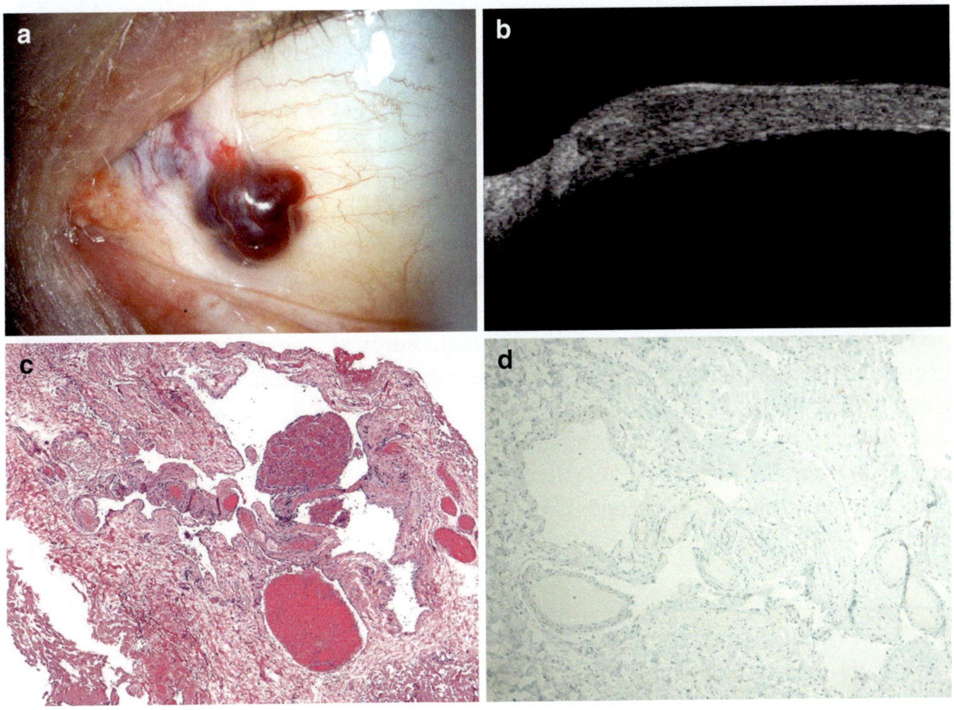

Fig. 11.11 Racemose hemangioma. (**a**) A multilobulated vascular lesion was identified in the medial canthal region that was extending posteriorly along the anterior margin of the caruncle. (**b**) The lesion consisted of highly reflective portions with well-defined, low-reflective channels on ultrasonography. (**c**) Vascular proliferation composed of a mixture of thick-walled arteries and thin-walled veins within a fibrotic conjunctival stroma (H&E, ×4). (**d**) The endothelial cells were negative for lymphatic marker D2–40 (×10)

movable over the sclera, and thrombosis is frequent. When asymptomatic, varix can be observed, but if symptomatic, surgical excision should be considered, bearing in mind prolonged bleeding.

Conjunctival racemose hemangioma is a lesion of dilated arteries and veins communicating directly without capillaries between them (Fig. 11.11). It appears as a loop of dilated vessels. It should be managed by observation. Wybrun-Mason syndrome should be ruled out in such cases.

11.4.1.5 Lymphangiectasia

This is a phenomenon of dilated and prominent lymphatic conjunctival channels that can be unilateral or bilateral with focal or diffuse bulbar chemosis. Conjunctival lymphangiectasia can occur spontaneously, after trauma or inflammation, or with systemic disease [24]. When filled with blood, they are termed "hemorrhagic lymphangiectasia" [25]. Subconjunctival hemorrhage may occur. Congenital cases have been reported.

Histologically, the lesion shows marked dilated lymphatics, which may be filled with blood. The phenomenon is intermittent, with a resolution of the channels' congestion and the chemosis between episodes.

Usually, no treatment is needed, although various methods of treatment, such as surgical excision and treatment by liquid nitrogen cryotherapy, high-frequency wave electro surgery, surgical drainage, and subconjunctival injection of bevacizumab were reported [24, 26–29].

11.4.1.6 Lymphangioma

Conjunctival lymphangioma is a benign lesion of lymphatic vessels that usually appears in the first decade of life. It can occur as an isolated conjunctival lesion, but it often represents an anterior component of an orbital lymphangioma [19].

It appears as a multiloculated lesion composed of dilated cystic spaces containing either clear fluid or blood ("chocolate cysts"). The spaces may be congested and dilated following inflammation in the surrounding area. When the orbital part is congested, the eye may become proptotic. Histologically, it shows dilated lymphatic channels filled with lymph and/or blood, lined by endothelium, and separated by thin septa.

The treatment of lymphangioma is difficult. Surgical excision and radiotherapy do not eradicate the lesions. Carbon dioxide laser, brachytherapy, and drainage with sclerotherapy have been used with partial success. When orbital pressure is raised and threatens the optic nerve, percutaneous drainage of blood may offer temporary relief [30–34].

11.5 Fibrous Lesions

Fibrous lesions of the conjunctiva are very rare in children; most of them were reported as case reports or small case series.

11.5.1 Fibrous Histiocytoma

Among known fibrous lesions of the conjunctiva, only fibrous histiocytomas (FH) were reported in children, most of them of the benign type [35–38], but a case of malignant FH was described in a child with xeroderma pigmentosum [39].

Clinically, conjunctival FH appears as an amelanotic mass that can range from a well-circumscribed to diffuse mass, often in the limbal area.

Histopathologically, FH shows a mixture of spindle-shaped fibroblasts, often arranged in a storiform pattern and lipid-laden histiocytes. Malignant FH shows marked pleomorphism, many mitotic figures, and multinucleated giant cells.

Benign FH can be treated by complete surgical excision alone. Since malignant FH can metastasize to regional lymph nodes and hematogenously to distant organs, it should be treated by radical surgery that may include exenteration and radical dissection of regional lymph nodes.

11.6 Neural Lesions

11.6.1 Neurofibroma

Conjunctival neurofibromas are rare and only a few such cases were reported in children [1, 2]. These are peripheral nerve sheath tumors that can occur as a solitary circumscribed or as a diffuse lesion; the latter is usually associated with neurofibromatosis type 1.

Clinically, it appears as an amelanotic translucent gelatinous mass. Histopathologically, neurofibroma demonstrates benign proliferation of Schwann cells, axons, and endoneurial fibroblasts, which may be difficult to differentiate from other spindle cell tumors.

Solitary tumors can be treated by complete surgical excision. However, plexiform neurofibroma may be difficult to excise completely.

11.6.2 Neurilemmoma (Schwannoma)

Neurilemmoma of the conjunctiva is a benign rare tumor that can arise from any part of the conjunctiva—bulbar, forniceal, or palpebral [40]. They are very rare in children [41, 42].

Clinically, it appears as a pink-yellow elevated conjunctival mass. Histopathologically, the tumor is the result of the proliferation of Schwann cells of a peripheral nerve sheath and is composed of spindle cells that may be arranged in an Antoni A or Antoni B pattern.

Conjunctival neurilemmoma is treated by complete excision within the tumor capsule. Incomplete excision may lead to recurrence. Malignant neurilemmoma has not been reported in the conjunctiva.

11.7 Histiocytic Lesions

Among histiocytic lesions in the conjunctiva, only juvenile xanthogranuloma is found in children.

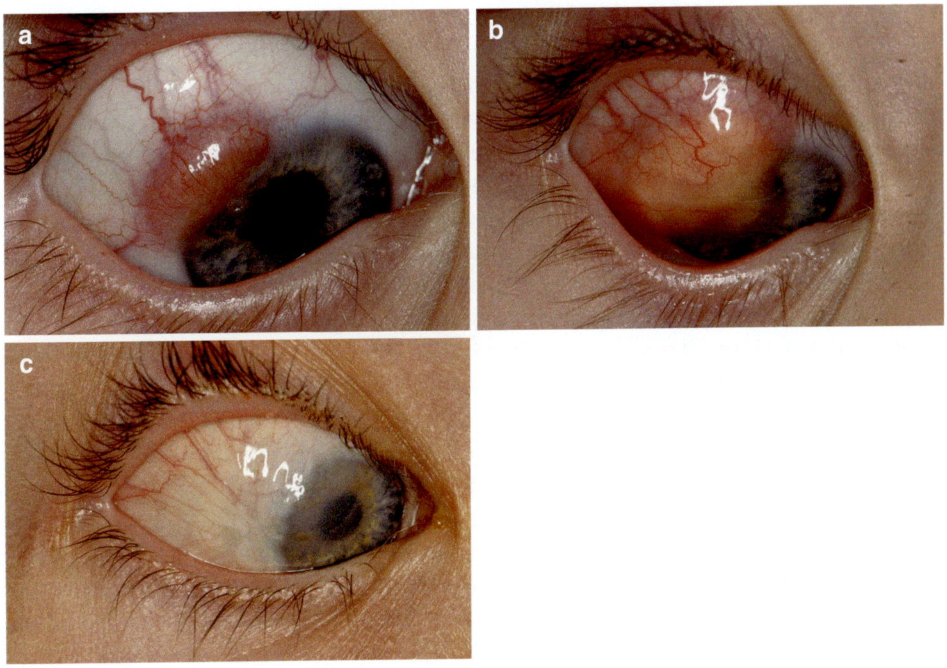

Fig. 11.12 Juvenile xanthogranuloma (JXG). (**a**) After a minor trauma, a 5-year-old boy was noted to have a reddish limbal lesion that did not respond to 3 weeks of topical steroids. An incisional biopsy was suspicious of JXG. (**b**) The lesion grew rapidly over the next 4 months, sprouting vessels toward the center of the cornea causing edema and a reduction in the visual acuity. The lesion was excised and immediately treated with Ru-106 plaque brachytherapy. (**c**) Ten years later, there was no sign of recurrence

11.7.1 Juvenile Xanthogranuloma

Juvenile xanthogranuloma (JXG) is a systemic, mostly cutaneous, disease that is generally present in young children. Conjunctival involvement occurs as a solitary orange-pink stromal mass, usually near the limbus (Fig. 11.12) [43, 44]. Sometimes, associated systemic findings may not be present.

Histologically, the lesions show typical findings of histiocytes and Touton giant cells. Lymphocytes, plasma cells, and eosinophils can also be found. Immunohistochemical staining is positive for CD68 (histiocytic marker) and negative for CD1a and S-100 (Langerhans cell markers) [45].

When xanthogranuloma is suspected clinically, it may be observed for spontaneous resolution. However, most lesions in the conjunctiva are treated by excision or can be treated by topical or systemic corticosteroids. In resistant cases, brachytherapy has been successfully applied.

11.8 Myogenic Lesions

Myogenic conjunctival tumors in children are very rare.

11.8.1 Rhabdomyosarcoma

Rhabdomyosarcoma (RMS) is the most common primary orbital tumor in childhood. However, its occurrence in the conjunctiva alone is rare. RMS appears as a pink, rapidly growing conjunctival mass that presents as a non-inflamed pedicle of soft tissue, but occasionally swelling and erythema precede visible tumor formation [46].

Histopathologically, most conjunctival RMS are of the embryonal type, and as a submucosal tumor, some call it "botryoid" RMS (sarcoma botryoides) [46, 47]. Prognosis used to rely on the histopathologic type of the tumor with the alveolar type having the worst prognosis. Recently, a molecular subclassification of these worse tumors identified alveolar RMS with fusion genes involving forkhead box protein O1 (FOXO1) to have a worse prognosis [48].

Complete surgical excision is recommended when this is possible without affecting ocular function. In most cases, the treatment includes chemotherapy and radiotherapy.

Other myogenic tumors of the conjunctiva were reported, although mainly in adults [49].

11.9 Lipomatous Lesions

Lipomatous tumors of the conjunctiva are very rare, and lipoma, liposarcoma, and fibrolipoma occur mainly in adults, although were reported also in children [1–3]. On the other hand, herniated orbital fat under the conjunctiva is not rare and may be mistaken for a lipomatous tumor. Dermolipoma, commonly seen in children, is discussed later in this chapter.

11.10 Lymphoproliferative Lesions

Most conjunctival lymphoid tumors occur in adults, commonly manifested in individuals aged 60–70 years [50], but, although not common, occurrence in children and adolescents has also been reported [2, 3, 51, 52]. These lesions in children are usually limited to the conjunctiva and are low-grade, without association with systemic disease.

Lymphoproliferative tumors of the conjunctiva, benign and malignant, appear as elevated pink masses resembling smoked salmon. Hence, it is termed a "salmon patch." It may appear in any part of the conjunctiva but almost never in the palpebral conjunctiva. In children and adolescents, they often present in the nasal bulbar conjunctiva near or connected to the plica semilunaris [51]. It is not possible to differentiate clinically between a benign and a malignant lymphoid tumor; therefore, a biopsy is necessary to establish the diagnosis. Analysis of the biopsy always requires immunohistochemistry and often also a molecular analysis to differentiate between benign reactive lymphoid hyperplasia and lymphoma.

11.10.1 Benign Reactive Lymphoid Hyperplasia

Benign reactive lymphoid hyperplasia (BRLH) is the most common conjunctival lymphoproliferative lesion in children [2, 3, 51]. Although usually benign, it may rarely be a premalignant condition, leading to lymphoma. It presents clinically as a slowly progressive pink fleshy mass over the nasal bulbar conjunctiva, indistinguishable from lymphoma.

Histopathologically, sometimes it may be difficult to distinguish between BRLH and lymphoma. These lesions show subepithelial chronic inflammatory infiltrate arranged in follicles of B-cells (stained with anti-CD-20) surrounded by T-cells (CD3+) with no staining of malignant B-cells (CD43+). Molecular analysis for B-cell clonality shows a polyclonal B-cell population [51].

Since it is impossible to differentiate clinically between BRLH and lymphoma, the treatment is usually complete surgical excision. No local recurrence has been documented. Such lesions may respond to topical anti-allergic drugs or corticosteroids without the need to excise them, also saving them general anesthesia [51]. Therefore, in this age group, it seems reasonable to carry out a treatment trial with topical treatment in the diagnosis process before taking the young patient to the operating room. Such a trial would not be harmful even if the lesion is a conjunctival lymphoma since a few weeks of delay of surgical excision of conjunctival lymphoma does not seem to cause clinically significant tumor growth or dissemination in any age group, especially in the young age group where it is usually a low-grade lymphoma.

11.10.2 Lymphoma

Conjunctival lymphomas belong to the group of ocular adnexal lymphomas, which are defined as lymphomas originating from the ocular adnexa—the eyelids, conjunctiva, orbit, lacrimal gland, and lacrimal sac.

Conjunctival lymphoma is rare in children. The vast majority of conjunctival lymphomas are non-Hodgkin's B-cell lymphoma of the extranodal marginal zone B cell lymphoma of mucosa-associated lymphoid tissue—EMZL type, also termed "MALT lymphoma." These are low-grade lymphoma of B-cell type, usually involving only the conjunctiva, without extension to neighboring tissues. T-cell lymphoma is extremely rare in the conjunctiva.

Histopathologically, the findings are similar to BRLH, and it may be difficult to distinguish between them. Polymerase chain reaction (PCR) testing of immune globulin heavy chain (IgH) gene rearrangement is helpful, showing monoclonality in most of these cases.

Since the MALT lymphoma of the conjunctiva is usually a local low-grade type of lymphoma, especially in children, surgical excision may be curative with no recurrence. Systemic evaluation should be considered, although systemic involvement is very rare in the young age group. Systemic chemotherapy, intravenous or local anti-CD20 monoclonal antibody (rituximab), interferon alpha (IFNa) injections, or external or local radiation, which are applied in conjunctival lymphoma in adults, is usually not needed in children and adolescents.

11.10.2.1 Pediatric-Type Follicular Lymphoma

In recent years, cases of conjunctival "pediatric-type follicular lymphoma" have been reported [53–55]. This is an uncommon type of B-cell lymphoma, which primarily involves the lymph nodes of the head and neck of children and young adults, all males. Ocular involvement is rare, and only a few cases were documented, all occurring in the conjunctiva (Fig. 11.13).

These tumors are clinically similar to EMZL lymphoma; both behave as low-grade lymphoma but have distinct histo-

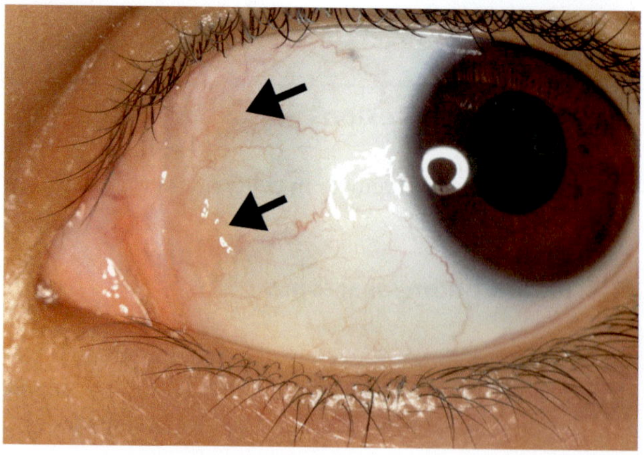

Fig. 11.13 Conjunctival lymphoma. An 8-year-old boy had a semi-transparent pink conjunctival lesion irresponsive to topical steroids. An incisional biopsy reveals a B cell follicular lymphoma grade 3A

logical and molecular features. In one case series [55], Lee et al. found overlapping morphological features of these two types of lymphomas. Hence, they were classified as a "mixed type." They suggested the possibility that pediatric-type follicular lymphoma and pediatric marginal zone lymphoma are single-entity pediatric B-cell lymphoma with a broad morphological spectrum.

11.10.3 Leukemic Infiltrates

Acute lymphoblastic leukemia (ALL) is the most common malignancy in children, and ocular manifestations of leukemia are well known [2, 3]. Conjunctival masses were reported as the presentation of acute lymphoblastic leukemia relapse in children [56–59]. It may indicate a poor prognosis.

Conjunctival involvement in leukemia shows various clinical presentations, either as hemorrhages from associate anemia or thrombocytopenia or as leukemic infiltrates. It can involve one or both eyes and have focal or diffuse infiltration of the conjunctival substantia propria. It may appear in any part of the conjunctiva as a pink and smooth stromal mass, similar to a lymphoid tumor, often with areas of hemorrhage.

Granulocytic sarcoma (chloroma) may appear in the ocular adnexa in the course of acute myelogenous leukemia (AML) as a gray-green mass in the eyelid or the forniceal or tarsal conjunctiva [60].

Histopathological studies show that conjunctival leukemic lesions are cellular infiltrates in all levels of the substantia propria. They can be diffuse or patchy and are generally localized along blood vessels.

The treatment includes various combinations of chemotherapy with secondary resolution of the conjunctival infiltration. Local radiotherapy may be added sometimes. Usually, there is a good local response; however, many of the patients eventually die of the systemic disease.

11.11 Choristomas

Choristomas are congenital lesions representing normal tissue in an abnormal location. When the lesion is composed of one type of tissue, it is considered to be a simple choristoma. When the choristoma is composed of variable combinations of ectopic tissue, such as bone, cartilage, and lacrimal gland, it is termed "complex choristoma."

Choristomas are the most common epibulbar lesions in children. Among them, dermoids and dermolipomas are very common [1–3, 61]. Epibulbar choristomas may affect the cornea, limbus, or subconjunctival space and range from a small, flat lesion to large masses filling most of the epibulbar region. They can often cause astigmatism. Epibulbar choristomas can affect other parts of the eye and orbit and may be associated with coloboma, Goldenhar syndrome, or organoid nevus syndrome [61].

11.11.1 Dermoid

Epibulbar dermoid is the most common choristoma of the ocular surface [1–3]. It is a well-circumscribed, firm, solitary congenital mass that involves the bulbar conjunctiva, adhered to the sclera under it, and often involves the corneoscleral limbus (Fig. 11.14). Rarely more than one lesion is found.

Epibulbar dermoid is usually a solid yellow-white mass, often with fine white hair protruding from its surface. Typically, it occurs in the inferotemporal limbus. The size of

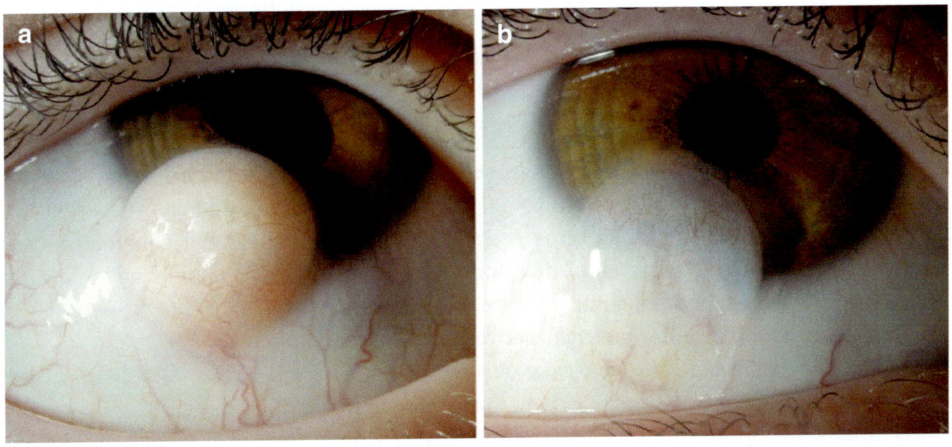

Fig. 11.14 *Limbal dermoid* in the lower temporal aspect of the cornea and conjunctiva. (**a**) Note hair growing from the middle of the lesion. (**b**) A residual corneal scar remains after surface excision

epibulbar dermoid is variable, from a more common small limbal dermoid through a large dermoid involving most or the entire corneal surface to extensive dermoids that involve the anterior chamber and iris. A grading system was suggested according to the scoring of the corneal area involved, surface shape and elevation, and area of conjunctival involvement [62]. Epibulbar dermoid, in addition to being cosmetically blemish, can cause severe astigmatism and amblyopia, affecting the vision according to the extent of corneal involvement.

Epibulbar dermoid can be associated with Goldenhar syndrome. In this syndrome, one can find, in addition to the epibulbar dermoid, preauricular skin appendages, eyelid coloboma, mandibular hypoplasia, vertebral anomalies, and hearing loss. It is also important to search for cardiovascular malformations, which have been reported in 5–58% of patients with Goldenhar syndrome. The most frequent is tetralogy of Fallot (TOF), followed by septal defects and situs inversus [63]. This syndrome is due to an abnormal development of first and second branchial arches derivatives during embryogenesis [64]. For more details, see Chap. 16.

Histopathologically, epibulbar dermoid is a simple choristoma that consists of dense fibrous tissue covered by stratified squamous epithelium. It usually contains dermal elements such as hair follicles, sebaceous glands, sweat glands, and sometimes adipose connective tissue.

When the epibulbar dermoid is small and visually asymptomatic, it can be managed by observation alone. When the dermoid is large, it can be managed by excision (lamellar keratosclerectomy) with or without a conjunctival flap in order to try to treat the astigmatism and/or amblyopia. Excision can leave an opaque or semi-opaque corneal scar. In advanced cases, usually with the involvement of the corneal center, lamellar or penetrating keratoplasty may be needed, sometimes with a staged technique, using amniotic membrane or limbal cell transplantation [65].

11.11.2 Dermolipoma

Epibulbar dermolipoma is a yellow-tan, soft, fusiform fluctuant mass, often with fine white hair on its surface, usually localized to the temporal or superotemporal aspect of the conjunctiva (Fig. 11.15). Although it is congenital, it may remain asymptomatic for years until detected when it protrudes from the superotemporal conjunctival fornix. Epibulbar dermolipoma often extends between the lateral rectus and superior rectus muscles to lie close to the lacrimal gland. They may extend posteriorly to the orbit or anteriorly toward the limbus. It should be differentiated from subconjunctival orbital fat prolapse, with the help of computed tomography (CT) and magnetic resonance (MR) imaging, which demonstrate that herniated fat is continuous with the intraconal orbital fat, while dermolipoma lies on the lateral wall of the globe without connection to the intraconal fat [66].

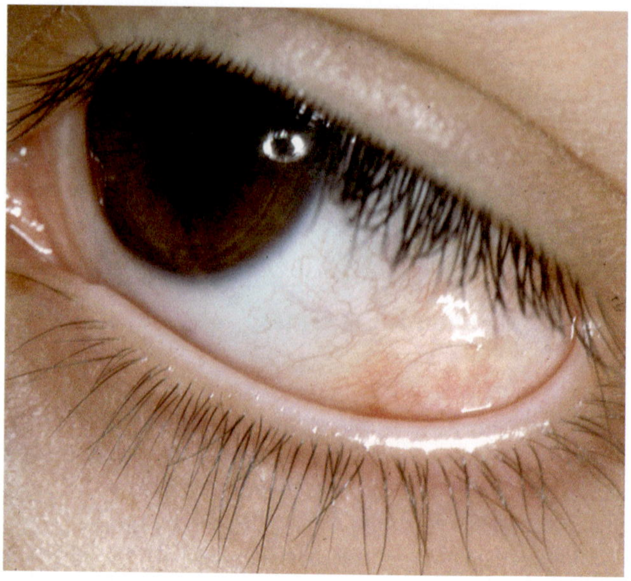

Fig. 11.15 *Dermolipoma* in the temporal part of the bulbar conjunctiva

Although epibulbar dermolipoma can be asymptomatic, the commonest symptom is the increasing size of a known peribulbar mass. Other symptoms are ocular irritation, episodic localized conjunctival injection, and mucoid discharge [67]. An examination may show, in some of the patients, lateral canthal widening, aberrant lacrimal gland ductules opening onto skin, and a complex lateral canthal anomaly, with both an external dermoid and an internal dermolipoma [67].

Histopathologically, the epithelium on the surface of the dermolipoma is stratified squamous epithelium that may be partially keratinized. The stroma contains variable quantities of dense collagenous tissue and a large amount of adipose tissue, mainly in the deeper aspects of the lesion. Pilosebaceous units and lacrimal gland tissue may be present.

The majority of the dermolipomas require no treatment, but when symptomatic or cosmetically blemished, it can be managed by excision of the entire lesion or by simple excision of the anterior portion of the lesion through a conjunctival forniceal approach. When the conjunctiva over the dermolipoma is adherent to the lesion and has to be excised, a rotational conjunctival flap or free conjunctival autograft have been applied to cover the conjunctival defect [68, 69].

11.11.3 Osseous Choristoma

Epibulbar osseous choristoma is a rare solitary firm congenital lesion that most typically presents as an isolated epibulbar lesion in the superotemporal quadrant, although it may occur in other locations on the surface of the globe. It may be associated with another epibulbar choristomatous lesion, such as dermolipoma and dermoid, but there are no related systemic syndromes [70, 71]. Bilateral lesions have been reported.

Although congenital, osseous choristoma typically remains undetectable until palpated by the patient who feels the hard lesion. It may appear pink or yellow or white in color, with a mean basal diameter of about 10 mm and a mean thickness of about 4 mm [70]. It may be freely movable or adherent to the bulbar conjunctiva and sclera or involves the extraocular muscle sheath. The diagnosis can be confirmed by ultrasonography or CT that demonstrates the calcifications. Usually, the lesion does not affect the visual acuity. It may cause foreign body sensation, ocular inflammation, and tearing [3, 70].

Histopathologically, osseous choristoma is composed of mature, compact bone surrounded by connective tissue. Occasionally, other choristomatous elements may be found.

The lesion can be managed by periodic observation, but if symptomatic or cosmetically blemished, it may be treated by surgical excision. If the lesion adheres to the sclera, as can be demonstrated by imaging, a superficial sclerectomy may be needed.

11.11.4 Lacrimal Gland Choristoma (Ectopic Lacrimal Gland)

Ectopic lacrimal glands are rare and have been described in various parts of the ocular adnexa and intraocularly, but the most common location is in the epibulbar conjunctiva [72]. It is a simple choristomatous lesion that presents usually as an asymptomatic unilateral pink to orange, well-circumscribed stromal mass [73]. It is typically located in the superotemporal or temporal parts of the conjunctiva, but it has also been described in other parts, including the limbal area [3, 72, 73]. Rarely, the lesion can be cystic due to ongoing secretions if there is no connection to the conjunctival surface. Neoplastic transformation of the lacrimal tissue has been reported [72].

Histopathologically, the isolated epibulbar ectopic lacrimal gland can be similar to normal lacrimal tissue in the conjunctival stroma or composed of variably dilated, branching tubular structures, with or without ducts and rare acinar zymogen granules [73]. Epibulbar complex choristoma may contain lacrimal gland tissue together with other tissue elements [74].

Most lacrimal gland choristomas are treated with complete excision.

11.11.5 Complex Choristoma

Complex choristoma is a congenital unilateral lesion that contains tissue derived from two germ layers—ectoderm and mesoderm.

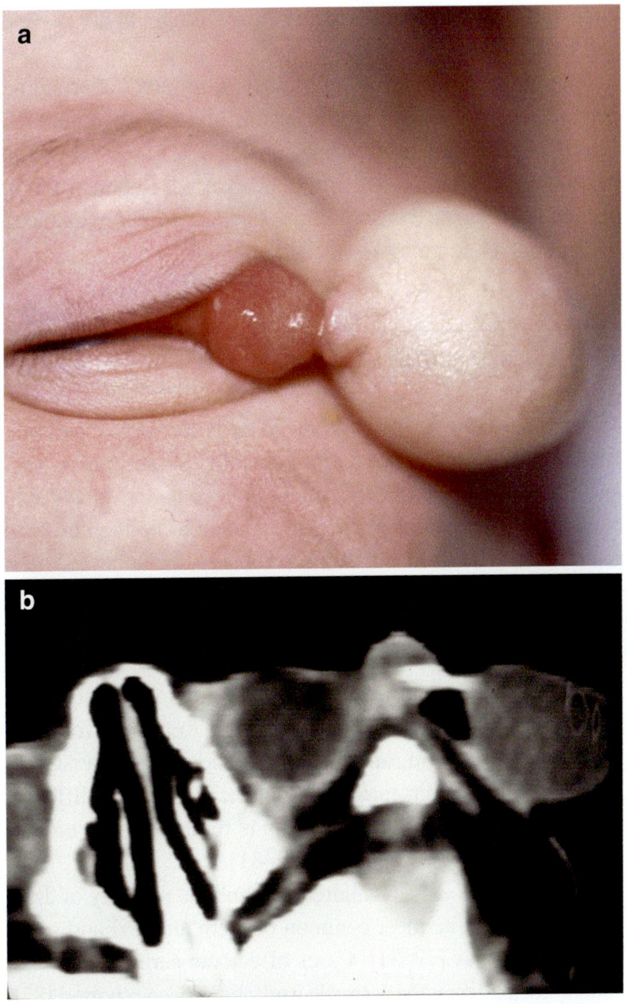

Fig. 11.16 Epibulbar complex choristoma in a 5-day-old child, associated with linear nevus sbaceous. A large pedunculated mass protrudes temporally through the left eyelid aperture (**a**). CT scan shows calcifications (bone) in the tumor base and cyst-like structure in the polypoid mass (**b**)

Epibulbar complex choristomas are rare [1–3]. They may have other ophthalmic manifestations and may be associated with systemic conditions, such as Goldenhar syndrome and organoid nevus syndrome, of which the most frequent feature is the sebaceous nevus of Jadassohn [75, 76] (Fig. 16). It has a variable clinical appearance, ranging from a small, localized lesion to a lesion that covers much of the epibulbar surface. A large pedunculated mass protruding through the eyelid aperture has been reported [76]. The choristoma may invade the cornea. The consistency and color depend on the type of tissue present in the choristoma. For example, when dermal elements contain adipose, the lesion appears yellowish, while lacrimal tissue appears pink, and when it contains bone or cartilage, it will be hard.

Histopathologically, complex choristoma may include a variable combination of ectopic tissue, such as dermal tissue containing adipose tissue, collagen and pilosebaceous structures, lacrimal gland, smooth muscle, cartilage, bone, nerves, and blood vessels [75–77].

The management of epibulbar complex choristoma depends on the extent of the lesion and the symptoms it causes. Asymptomatic small lesions can be observed, while large symptomatic lesions should be excised. Reconstruction of the ocular surface is sometimes needed. In very advanced cases, enucleation may be needed.

11.12 Caruncular Lesions

The caruncle is a fleshy, pink, ovoid body located in the inner canthus, measuring about 5 mm vertically, 3 mm transversely, and 1.5 mm in thickness. It contains both conjunctival and skin elements. It is covered by stratified squamous epithelium with goblet cells. The stroma contains fibroblasts, melanocytes interspersed with collagen, adipose tissue, sebaceous glands, hair follicles, striated muscle fibers, and inflammatory cells and may contain sweat glands and accessory lacrimal glands [78].

Lesions of the caruncle are uncommon. Because of its histological composition, it can give rise to tumors found in the conjunctiva, skin, and lacrimal glands. The diversity of the caruncular lesions makes their clinical diagnosis difficult, and preoperative clinical diagnosis is reported to be correct only in about half of the cases [79–81].

Caruncular lesions in children are rare; the majority of them are benign, and the most common of them are nevi and squamous papillomas [79–81]. Cases of ectopic caruncular tissue, usually located near the caruncle itself, have been reported [82].

For more details on caruncular tumors, see Chap. 10.

11.13 Xeroderma Pigmentosum

Xeroderma pigmentosum (XP) is a rare genetic, usually autosomal recessive disease, with clinical and cellular hypersensitivity to UV radiation and defective DNA repair. Patients with XP experience cutaneous, ocular, and neurological abnormalities, including neoplasia [83].

Ophthalmic findings are present in 20–90% of cases, due to the high exposure of the eye to UV radiation and are confined mainly to the eyelids and ocular surface [4, 84, 85]. They may start in early childhood, and the main initial symptom is an abnormal reaction to sun exposure. Tumors of the eyelids and ocular surface are diagnosed in many of the cases during childhood and adolescence. The most common tumors of the eyelid skin are basal cell carcinoma and squamous cell carcinoma, followed by malignant melanoma.

As opposed to most conjunctival tumors at this young age group, in XP patients, the ocular surface tumors are often malignant. They are usually present in the bulbar conjunctiva and limbus, often with corneal involvement, as unilateral or bilateral disease [4, 84, 85]. The most common tumors of the ocular surface are ocular surface squamous neoplasia (Fig. 11.17), ranging from epithelial dysplasia to invasive squamous cell carcinoma [4, 86]. Other ocular surface tumors that were reported in XP are melanocytic lesions, including malignant melanoma [87], and stromal tumors, such as angiosarcoma and malignant fibrous histiocytoma [4, 39].

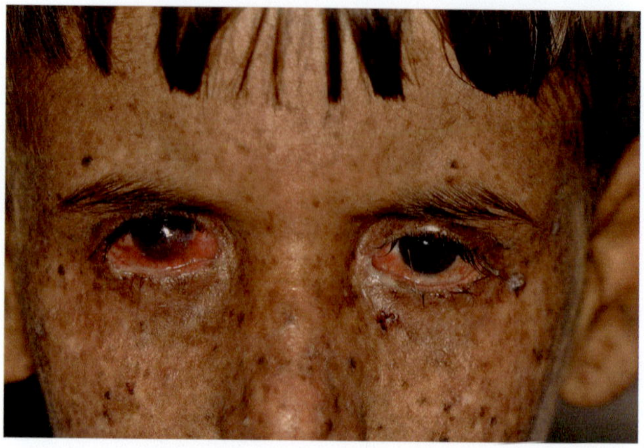

Fig. 11.17 Ocular surface squamous neoplasia in a child with xeroderma pigmentosa. This 9-year-old boy has a right eye inferior limbus pinkish epithelial lesion that was excised and diagnosed as corneal-conjunctival intraepithelial neoplasia (CCIN) grade 3 (carcinoma in situ). Notice the solar skin damage over the sun-exposed face

Malignant conjunctival tumors in XP patients are treated, as in other patients, by a wide excisional biopsy, with or without cryotherapy, topical chemotherapy, and immunotherapy, and, when very extensive, by extended enucleation or orbital exenteration. Despite the treatment, and because of the aggressiveness of many of the tumors in XP, local tumor recurrence happens in more than half of the cases [4, 86].

For more details on XP, see Chap. 16.

References

1. Elsas FJ, Green WR. Epibulbar tumors in children. Am J Ophthalmol. 1975;79:1001–7.
2. Cunha RP, Cunha MC, Shields JA. Epibulbar tumors in children: a survey of 282 biopsies. J Pediatr Ophthalmol Strabismus. 1987;24:249–54.
3. Shields CL, Shields JA. Conjunctival tumors in children. Curr Opin Ophthalmol. 2007;18:351–60.
4. Kaliki S, Jajapuram SV, Maniar A, Mishra DK. Ocular and periocular tumors in xeroderma pigmentosum: a study of 120 Asian Indian patients. Am J Ophthalmol. 2019;198:146–53.
5. Lass JH, Jenson AB, Papale JJ, et al. Papillomavirus in human conjunctival papillomas. Am J Ophthalmol. 1983;95:364–8.
6. Sjo NC, von Buchwald D, Cassonnet P, et al. Human papillomavirus in normal conjunctival tissue and in conjunctival papilloma: types and frequencies in large series. Br J Ophthalmol. 2007;91:1014–5.
7. Malakar J, Kocjan BJ, Hosnjak L, et al. Morpholoical characteristics of conjunctival squamous papillomas in relation to human papillomavirus infection. Br J Ophthalmol. 2015;99:431–6.

8. Schechter BA, Rand WJ, Velazquez GE, et al. Treatment of conjunctival papillomata with topical interferon Alpha-2b. Am J Ophthalmol. 2002;134:268–70.
9. Rodriguez-Cabrera L, Garcia-Regil P, Velasco-Levy A, Serna-Ojeda J. Conjunctival papillomatosis in children treated with co-adjuvant interferon Alpha-2b. Arch Soc Esp Oftalmol. 2019;94:352–4.
10. Hawkins AS, Yu J, Hamming NA, et al. Treatment of recurrent conjunctival papillomatosis with mitomycin C. Am J Ophthalmol. 1999;128:638–40.
11. Shields CL, Lally MR, Singh AD, et al. Oral cimetidine (Tagamet) for recalcitrant, diffuse conjunctival papillomatosis. Am J Ophthalmol. 1999;128:362–4.
12. Kalantzis GK, Verity DH, Rose GE. Periocular implantation cysts: a late complication of ophthalmic surgery. Eye (Lond). 2014;28:1004–7.
13. Zamir E, Mechoulam H, Micera A, et al. Inflamed juvenile conjunctival nevus: clinicopathological characterization. Br J Ophthalmol. 2002;86:28–30.
14. Maly A, Epstein D, Meir K, Pe'er J. Histological criteria of atypia in melanocytic conjunctival lesions. Pathology. 2008;40:676–81.
15. Choi EK, Chevez-Barrios P. Inflamed juvenile nevi: histopathological criteria. Arch Pathol Lab Med. 2014;138:1242–6.
16. Levi-Schaffer F, Micera A, Zamir E, et al. Nerve growth factor and eosinophils in inflamed juvenile conjunctival nevus. Invest Ophthalmol Vus Sci. 2002;43:1850–6.
17. Strempel I, Kroll P. Conjunctival malignant melanoma in children. Ophthalmologica. 1999;213:129–32.
18. Mehran T, Traboulsi EI. Malignant melanoma of the conjunctiva in children: a review of the international literature 1965–2006. J Pediatr Ophthalmol Strabismus. 2007;44:277–8.
19. Shields JA, Mashayekhi A, Kligman BE, et al. Vascular tumors of the conjunctiva in 140 cases. Ophthalmology. 2011;118:1747–53.
20. Ferry AP. Pyogenic granuloma of the eye and ocular adnexa: a study of 100 cases. Trans Am Ophthalmol Soc. 1989;87:327–43.
21. Oke I, Alkharashi M, Petersen RA, et al. Treatment of ocular pyogenic granuloma with topical timolol. JAMA Ophthalmol. 2017;135:383–5.
22. Chang TC, Estes R. Beta blocker treatment of infantile conjunctival hemangioma—observation from 2 cases. J AAPOS. 2014;18:80–2.
23. Kiratli H, Uzun S, Tarlan B, et al. Recurrent subconjunctival hemorrhage due to cavernous hemangioma of the conjunctiva. Can J Ophthalmol. 2012;47:318–20.
24. Welch J, Srinivasan S, Lyall D, et al. Conjunctival lymphangiectasia: a report of 11 cases and review of the literature. Surv Ophthalmol. 2012;57:136–48.
25. Awdry P. Lymphangiectasia hemorrhagica conjunctivae. Br J Ophthalmol. 1969;53:274–8.
26. Fraunfelder FW. Liquid nitrogen cryotherapy for conjunctival lymphangiectasia: a case series. Trans Am Ophthalmol Soc. 2009;107:229–32.
27. Goshe JM, Platt S, Yeaney G, et al. Surgical drainage of lymphangiectasia haemorrhagica conjunctivae. Cornea. 2017;36:116–8.
28. Han KE, Choi CY, Seo KY. Removal of lymphangiectasia using high-frequency radio wave electrosurgery. Cornea. 2013;32:547–9.
29. Tan JC, Mann S, Coroneo MT. Successful treatment of conjunctival lyphangiectasia with subconjunctival injection of bevacizumab. Cornea. 2016;35:1375–7.
30. Spector JA, Zide BM. Carbon dioxide laser ablation for treatment of lymphangioma of the conjunctiva. Plast Reconstr Surg. 2006;117:609–12.
31. Behrendt S, Bernsmeier H, Randzio G. Fractionated beta-irradiation of conjunctival lymphangioma. Ophthalmologica. 1991;203:161–3.
32. Baracle AM, Theodorou M, Maling SJ, et al. Sclerotherapy treatment of orbital lymphatic malformation: a large single-centre experience. Br J Ophthalmol. 2016;100:204–8.
33. Gandhi NG, Lin LK, O'Hara M. Sildenafil for pediatric orbital lymphangioma. JAMA Ophthalmol. 2013;131:1228–30.
34. Foster JA, Czyz CN, Stacey A, et al. Percutaneous drainage and ablation as first line therapy for macrocystic and microcystic orbital lymphatic malformations. Ophthalmic Plast Reconstr Surg. 2012;28:119–25.
35. Kim HJ, Shields CL, Eagle RC, et al. Fibrous histiocytoma of the conjunctiva. Am J Ophthalmol. 2006;142:1036–43.
36. Knapp AN, Samara WA, Shields CL, et al. Conjunctival fibrous histiocytomaa in an 8-year-old boy. J AAPOS. 2016;20:368–70.
37. Ali-Ridha A, Brownstein S, O'Connor M, et al. Benign solitary fibrous histiocytoma of xanthomathous subtype of the perilimbal conjunctiva and adjacent sclera in a youth. Ocul Oncol Pathol. 2018;4:341–4.
38. Tieger MG, Jakobiec FA, Ma L, et al. Small benign storifoem fibrous tumor (fibrous histiocytoma) of the conjunctival substantia propria in a child: review and clarification of biologic behavior. Ophthal Plasr Reconstr Surg. 2019;35:495–502.
39. Pe'er J, Levinger S, Chirambo M, et al. Malignant fibrous histiocytomaof the skin and conjunctiva in xeroderma pigmentosum. Arch Pathol Lab Med. 1991;115:910–4.
40. Charles NC, Fox DM, Avendano JA, et al. Conjunctival neurilemmoma. Report of 3 cases. Arch Ophthalmol. 1997;115:547–9.
41. Nair AG, Kaliki S, Mishra SK, et al. Epibulbar schwannoma in a 12-year-old boy: a case report and review of literature. Indian J Ophthalmol. 2015;63:620–2.
42. Demrici H, Shields CL, Rc E, et al. Epibulbar schwannoma in a 17-year-old boy and review of the literature. Ophthalmic Reconstr Surg. 2010;26:48–50.
43. Chaudhry IA, Al-Jishi Z, Shamsi FA, et al. Juvenile xanthogranuloma of the corneoscleral limbus: case report and review of the literature. Surv Ophthalmol. 2004;49:608–14.
44. Samara WA, Khoo CTL, Say EAT, et al. Juvenile xanthogranuloma involving the eye and ocular adnexa: tumor control, visual outcome, and globe salvage in 30 patients. Ophthalmology. 2015;122:2130–8.
45. Lee KM, Wee WR, Lee JH, et al. Juvenile xanthogranuloma presenting as infiltrative conjunctival mass in an adult. Cornea. 2012;31:447–9.
46. Cameron JD, Wick MR. Embryonal rhabdomyosarcoma of the conjunctiva. A clinicopathologic and immunohistochemical study. Arch Ophthalmol. 1986;104:1203–4.
47. Polito E, Pichierri P, Loffredo A, et al. A case of primary botryoid conjunctival rhabdomyosarcoma. Graefes Arch Clin Exp Ophthalmol. 2006;244:517–9.
48. Gallego S, Zanetti I, Orbach D, et al. Fusion status in patients with lymph node-positive (N1) alveolar rhabdomyosarcoma is a powerful predictor of prognosis: experience of the European Paediatric Soft Tissue Sarcoma Study Group (EpSSG). Cancer. 2018;124:3201–9.
49. Park R, Centeno MG, Shnider R. Ocular surface leiomyoma in a child after strabismus repair. Ophthalmology. 2018;125:1968.
50. Kirkegaard MM, Rasmussen PK, Coupland SE, et al. Conjunctival lymphoma—an international multicenter retrospective study. JAMA Ophthalmol. 2016;134:406–14.
51. Beykin G, Pe'er J, Amir G, et al. Pediatric and adolescent elevated conjunctival lesions in the plical area: lymphoma or reactive lymphoid hyperplasia? Br J Ophthalmol. 2014;98:645–50.
52. Moustafa GA, Topham AK, Aronow ME. Paediatric ocular adnexal lymphoma: a population-based analysis. BMJ Open Ophthalmol. 2020;5(1):e000483.
53. Okudolo JO, Bagg A, Meghpara BB, et al. Conjunctival pediatric-type follicular lymphoma. Ophthalmic Plast Reconstr Surg. 2020;36:e46–9.
54. AlSemari MA, Maktabi A, AlSamnan MS, et al. Conjunctival pediatric follicular lymphoma: case report and literature review. Ophthalmic Plast Reconstr Surg. 2020;36:e14–5.
55. Lee J, Han JH, Lee CH, et al. Comparison of histological and molecular features of pediatric-type follicular lymphoma and pediatric marginal zone lymphoma. Vitchow Arch. 2023;482:849–58.

56. Campagnoli MF, Parodi E, Linari A, et al. Conjunctival mass: an unusual presentation of acute lymphoblastic leukemia relapse in children. J Pediatr. 2003;142:211.
57. Bakhshi S, Arya LS. Conjunctival mass: rare site of extramedually relapse in childhood acute lymphoblastic leukemia. J Assoc Physicians India. 2005;53:160–1.
58. Javadi MA, Kanavi MR, Faramarzi A, et al. Relapse of acute lymphoblastic leukemia as a conjunctival mass in a 9-year-old girl. J Pediatr Ophthalmol Strabismus. 2009;47:PMID 19645387.
59. Chocron IM, Morrison DG, Friedman DL, et al. Ophthalmic manifestations of relapsing acute childhood leukemia. J AAPOS. 2015;19:284–6.
60. Rosenberg C, Finger PT, Furlan L, et al. Bilateral epibulbar granulocytic sarcomas: a case of an 8-year-old girl with acute myeloid leukemia. Graefes Arch Clin Exp Ophthalmol. 2007;245:170–2.
61. Mansour AM, Barber JC, Reinecke RD, et al. Ocular choristomas. Surv Ophthalmol. 1989;33:339–58.
62. Zhong J, Deng Y, Zhang P, et al. New grading system for limbal dermoid: a retrospective analysis of 261 cases over a 10-year period. Cornea. 2018;37:66–71.
63. Choudhury M, Kapoor PM. Goldenhar syndrome: cardiac anesthesiologist's perspective. Ann Card Anaesth. 2017 Jan;20(Supplement):S61–6.
64. Tingaud-Sequeira A, Trimouille A, Sagardoy T, et al. Oculo-auriculo-vertebral spectrum: new genes and literature review on a complex disease. J Med Genet. 2022;59:417–27.
65. Franco E, Gagrani M, Lalgudi VG, et al. Technique for the management of extensive ocular surface lipodermoid involving the cornea in children. Cornea. 2023;42:770–5.
66. Kim E, Kim HJ, Kim YD, et al. Subconjunctival fat prolapse and dermolipoma of the orbit: differentiation on CT and MR imaging. AJNR Am J Neuroradiol. 2011;32:465–7.
67. Vahdani K, Rose GE. The presentation and surgical treatment of peribulbar dermolipoma. Ophthalmic Plast Reconstr Surg. 2021;37:226–9.
68. Sa HS, Kim HK, Shin JH, et al. Dermolipoma surgery with rotational conjunctival flaps. Acta Ophthalmol. 2012;90:86–90.
69. Choi YJ, Kim IH, Choi JH, et al. Early results of surgical management of conjunctival dermolipoma: partial excision and free conjunctival autograft. Br J Ophthalmol. 2015;99:1031–6.
70. Shields CL, Qureshi A, Eagle RC, et al. Epibulbar osseous choristoma in 8 patients. Cornea. 2012;31:756–60.
71. Vachette M, Moulin A, Zografos L, et al. Epibulbar osseous choritoma: a clinicopathological case series and review of the literature. Klin Monatsbl Augenheilkd. 2012;229:420–3.
72. Nagendran S, Alsamnan M, Strianese D, et al. Ectopic lacrimal gland tissue: a systematic review. Ophthalmic Plast Reconstr Surg. 2020;36:540–4.
73. Milman T, Jakobiec FA, Lally SE, et al. Lacrimal gland hamartoma (formerly termed dacryoadenoma). Am J Ophthalmol. 2020;217:189–97.
74. Pokorny KS, Hyman BM, Jakobiec FA, et al. Epibulbar complex choristomas containing lacrimal tissue. Clinical distinction from dermoids and histologic evidence of an origin from palpebral lobe. Ophthalmology. 1987;94:1249–57.
75. Aldossary MM, Alkatan HM, Maktabi A. Epibulbar complex and osseous choristoma: clinicopathological study with interesting associations. Ann Med Surg. 2018;31:135–41.
76. Pe'erJ IM. Epibulbar complex choristoma associated with nevus sebaceous. Arch Ophthalmol. 1995;113:1301–4.
77. Zhang Z, Yang Z, Pan Q, et al. Epibulbar complex cartilaginous choristoma: a distinctive clinicopathological case series and literature review. Medicine (Baltimore). 2018;97:e9902.
78. Kathuria SS, Howarth D, Huewitz JJ, et al. Anatomic and histologic study of the caruncle. Ophthalmic Plast Reconstr Surg. 1999;15:407–11.
79. Shields CL, Shields JA, White D, et al. Types and frequency of lesions of the caruncle. Am J Ophthalmol. 1986;102:771–8.
80. Ostegard J, Prause JU, Heegaard S. Caruncular lesions in Denmark 1978–2002: a histopathological study with correlation to clinical referral diagnosis. Arch Ophthalmol Scand. 2006;84:130–6.
81. Levy J, Illsar M, Deckel Y, et al. Lesions of the caruncle: a description of 42 cases and a review of the literature. Eye (Lond). 2009;23:1004–18.
82. Zamir E, Banin E, Chowers I, et al. Ectopic caruncle. Arch Ophthalmol. 1999;117:1446–7.
83. Kraemer KH, Lee MM, Scotto J. Xeroderma pigmentosum. Cutaneous, ocular, and neurological abnormalities in 830 published cases. Arch Dermatol. 1987;123:241–50.
84. Dolfus H, Porto F, Caussade P, et al. Ocular manifestations in inherited DNA repair disorders. Surv Ophthalmol. 2003;48:107–22.
85. Lim R, Sethi M, Morley AMS. Ophthalmic manifestations of xeroderma pigmentosum: a perspective from United Kingdom. Ophthalmology. 2017;124:1652–61.
86. Gupta N, Sachdev R, Tandon R. Ocular surface squamous neoplasia in xeroderma pigmentosum: clinical spectrum and outcome. Graefes Arch Clin Exp Ophthalmol. 2011;249:1217–21.
87. Vasanthapuram VH, Kaliki S. Conjunctival melanoma in patients with xeroderma pigmentosum: a series of four cases. Int Ophthalmol. 2020;40:1143–6.

Conjunctival Tumors: Pharmacotherapy

12

Diego Alba, Michael Antonietti, Anat Galor, Jacob Pe'er, and Carol L. Karp

12.1 Ocular Surface Squamous Neoplasia

12.1.1 Introduction

Ocular surface squamous neoplasia (OSSN) involves a broad spectrum of neoplastic squamous epithelial abnormalities from squamous dysplasia to intraepithelial neoplasia in situ to squamous cell carcinoma (SCC). OSSN is usually slow-growing and remains localized. However, SCC has the ability to invade the eye, orbit, or rarely even metastasize [1, 2]. Exposure to ultraviolet (UV) radiation in sunlight is the strongest risk factor [3]. Other environmental risk factors include human immunodeficiency virus (HIV), human papillomavirus (HPV), smoking, and immuno-suppression [4]. Features of OSSN can include a fleshy gelatinous mass, leukoplakia, abnormal vascularity, and irregular corneal borders, and these features can be seen in isolation or combination [5, 6]. A wide variety of lesions can be confused with OSSN including pterygium, corneal pannus, pyogenic granuloma, sebaceous cell carcinoma, and amelanotic melanoma, but recent diagnostic tools like the anterior-segment high-resolution optical coherence tomography (HR-OCT) offer optical visualization to differentiate and monitor OSSN progression [5]. In many parts of the world, the pendulum has now shifted from surgical resection to a medical approach in OSSN [7]. Surveys done by Adler et al. have shown increased use of medical therapies for OSSN [8] (see Chap. 5).

D. Alba · M. Antonietti · A. Galor · C. L. Karp (✉)
Department of Ophthalmology, Bascom Palmer Eye Institute, Miami, FL, USA
e-mail: ckarp@miami.edu

J. Pe'er
Ocular Oncology Service and Ophthalmic Pathology Laboratory, Department of Ophthalmology, Hadassah—Hebrew University Medical Center, Jerusalem, Israel

12.1.2 Treatment

Traditionally, the gold standard for the diagnosis and treatment of OSSN was surgical removal, but topical chemotherapeutic drugs are becoming a viable alternative [8, 9]. The advantages of surgery are that it is both diagnostic and therapeutic and it provides rapid resolution. It is covered by insurers in the United States and is a readily available modality for most patients. The disadvantages to a surgical approach include residual tumor from positive margins, limbal stem cell deficiency from extensive excisions, symblepharon, and other severe ocular surface complications. Medical therapy has the advantage of treating the entire ocular surface, including any subclinical disease. Especially in cases of extensive, annular, recurrent OSSN, topical therapies can cure the neoplasia with minimal sequelae to the ocular surface. Due to the mostly superficial effect of topical chemotherapy, their use for invasive SCC as primary treatment is uncertain.

12.2 5-Fluorouracil

12.2.1 Pharmacology

5-Fluorouracil (5-FU) is an analog of uracil and works by being converted into 5-fluorouracil deoxynucleotide (5-FdUMP) which inhibits the thymidylate synthase (TS) leading to inhibition of DNA purine synthesis, essential for replication and repair [10]. Additionally, it has been shown to interfere with protein synthesis by incorporating it into the RNA [11]. These processes, subsequently, inhibit the growth of tumor cells [12].

12.2.2 Role in the Treatment of OSSN

5-FU is an agent available as a primary treatment in OSSN. It is one of our preferred options when treating OSSN given its high efficacy, low cost, easy drop cycling schedule, and gen-

© The Author(s), under exclusive license to Springer Nature Switzerland AG 2024
J. Pe'er et al. (eds.), *Clinical Ophthalmic Oncology*, https://doi.org/10.1007/978-3-031-72443-5_12

erally tolerable side effect profile [13–19]. Since its FDA approval in 1962 for the treatment of adenocarcinoma of the colon, rectum, breast, stomach, and pancreas, this medication has been extensively studied in various types of cancer and is administered intravenously for these indications. Its topical application in ophthalmology has gained attention since 1986, making it a key agent in the treatment of OSSN [13, 18, 20] as well as basal cell and SCC of the skin [21–24].

Compared to mitomycin C (MMC) and interferon alpha-2b (IFNα-2b), 5-FU is usually the least expensive topical treatment. As interferon is currently not available in the United States, we utilize topical 5-FU in most cases where treatment with topical medical therapy for OSSN is indicated.

12.2.3 Dosage

Several dosing regimens have been reported for the primary treatment of OSSN [13, 14, 19, 25]. Our protocol is to use compounded 1% 5-FU drops four times daily for 1 week, followed by 3 weeks off the medication [13, 19] (Fig. 12.1). This schedule is generally repeated until complete resolution is seen (typically 4–6 cycles). Other protocols have used 5-FU cycles four times a day for 4 days followed by 30–45 days of no treatment [17, 25, 26] or four times a day for 4 weeks [14]. Its efficacy as a primary treatment for OSSN has been well studied, and recent studies achieve resolution from 82% up to 100% with very low recurrence (about 0–11% after 1 year of resolution) [18]. We advocate refrigeration of the 5-FU, but it has also been used at room temperature [13].

12.2.4 Side Effects

5-FU side effect profile is considered moderate. It affects the synthesis of DNA and RNA of epithelial cells on the ocular surface, and ocular surface symptoms are not uncommon [14]. Side effects include lid edema, conjunctival hyperemia, filamentary keratitis, superficial keratitis, and on rare occasions superficial stromal melting [14]. Punctal stenosis has been reported in rabbits after topical 5-FU; thus, manual occlusion of the lacrimal canaliculus after a drop is applied is recommended to lower this risk [27]. Preservative-free artificial tears are recommended to decrease discomfort, and the application of petroleum jelly on the eyelids is advised to

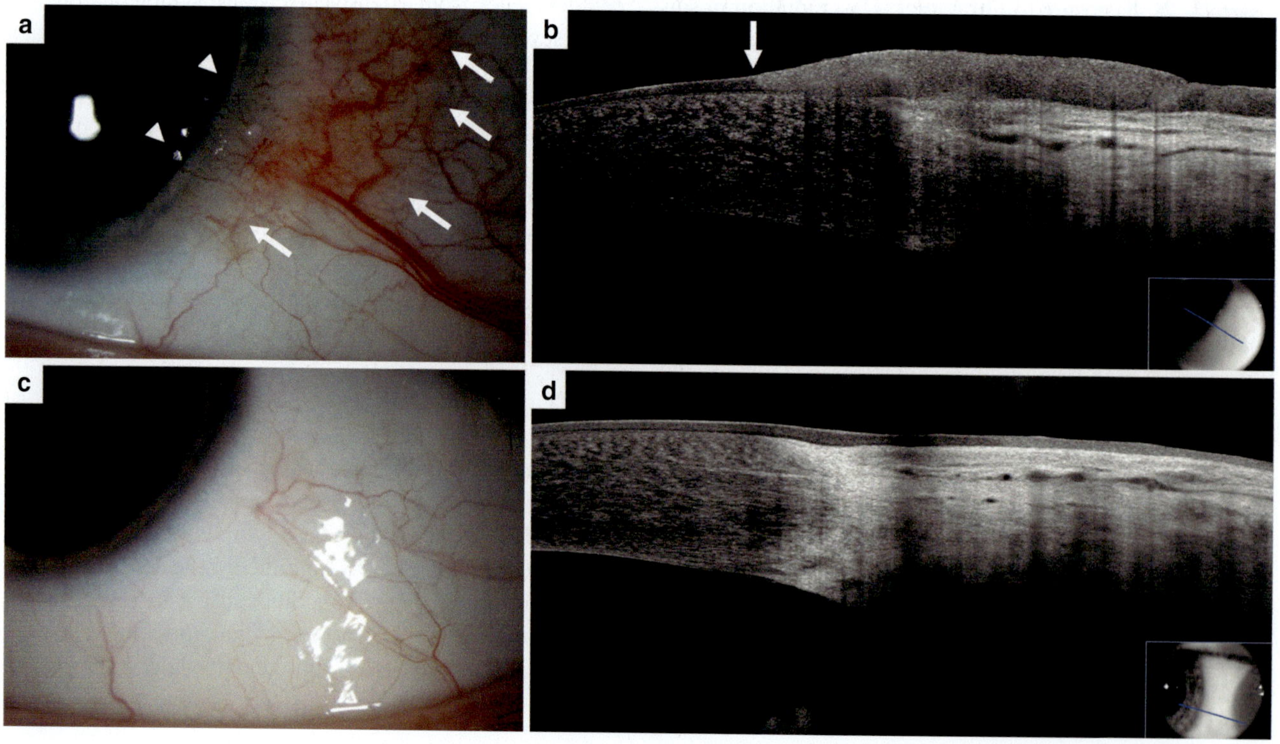

Fig. 12.1 Slit-lamp photography and HR-OCT imaging of an ocular surface squamous neoplasia lesion before and after topical treatment with 5-FU. (**a**) Slit lamp photography demonstrates temporal limbal gelatinous lesion with corneal (arrowheads) and conjunctival involvement (arrows) with injection and inferotemporal adjacent feeder vessels in the left eye, prior to treatment. (**b**) HR-OCT image of the temporal conjunctiva and cornea demonstrates hyperreflective epithelial lesion with epithelial thickening along with an abrupt transition between normal and abnormal epithelium (arrow). The lower right inset represents the anatomical location of the OCT raster section. (**c**) Slit lamp photography demonstrates resolution of the temporal limbal lesion after treatment with 6 cycles of 1% 5-FU. (**d**) HR-OCT image shows normalized, thin, and dark epithelium consistent with tumor resolution. The lower right inset represents the anatomical location of the OCT raster section

avoid irritation that might occur [18, 19]. Topical corticosteroid eyedrops such as prednisolone acetate 1% one drop every 6 h can be used if side effects following the 5-FU administration appear [13, 28] (Table 12.1).

12.3 Interferon Alpha-2b

12.3.1 Pharmacology

Interferons are a group of pleiotropic proteins produced by several immune and nonimmune cell types in response to infection (virus, bacteria, fungi, and parasites) and neoplasia [29]. There are six main types of interferons present in humans: alpha (α), beta (β), gamma (γ), epsilon (ε), kappa (κ), and omega (ω) based on their antigenic specificities [30]. Interferon alpha-2b is an immunomodulatory cytokine consisting of 165 amino acid residues, with arginine in position 23 [31]; it triggers the transcription of specific genes, known as interferon-stimulated genes (ISGs) responsible for antiviral and antineoplastic cascades involving target and host immune cells [32, 33]. The effects of interferons include the inhibition of biosynthetic enzymes, induced apoptosis to cells, decreased blood vessel proliferation, inactivation of viral RNA, and enhanced phagocytic and cytotoxic mechanisms. Interferon alpha is well absorbed via intramuscular and subcutaneous routes. Peak concentrations occur at about 2 h following the intramuscular injection and 4 h following the subcutaneous route [31].

12.3.2 Role in OSSN

In cancer, interferon alpha has been identified to play a key role in immunity. It upregulates the class I and class II major histocompatibility complex (MHC)-mediated antigen presentation, triggers apoptosis by interfering in the phases of the tumoral cell cycle, and downregulates immunosuppressive regulatory T-cells and angiogenic growth factors such as vascular endothelial growth factor (VEGF) and fibroblast growth factor 2 (FGF2) [34]. These processes help in the elimination of tumor cells.

Interferon in the form of topical eye drops and intralesional IFNα-2b have been used in the treatment of OSSN, both as primary therapy (Fig. 12.2) and as an adjuvant after

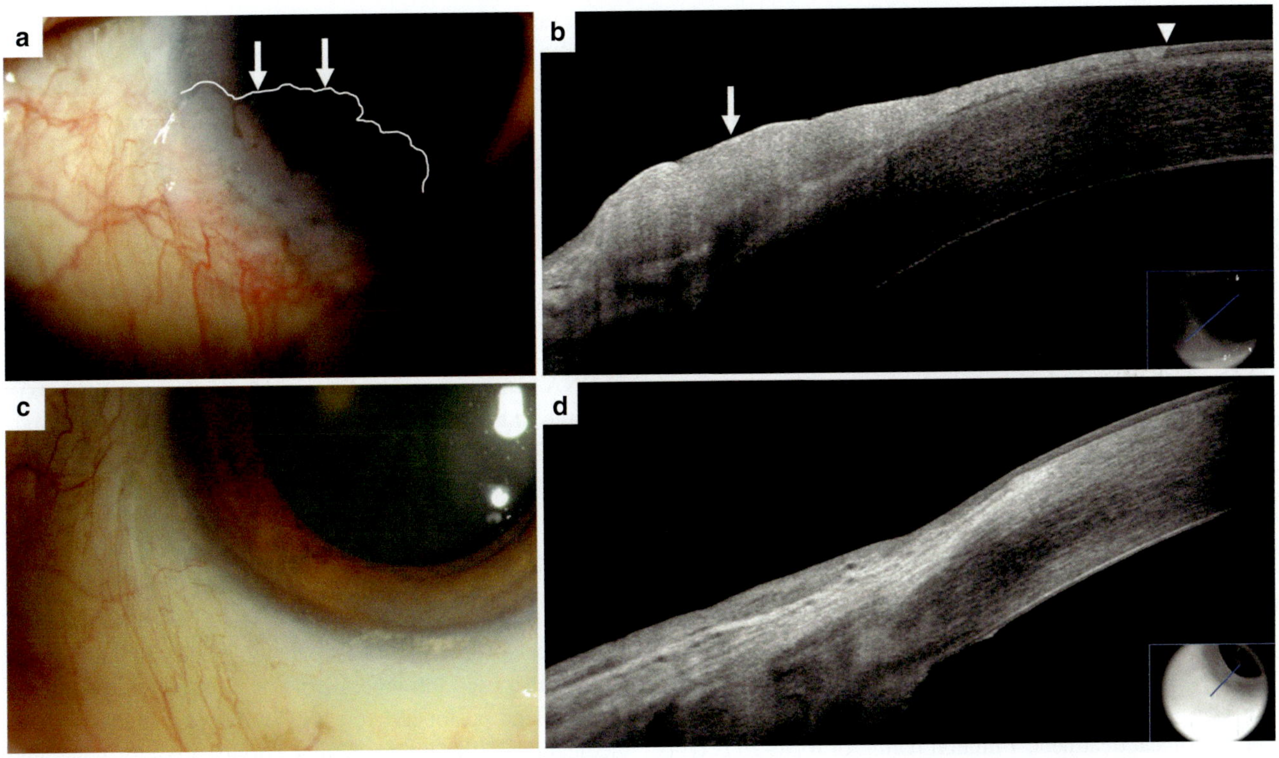

Fig. 12.2 Slit-lamp photography and HR-OCT imaging of an ocular surface squamous neoplasia lesion before and after topical treatment with IFNα-2b. (**a**) Slit lamp photography demonstrates a nasal gelatinous lesion of the left eye. Note the opalescent and fimbriated extension onto the cornea (white outline and arrows). (**b**) HR-OCT image of the nasal conjunctiva and cornea demonstrates a hyperreflective thick epithelial lesion (arrow) with a zone of abrupt transition between normal and abnormal epithelium (arrowhead). The lower right inset represents the anatomical location of the OCT raster section. (**c**) Slit lamp photography demonstrates quiet conjunctiva with a resolution of the nasal lesion shortly after completing a 6-month course of daily topical IFNα-2b 1 million IU. **D** HR-OCT image shows normalized, thin epithelium consisting of tumor resolution. The lower right inset represents the anatomical location of the OCT raster section

surgery [35–48]. In our practice, IFNα-2b was one of our preferred treatments for OSSN since it has comparable levels of tumor resolution to MMC and 5-FU with far less side effects and toxicity. Studies have shown the resolution rate of OSSN ranging from 81% to 100% when IFNα-2b is used as a primary treatment [16, 18, 35–48]. It is a versatile medication: besides the regular eye drops, it can be administered as a subconjunctival injection in patients with low treatment adherence [37, 43, 46, 47, 49, 50].

As a neoadjuvant and adjuvant, it has shown good results and is recommended in aggressive cases of high-grade lesions, tarsal involvement, and recurrent disease and particularly when margins are positive after surgical excision [44, 45]. In a case series of 18 patients with giant OSSN (median diameter of 20 mm and median clock-hour span of 6), IFNα-2b was administered in various forms: topically ($n = 12$), via intralesional injection ($n = 3$), or both ($n = 3$). The results showed that 72% of the patients experienced complete resolution solely with the use of IFNα-2b. However, for the remaining 28% of patients, IFNα-2b resulted in a median reduction in tumor size of 74% after 6 months. This remaining group required additional treatments such as surgical excision, cryotherapy, or photodynamic therapy to achieve complete resolution [46]. It has also been reported the complete resolution of a giant OSSN in a patient where IFN α-2b was initially intended only as a neoadjuvant, and this was maintained for more than 7 years without signs of recurrence [47]. Additionally, recurrence of OSSN might depend on environmental factors as well. A recent interventional cohort study ($n = 192$) found recurrence being more frequent in smokers than in nonsmokers (23% vs. 13%, $p = 0.04$) [48]. Pegylated interferon has also been used in small series [51, 52]. Interferon alpha 2a (IFNα-2a) has also been tried subconjunctivally and intralesional and in drops in limited cases [49, 53].

The high costs and daily usage requirements can make it a less optimal alternative in some countries compared to others [54, 55]. Regrettably, the manufacturer in the United States ceased production of the interferon alpha 2b product for business reasons in February 2016, making it unavailable in any form in the United States. Hopefully, it will be manufactured again soon for the US market.

12.3.3 Dosage

For the topical treatment, 1 million IU/mL of IFNα-2b is typically dosed four times daily continuously until resolution of the tumor, followed by 1 or 2 more months of treatment even after clinical resolution (Fig. 12.2). Higher doses of 3 million IU/mL have also been used but seem similar in effect without a therapeutic advantage over 1 million IU/mL dose [55]. The average time from the start of treatment to resolution is about 4 months [6, 36, 55]. The dose for subconjunctival injection varies. Some clinicians use 3 million IU in 0.5 cc given weekly, others 10 million IU/0.5 cc monthly of interferon IFNα-2b [36, 37, 50]. Others have used 1.5–3 million IU/0.5 cc of IFNα-2a 3 times weekly for 4 weeks or as a single dose when used as neoadjuvant [49]. Little data exists on pegylated interferon, but in case series, it has been used in doses of 20–36 μg/mL of pegylated IFNα-2a 4 times a day until tumor resolution [52, 53, 56].

12.3.4 Side Effects

Topical IFNα-2b eye drops are very well tolerated with minimal to no side effects [39]. Unlike other topical agents like mitomycin C and 5-fluorouracil, there is rarely hyperemia, but occasional follicular conjunctivitis and rare corneal microcysts have been reported [6, 36, 55, 57]. The use of IFNα-2a is very limited but also appears well tolerated. When injected subconjunctivally, patients do experience systemic side effects [52, 53]. These include a "flu-like" syndrome that may ensue after each injection. Pretreatment with oral antipyretic (e.g., acetaminophen, ibuprofen) is typically used to mitigate post-injection symptoms. Our protocol is to administer 1000 mg of acetaminophen prior to the injection and then every 4–6 h as needed (maximum daily dose: 4 g/day) (Table 12.1).

12.4 Mitomycin C

12.4.1 Pharmacology

Mitomycin C is an antibiotic with antimetabolite activity isolated in 1958 from the bacterium *Streptomyces caespitosus* and other *Streptomyces* bacterial species. It acts as an alkylating agent leading to irreversible cross-linking, impairment of DNA synthesis, and apoptosis. MMC also generates oxygen free radicals, causing cytotoxicity through lipid peroxidation. Therefore, it is toxic to both proliferating and nonproliferating cells [58, 59].

12.4.2 Role in Treatment of OSSN

As topical drops, MMC is a potent medical therapy for OSSN, also used intraoperatively as an adjuvant to surgical excision and postoperatively. A significant downside of this medication is the higher ocular surface toxicity generated compared to the other agents, mainly when using the highest concentration [60–62]. It is also used intraoperatively as an adjunct to surgical tumor removal [63]. In terms of topical use as a primary treatment modality, we typically do not use MMC as a first-line therapy for OSSN. Instead, we use it as a secondary agent when individuals fail treatments such as 5-FU (Fig. 12.3).

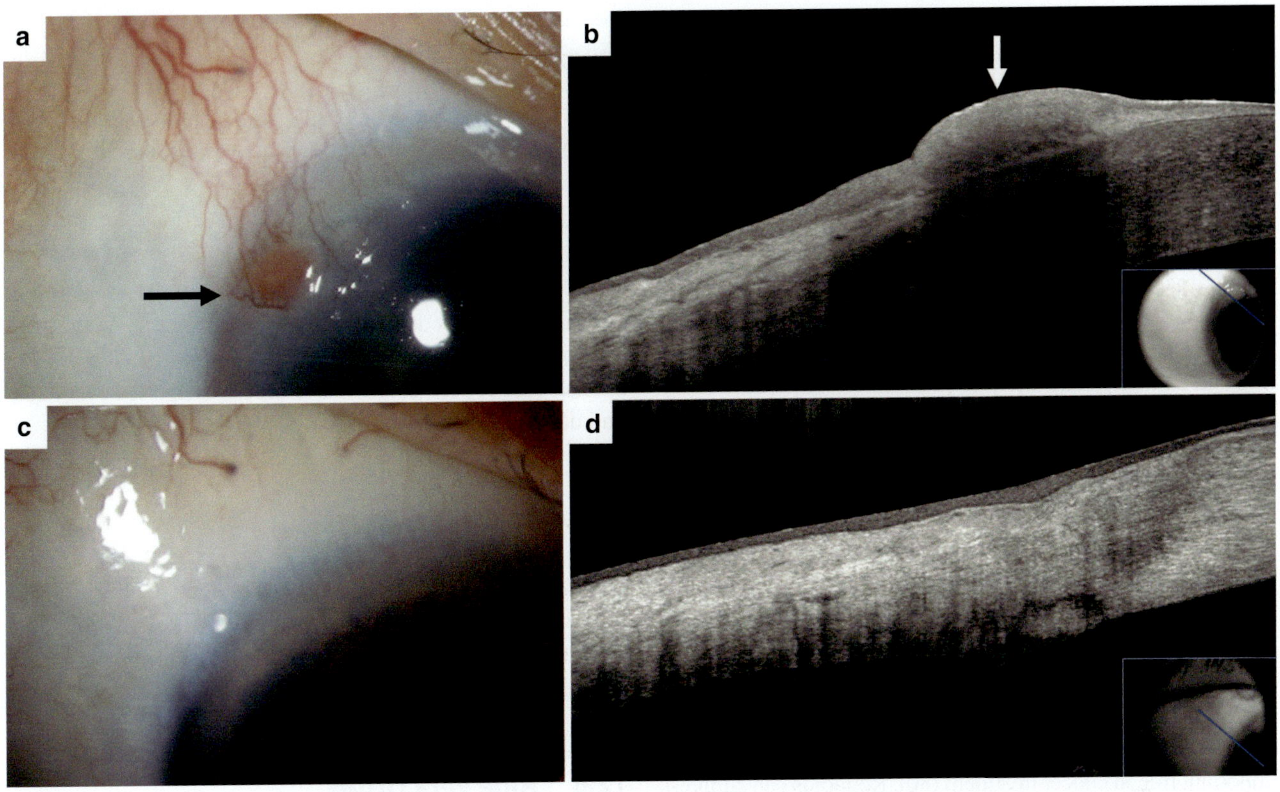

Fig. 12.3 Slit-lamp photography and HR-OCT imaging of an ocular surface squamous neoplasia lesion before and after topical treatment with MMC. (**a**) Slit lamp photography demonstrates discrete and elevated temporal nodule (arrow) with adjacent feeder vessels and subepithelial haze in right eye, after recurrence following 6 cycles of topical 5-FU. (**b**) HR-OCT image of the temporal conjunctiva and cornea demonstrates hyperreflective thick epithelial lesion (arrow). The transition zone in the cornea is not imaged in this cut. Lower right inset represents anatomical location of OCT raster section. (**c**) Slit lamp photography demonstrates quiet conjunctiva with resolution of the temporal lesion after 3 one-week cycles of topical 0.04% MMC. (**d**) HR-OCT image shows normalized, thin, and dark epithelium confirming tumor resolution. Lower right inset represents anatomical location of OCT raster section

12.4.3 Dosage

Several dosing regimens, using primarily 0.02–0.04% concentrations, have been reported for the primary treatment of OSSN concentration [6, 60–62]. Very low dose (0.002%) has also been reported [64]. Several protocols have been used for MMC administration, including four times daily for 2 weeks, 1 week with 2–3 weeks off, 7 days on and 7 days off, and variable regimens depending on the severity of the disease [60–62, 64, 65]. The optimal regimen in terms of length of time, number of cycles, and dose for MMC use is yet to be determined. Our recommended regimen is to administer 0.02–0.04% MMC four times daily for a week followed by 2–3 weeks off until the eye is white and quiet. Then, repeat this cycle until complete tumor resolution is achieved [18, 66]. MMC has to be refrigerated at 4 °C to prevent loss of activity of the molecule [67].

When used intraoperatively as an adjuvant to surgical removal, different approaches have been used, one protocol involves applying 0.02% MMC soaked on a surgical sponge to only the conjunctival margins, and some place the MMC directly on the scleral bed, followed by closure of the conjunctiva [63]. Postoperatively, topical MMC has been used in patients with positive surgical margins [68, 69]. Topical 0.04% was used four times a day for a week after epithelial healing followed by a week off and then repeated [68].

12.4.4 Side Effects

Topical eye drops of MMC have more side effects compared to IFNα-2b and 5-FU. The most common reported side effects are hyperemia, superficial punctate epithelial erosions, allergic conjunctivitis, photophobia, pain, and blepharospasm [60, 65, 70–75]. Especially when using high concentration of 0.04% MMC, limbal cell deficiency may occur [76]. Alternating weeks of topical MMC increase patient comfort and compliance. Topical steroids are very helpful to mitigate the inflammation from the MMC. Some have advocated also using cyclosporine 0.05% combined with the MMC therapy [77], and like with 5-FU, petroleum

Table 12.1 Common topical treatment drops for ocular surface squamous neoplasia

OSSN- preferred treatment options	Most common dosage	Main side effects
IFNα-2b	1 million IU/mL 4 times daily continuously	Minimal side effects
5-FU	1% 4 times a day for 1 week with 3 weeks off, cycled	Mild pain, lid edema, epitheliopathy
MMC	0.02% to 0.04% 4 times a day for of 1–2 weeks, 2–3 weeks off, cycled	Hyperemia, keratopathy, pain photophobia

IFNα 2b interferon alpha-2b, *5-FU* 5-fluorouracil, *MMC* mitomycin C, *LSCD* limbal stem cell deficiency

jelly is recommended to minimize the risk of eyelid irritation. Punctal stenosis has been reported; therefore, punctal plugs are typically placed before treatment to prevent scarring and damage to the lacrimal canaliculus [78] (Table 12.1).

12.5 Retinoic Acid

12.5.1 Pharmacology

Retinoic acid is a metabolite of vitamin A and is involved in several important physiological processes such as cell reproduction, proliferation, differentiation, and growth [79]. There is also evidence that retinoids have potent growth-inhibiting effects on malignant and non-malignant cells, giving them an important role in cancer treatment [80]. Retinoids can suppress the proliferation of cells by blocking the cell cycle or by inducing apoptosis [79, 81]. These molecules also regulate the activity of signaling pathways involved in either cellular growth or differentiation, being a key component in acute promyelocytic leukemia (APL) treatment for more than 20 years [82, 83].

12.5.2 Role in Treatment of OSSN

Retinoic acid has been used as an adjuvant therapy for the treatment of OSSN alone [84] and, in most cases, in combination with IFNα-2b [85]. More studies are needed to establish its efficacy as a sole treatment for OSSN. However, in theory, combination treatment may lead to more rapid tumor resolution based on synergistic mechanisms of action [85–87]. Combined therapy has been proposed for other conditions such as T-cell lymphoma [88, 89]. Given its strong evidence in dermatologic conditions [90–94] and its well-studied antineoplastic profile [95–99], it remains a valid medication to consider and further study [100].

12.5.3 Dosage

Retinoic acid can be prepared into a 0.01% drop and is administered once every 2 days, and when used in combination with topical IFNα-2b drops of 1 million IU/mL four times daily for an average of 3–12 months, it has shown complete clinical resolution in up to 98% of the cases [85]. Herbort et al. described retinoic acid 0.05% ointment, 1–3 times a day for 1–2 weeks, reporting complete resolution, but some cases needed to be treated for a month, so the dose was then lowered to 0.01% to decrease skin irritation [84]. In another case report, 0.01% 1 eye drop was applied every second day for 9 months [86].

12.5.4 Side Effects

Topical retinoic acid is generally well tolerated but can cause lid irritation, papillary conjunctivitis [84], and epithelial microcysts, and in one case marginal keratitis has been described with its use [85].

12.6 Aloe Vera Drops

12.6.1 Pharmacology

Aloe plants exhibit antineoplastic properties through three important mechanisms: antiproliferative, immunostimulatory, and antioxidant. Aloe antiproliferative actions are mediated by anthraquinone molecules such as aloin and aloe emodin [101–103]. The aloe emodin has been shown to induce apoptosis in vitro in multiple cell lines. Aloe's immunostimulating effects are thought to be driven by acemannan and aloemannan [104].

12.6.2 Role in Treatment of OSSN

In a case study, a 64-year-old female patient diagnosed with OSSN exhibited total remission with no recurrence after 6 years following a 3-month regimen of three times daily administration of a concentrated topical aloe vera ocular solution, as per a homeopathic recommendation [105]. To our knowledge, this is the only use of aloe vera for ocular neoplasia reported in literature, and therefore more studies are needed to understand its role in OSSN.

12.6.3 Dosage

In the only reported case, aloe vera oil drops (Aloe Fleur de Jouvence® [Forever Living Products®; Scottsdale, Arizona]) three times daily for 3 months were used [105].

12.6.4 Side Effects

The drops were well tolerated without side effects [105].

12.7 Cidofovir

12.7.1 Pharmacology

Cidofovir is a monophosphate nucleotide analogue that inhibits viral replication with its activity against a broad spectrum of DNA viruses such as HPV [106, 107]. As HPV has been implicated as a likely etiologic agent in the pathogenesis of SCC of the conjunctiva, this is possibly its therapeutical effect [107–109].

12.7.2 Role in Treatment of OSSN

In a case series of six patients (five males, one female; mean age approximately 82.1 years) diagnosed with OSSN unresponsive to standard therapies, a therapeutic regimen of 2.5 mg/mL topical cidofovir was initiated, dosed three times daily over a duration of 4 to 9 weeks. The interval to initial discernible tumor eradication ranged between 24 and 60 days, necessitating an extension of therapy until 1 week post the initial observation of clearance [110]. Another case reported an OSSN treated with 2.5 mg/mL topical cidofovir for 6 weeks followed by cryotherapy, and no recurrence was observed [111]. While limited experience with OSSN, it has been used for vulvar [112] and high-grade anal intraepithelial neoplasia [113] as well as respiratory papillomas [114].

12.7.3 Dosage

Topical cidofovir has been used in eye drops (2.5 mg/mL) at a frequency of 1 drop every 2 h for 2 weeks, then four times daily for 2 weeks, and then thrice daily for 2 weeks. In a case report, most of the superior tarsal lesions resolved with this therapy [111]. In the case series of six patients mentioned above, the concentration was 2.5 mg/mL, but the frequency was three times daily over 4–9 weeks, and this achieved tumor resolution in five of the six patients [110].

12.7.4 Side Effects

In one case, 6 months after treatment with cidofovir and cryotherapy, the patient developed scarring of the inferior punctum [111]. One adverse reaction also reported was conjunctivitis accompanied by punctal stenosis, which ameliorated upon cessation of cidofovir. Moreover, a pre-treatment assessment for high-risk HPV in five samples revealed the presence of HPV-16 in a solitary instance [110, 111, 115]. In our experience, topical cidofovir causes significant ocular surface irritation, which resolves with drop cessation.

12.8 Anti-vascular Endothelial Growth Factor Therapy

12.8.1 Pharmacology

Anti-VEGF medications are monoclonal antibodies that block the VEGFs, naturally occurring factors essential in the regulation of vasculogenesis and angiogenesis [116, 117]. Different types of VEGF and its receptors have shown to play a major role in the angiogenesis of glioblastoma [118], colorectal [119], breast [120], non-small cell type of lung [121], and kidney cancers [122], among others [123, 124]. Since the development of OSSN involves angiogenesis, the use of anti-VEGF has been studied as a treatment as well [116, 125–127].

12.8.2 Role in Treatment of OSSN

The role of anti-VEGF therapy in OSSN remains uncertain. It has been used in topical, subconjunctival, perilesional, and intralesional approaches. Studies had mixed results using ranibizumab and bevacizumab showing complete reduction in some cases and partial reduction in others which needed subsequent surgical intervention [126, 128–130].

12.8.3 Dosage

Topical bevacizumab (5–25 mg/mL) has been used as an eye drop four times a day for a period from 5 to 14 weeks [125, 126]. Perilesional/subconjunctival bevacizumab injections (2.5 mg in 0.1 mL) were given 1 week apart, with a total of two injections [130]. In another study, bevacizumab 1.25 mg in 0.05 mL was injected once [129]. In a case of a conjunctival papilloma with mild dysplasia, it was used as a single injection of 5 mg in 0.2 mL [127]. Ranibizumab 0.5 mg was injected perilesionally (0.05 mL of 10 mg/mL) monthly or twice monthly for refractory conjunctival squamous cell carcinoma with a mean of 22 injections [128].

12.8.4 Side Effects

No side effects have been reported with topical or perilesional/subconjunctival injections of bevacizumab [125–130].

12.9 Checkpoint Inhibitors and Other Targeted Therapies

12.9.1 Pharmacology

Checkpoint inhibitors and targeted therapies in cancer encompass a group of medications directed to specific cell division pathways, programmed cell death proteins, their ligands, and, in general, proteins involved in mechanisms related to cancer survival, including immune regulation, which has been found to play a role in neoplastic cells by avoiding the normal immune response to malignancy [131, 132]. Targeting these pathways with monoclonal antibodies has shown promising results in cancer treatment by inhibiting cell division and also activating immune responses against cancer directly overcoming tumoral immune tolerance.

Among the checkpoint inhibitors, pembrolizumab, nivolumab, and cemiplimab, are monoclonal antibodies directed against human cell surface receptor PD-1 (programmed cell death 1). In 2015, pembrolizumab was approved by the US Food and Drug Administration (FDA) for the treatment of metastatic cutaneous melanoma and of unresectable or metastatic solid tumor with certain genetic anomalies [133]. The checkpoint inhibitors directed toward the PD-ligand 1 (PD-L1) are involved in the same pathway as PD-1 and include atezolizumab, avelumab, and durvalumab [134–137]. Other checkpoint inhibitors such as ipilimumab are those which inhibit the cytotoxic T-lymphocyte-associated antigen 4 (CTLA-4), another signaling protein normally present in immune cells but involved in mechanisms of immune tolerance to malignancy [138, 139].

12.9.2 Role in Treatment of OSSN

Targeted therapies, particularly checkpoint inhibitors, have been extensively studied in cutaneous squamous cell carcinoma [140, 141]. Large-scale studies, including more than eight clinical trials, have highlighted their significant role in treating advanced cases [141, 142]. These therapies have induced high pathologic response rates, often leading to curative outcomes, and also made patients eligible for surgery in cases where surgery or radiotherapy was previously not possible. The pivotal trial leading to the approval of cemiplimab included phase I/II cohorts with patients with locally advanced and metastatic cutaneous SCC. This study demonstrated response rates of 47– 50% [143]. More recently, a phase II trial evaluated cemiplimab in patients with stage III and IV cutaneous SCC (n = 20), observing either a complete pathologic response or a major pathologic response (≤10% viable tumor) in 75% of patients, accompanied by a 12-month overall survival rate of 95% [142]. Another recent study, using cemiplimab as a neoadjuvant in 79 patients with stage III/IV cutaneous SCC, achieved complete pathologic responses in 51% of patients and major pathological responses in 13% [141].

Regarding OSSN, the invasive squamous cell conjunctival variant has shown a level of expression of PD-L1 in neoplastic cells that has been correlated with tumor invasion [144, 145]. A study of 18 cases of invasive ocular surface SCC and ocular adnexal SCC demonstrated different levels of expression of PD-L1 and PD-L2, with PD-L1 being expressed in 100%, and the level of expression directly correlated with the presence of CD8-positive T lymphocytes [144]. Another study of 31 patients with conjunctival SCC found expression of PD-L1 in 47% of the cases, and its expression was correlated with higher presence of CD3, CD8, and PD-1 expression in the tumor-associated immune infiltrate [145]. These findings are similar to studies in head and neck cancer, where PD-L1 expression was a predictor of response to checkpoint inhibitors [146–148]. Anti-PD1 and anti-PD-L1 medications like pembrolizumab, nivolumab, and cemiplimab have also been used both in OSSN as well as orbital and adnexal SCC [18, 149, 150].

In addition to the expression of PD-1 and PD-L1, the tumor mutational burden (TMB), a biomarker that indicates the number of mutations per megabase of DNA, has been studied as a predictor of response to immunotherapy. TMB has demonstrated predictive value in solid tumors such as melanoma, SCC, and non-small cell lung cancer [151]. The underlying rationale is that an increased number of mutations is likely to raise immunogenicity, thereby potentially improving T-cell response. However, additional studies are necessary to fully understand its capabilities and limitations [152].

A case series, consisting of five patients with conjunctival squamous cell carcinoma, investigated the efficacy of pembrolizumab and cemiplimab in treating biopsy-proven SCC/OSSN with orbital extension in patients who declined exenteration. TMB was measured in all cases; in four patients with a high TMB (61.5–109.6 mutations/Mb of DNA), one checkpoint inhibitor was administered, and one patient with low TMB (8.1 Mutations/Mb of DNA) received both pembrolizumab and chemotherapy. The patients with high TMB experienced complete tumor resolution; this included one patient treated with pembrolizumab and three with cemiplimab. This resolution was sustained throughout the follow-up period, which averaged 6 months. Conversely, the only patient with low TMB, initially treated with pembrolizumab and 5-FU and subsequently with carboplatin and docetaxel, exhibited disease progression which ultimately necessitated wide resection and subsequent radiotherapy

[149]. Additionally, a case report detailed the treatment of a patient with poorly differentiated conjunctival SCC/OSSN, exhibiting a 20% expression of PD-L1. This patient, having undergone repeated radiotherapy and experienced multiple recurrences, opted for cemiplimab therapy after declining the recommended exenteration. After 19 months on cemiplimab, both clinical evaluations and orbital magnetic resonance monitoring indicated that the tumor remained stable [153].

Targeted therapies for mTOR, NRAS, NF1, and TERT mutations are rapidly advancing. Studied in other types of cancers, some ocular surface cancer has also been already linked to these mutations [154–156]. Interestingly, targeted therapies anti EGFR (epidermal growth factor receptor) such as cetuximab and gefitinib have shown good results as neoadjuvants for cutaneous SCC facilitating surgical resectability and even complete pathologic response [157–161]. These may be future targets for OSSN therapies.

12.9.3 Dosage

Nivolumab 240 mg intravenously every 2 weeks or 480 mg intravenously every 4 weeks is infused over 30 min, until disease recurrence or unacceptable toxicity (OPDIVO® Bristol-Myers Squibb Company, Princeton, NJ, 2018).

Cemiplimab 350 mg intravenous infusion over 30 min every 3 weeks is given until disease recurrence or unacceptable toxicity (Product Information: LIBTAYO® intravenous injection, cemiplimab-rwlc intravenous injection. Regeneron Pharmaceuticals Inc. (per FDA), Tarrytown, NY, 2023).

Pembrolizumab 200 mg intravenous infusion over 30 min is given every 3 weeks or 400 mg intravenous over 30 min every 6 weeks for up to 24 months (Product Information: KEYTRUDA® intravenous injection, pembrolizumab intravenous injection. Merck Sharp & Dohme Corp (per FDA), Whitehouse Station, NJ, 2020).

12.9.4 Side Effects

Checkpoint inhibitors are known to cause systemic and ocular proinflammatory side effects such as uveitis, myocarditis, chemosis, and orbital myositis [162–164].

12.10 Lymphoma of the Conjunctiva

12.10.1 Introduction

Lymphomas are malignant neoplasms that arise from lymphocytes [165]. Around 5–15% of extranodal lymphomas occur in the ocular adnexal area, and of these, 25% are identified in the conjunctiva [166]. Extranodal marginal zone lymphoma (EMZL) is the predominant type of lymphoma seen in the conjunctiva [167, 168] of which mucosal-associated lymphoid tissue (MALT) is the most common. The systemic prognosis for conjunctival lymphomas varies with the cell type. It is best with EMZL and worse with mantle cell lymphoma (MCL) or diffuse B-cell subtypes [165–167]. Typically, conjunctival lymphoma presents as a subconjunctival salmon-pink, “fleshy” painless lesion that is seen in the bulbar conjunctiva (Fig. 12.4). Of note, the diffuse large B-cell lymphoma (DLBCL) may present with a grayer color rather than salmon-pink [167]. Conjunctival lymphoma typically presents with symptoms of irritation, dryness, tearing, ptosis, and redness but can be asymptomatic. Older age, exposure to radiation, and immunodeficiency are the principal risk factors associated with lymphoma. Bacterial and viral agents such as *Helicobacter pylori*, *Campylobacter jejuni*, *Chlamydophila psittaci*, EBV, and hepatitis C virus have all been associated with the pathogenesis of lymphomas as oncogenic microorganisms promoting carcinogenesis by hyperactivation of the immune system [169–175]. A well-known correlation is *Helicobacter pylori* with gastric MALT lymphoma [169, 170]. Lymphoma has a wide differential diagnosis ranging from benign lesions like reactive lymphoid hyperplasia, pyogenic granuloma, and lymphangiectasis to malignant tumors such as SCC and amelanotic melanoma [176, 177] (see Chap. 8).

12.10.2 Treatment

Radiation therapy (XRT) has been the mainstay for unilateral isolated conjunctival lymphoma, but the optimal radiation dose has not been established [178]. In a comprehensive Korean study examining radiation therapy for lymphoma in the conjunctiva, 121 eyes (from 79 patients) with a median age of 38 were treated with a total of 26 Gy delivered with 2 Gy per fraction and five fractions per week. After radiation, local control was 98.1%. The 5-year survival was 100%, with re-radiation used for nearly all relapsed cases [179]. Other study found similarly high control rates (98%) with doses of 25 Gy delivered over 10 fractions [180]. Regimes of “ultra-low dose” radiation therapies have gained popularity in conjunctival, orbital, and ocular adnexal lesions given the radiosensitivity of lymphomas and the non-inferiority demonstrated in some clinical trials [181–185]. Four Gy delivered in two consecutive fractions of 2 Gy (2 × 2 Gy) has been used for marginal zone B-cell lymphoma (MZL) and MALT lymphoma, mostly recommended in patients with a single lesion for curative purposes and for palliation in advanced stage and relapsed disease [181–185].

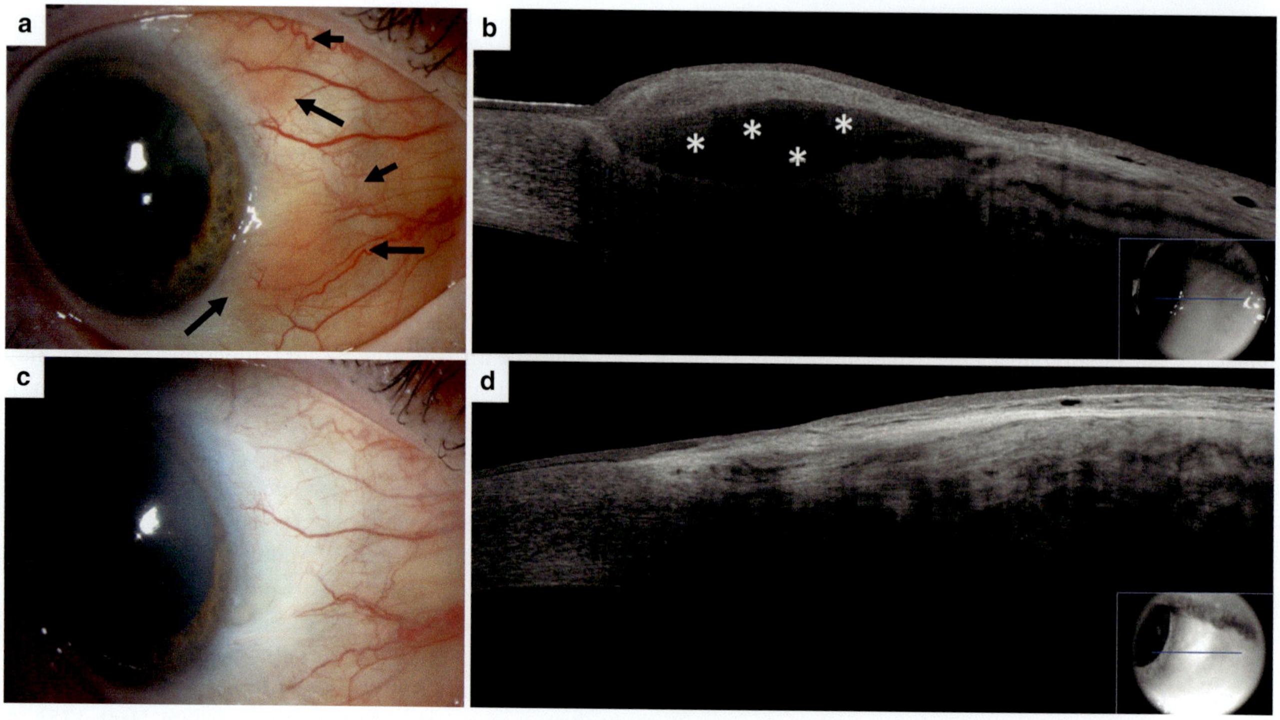

Fig. 12.4 Slit-lamp photography and HR-OCT imaging of a right eye with conjunctival lymphoma before and after treatment with radiotherapy. (**a**) Slit lamp photography demonstrates elevated salmon-colored lesions on the superior and nasal conjunctiva (arrows) of the right eye. (**b**) HR-OCT image of the nasal limbal conjunctiva demonstrates a subepithelial hyperreflective lesion with monomorphic "dot-like" accumulation (asterisks). The lower right inset represents the anatomical location of the OCT raster section. (**c**) Slit lamp photography demonstrates complete resolution of elevated lesions 1.5 years after ending 30.6 Gy delivered in 17 fractions. (**d**) HR OCT image shows complete regression of the conjunctival tumor. The lower right inset represents the anatomical location of the OCT raster section

Table 12.2 Common pharmacotherapeutic treatment options for ocular adnexal lymphoma

Lymphoma- preferred treatment options	Most common dosage	Main side effects
Rituximab	IV: 375 mg/mL rituximab every 3 weeks, maintenance dose every 2–3 months for 2 years. Subconjunctival injections: 1.5 cc of rituximab (10 mg/mL) with xylocaine 2% is received 4 times a week followed by a monthly injection for the next 6 months	IV: Fever, anemia, infusion-related reaction, neutropenia, lymphocytopenia, hypogammaglobulinemia, varicella-zoster virus infection or reactivation, hepatitis B virus reactivation, bacterial infection, herpes simplex infection and reactivation Subconjunctival injections: discomfort at site of injection
Ibritumomab tiuxetan	IV rituximab 250 mg/m^2 followed by an infusion of ^{90}Y ibritumomab tiuxetan with a dose that depends on the platelet count. For patients with a platelet count of 100,000/mm^3–149,000/mm^3, 0.3 mCi/kg was used and 0.4 mCi/kg for patients with counts of >150,000/mm^3	Thrombocytopenia, anemia, and neutropenia
IFNα	Subconjunctival injection: 1 MU or 1.5 MU of IFNα-2a or 2b is administered 3 times a week for a total of 4 weeks or more	Flu-like syndrome, discomfort at site of injection

IFN-α interferon alpha, *IV* intravenous

Medical therapies have been utilized as alternatives to radiation in cases of unilateral disease and in systemic disease (Table 12.2). Rarely, aggressive bilateral disease or conjunctival lymphoma accompanied by systemic lesions will be treated with CHOP (cyclophosphamide, doxorubicin, vincristine, prednisone), CVP (cyclophosphamide, vincristine, prednisolone), or chlorambucil [186–189]. Interferon, rituximab, and ibritumomab are more commonly used for local treatment [190, 191] (see also Chap. 8).

12.11 Interferon Alpha

12.11.1 Pharmacology

Discussed α-2b above in OSSN section.

12.11.2 Role in Lymphoma

The use of IFNα has been described as a possible alternative in patients with unilateral localized conjunctival lymphoma who are not amenable to radiation treatment. A study on the effects of intralesional interferon-alpha for conjunctival lymphoma was conducted. Here, 20 patients with localized conjunctival EMZL were treated with intralesional IFNα-2a. Nineteen patients had no systemic disease, and one patient had quiescent systemic disease (in remission at the time of conjunctival presentation). Treatment involved 12 doses of 1.5 million IU. For those with minimal response, another 12 doses of 1 million IU of interferon-alpha were given. Fifteen patients had complete resolution after the first 12 injections, and the other 5 patients resolved with the additional 12 injections. After a median follow-up period of 65 months, 85% were recurrence-free [192]. Other studies have also used IFN α-2a or IFNα-2b for primary therapy [192–195]. Since interferon was discontinued by its manufacturer in the United States in all its presentations, it is currently not available in the United States.

12.11.3 Dosage

The intralesional administration of IFNα-2a and 2b have been reported as 1–1.5 million IU of interferon in 0.25–1 mL subconjunctivally. The treatment can be given up to 3 times a week for 4–6 weeks, and additional cycles are suggested if there's an incomplete response [194–197].

12.11.4 Side Effects

For intralesional injections of IFNα, side effects are discussed above and include flu-like syndrome and malaise [192, 193](Table 12.2).

12.12 Rituximab

12.12.1 Pharmacology

Rituximab is an anti-CD20 monoclonal antibody that kills CD20-positive B cells via multiple mechanisms. These include direct effects on complement-mediated cytotoxicity and antibody-dependent cell-mediated and an indirect effect on cell structures, both of which lead to apoptosis. In addition, rituximab sensitizes cancer cells to other chemotherapy drugs [198, 199]. Since its approval, rituximab has dramatically changed the treatment of B-cell malignancies. Since most B-cells are CD20 positive (this excludes pro-B cells and plasma B cells) [200, 201], rituximab has become a standard component of care in several regimens for follicular lymphoma [201], large B-cell lymphoma [202], and chronic lymphocytic leukemia [203].

12.12.2 Role in Lymphoma

Since intravenous rituximab received approval for use 20 years ago, it has become a standard component of care for patients with non-Hodgkin lymphoma, follicular lymphoma, diffuse large B-cell lymphoma, chronic lymphocytic leukemia, EMZL (MALT) lymphoma, and mantle cell lymphoma [204–209]. Furthermore, systemic rituximab has also been used for bilateral ocular and adnexal lymphoma in patients with systemic disease. Annibali et al. carried out a retrospective analysis involving seven patients who had primary MALT ocular adnexal lymphomas. Among these individuals, six underwent single-agent rituximab treatment. All patients received six cycles of rituximab intravenously at a dosage of 375 mg/m^2 every 3 weeks [210]. The study yielded encouraging findings, demonstrating a 100% overall response rate. Furthermore, during a median follow-up period of 29 months (with a range of 8 to 34 months), there were no instances of recurrence or adverse effects [210]. Tuncer et al. reported a case series of 10 patients with biopsy-proven ocular adnexal lymphoma managed with rituximab intravenously observing complete regression in one-third of the patients; the remaining two-thirds showed only a partial response. Subsequent adjunctive radiotherapy was required for these patients to achieve a complete response [211].

In addition, there have been a few small studies using intralesional rituximab for isolated ocular adnexal lymphoma. The intralesional, localized ocular use of rituximab is an alternative in patients without systemic disease or those who refuse or are not candidates for radiation, as systemic use of rituximab or radiation is the current standard of care for ocular adnexal lymphoma. Yazicioglu et al. reported a case of a patient diagnosed with low-grade conjunctival extranodal marginal zone lymphoma and underwent successful and safe treatment with intralesional rituximab therapy. Initially, she received injections of undiluted rituximab (10–20 mg/mL) combined with 2% epinephrine-free lidocaine, with a volume of 1–2 mL. The treatment started with weekly injections, and after completing the fourth cycle, the patient received intralesional rituximab injections once a month for 6 months, totaling ten cycles [212]. Near complete regression of the condition was observed by the end of the tenth cycle. Furthermore, no recurrence was detected during the 20-month follow-up period [212]. Demirci et al. used intralesional rituximab for a patient with recurrent bilateral MALT lymphoma of the lacrimal glands who refused external beam radiation or further systemic treatment with rituximab. He injected 1 ml of rituximab 50 mg/mL into each lacrimal gland. This resulted in clinical resolution, and at 23 months after the last injection, there was no clinical evidence of recurrence. The CT scan confirmed left lacrimal gland atrophy and a stable and heterogeneous appearance of the right lacrimal gland [213]. Ferreri et al. also achieved full remission in a patient with marginal zone lymphoma of the conjunctiva following intralesional rituximab treatment [214].

12.12.3 Dosage

Intravenous rituximab has been administered in 6 cycles of 375 mg/m^2 every 3 weeks with a maintenance dose every 2–3 months for 2 years in EMZL of MALT tissue of the ocular adnexa [210]. EMZL bilateral cases without systemic involvement, can be managed by bilateral XRT or systemic medication. When selecting XRT, it is best tolerated with the ultralow dose regimes. Alternatively, intravenous rituximab 375mg/m^2 every week for 4 weeks may be used. When conjunctival lymphoma occurs with systemic involvement rituximab 375mg/m^2 may be combined with bemdamustine. Furthermore, rituximab may be used as R-CHOP (rituximab with cyclophosphamide, doxorubicin, vincristine, and prednisone) for more aggressive variants and is associated with better outcomes in follicular lymphoma (FL), MCL, and DLBCL [167].

When there is no systemic involvement and is isolated EMZL to the ocular adnexa, generally, radiation is the treatment of choice. However, in patients who refuse or have contraindications to radiation, intralesional (subconjunctival) rituximab administration for EMZL is an alternative option that may be used. However, this is not the preferred treatment. The dose reported is 1.5 mL of rituximab (10 mg/mL) with xylocaine 2%, given four times a week followed by a monthly injection for the next 6 months [167, 214]. As mentioned above, the protocol Demirci et al. used in a patient with bilateral MALT lymphoma of the lacrimal glands consisted of 1 mL of rituximab (50 mg/1 mL) injected into the left lacrimal gland with B-scan ultrasound guidance; this was followed by an injection in the right lacrimal gland 7 months later [213].

12.12.4 Side Effects

Side effects of systemic rituximab are rare but include varicella-zoster virus (VZV) reactivation following intravenous administration [210]. In addition, intravenous rituximab has been associated with hematologic side effects, such as neutropenia and thrombocytopenia [215, 216]. Following intralesional administration of rituximab, some patients have reported mild pain and local inflammation 24 h following injection [214] (Table 12.2).

12.13 Ibritumomab Tiuxetan

12.13.1 Pharmacology

While rarely used in conjunctival lymphomas, ibritumomab tiuxetan (Zevalin, Spectrum Pharmaceuticals, Henderson NV) is an approved medication for refractory B-cell lymphomas. It links the radioactive isotope yttrium-90(^{90}Y) to a monoclonal antibody that targets CD20 [217]. By targeting CD20 cells, it is able to deliver pure β radioactive emission to eliminate target cells and adjacent non-expressing cells through a bystander effect, operating independently of the host's immune system [217].

12.13.2 Role in Lymphoma

As ocular and adnexal EMZL is highly sensitive to radiotherapy, it is certainly possible that radio- immunotherapy may also be very effective in controlling the disease as well as preventing relapse [217, 218]. The only two studies showing the use of this monoclonal antibody for conjunctival lymphoma suggest that it can be an effective alternative for the treatment of conjunctival lymphoma. In a patient with MALT lymphoma refractory to rituximab treatment, complete resolution of the tumor was achieved using ibritumomab tiuxetan [217, 218].

12.13.3 Dosage

In the case reports available, it has been administered in combination with intravenous rituximab 250 mg/m^2 followed by an infusion of ^{90}Y ibritumomab tiuxetan with the dose adjusted according to the platelet count. For patients with a platelet count of 100,000/mm^3–149,000/mm^3, 0.3 mCi/kg is used, with 0.4 mCi/kg being administered to patients with platelet counts exceeding 150,000/mm^3, and contraindicated when the platelet count is below 100,000/mm^3 [217, 218].

12.13.4 Side Effects

Given its directed mechanism toward CD20 cells, the principal side effects are hematologic. Most patients present with severe and prolonged cytopenias, and it should not be given to patients with more than 25% of lymphoma marrow involvement or in patients with inadequate bone marrow reserve [219]. Close monitoring from the first 24 h is crucial since severe infusion reactions are not uncommon [220, 221]. Some other notable side effects include fatigue, nausea, and headache [166] (Table 12.2).

12.14 Clarithromycin

12.14.1 Pharmacology

Clarithromycin is a member of the macrolide antibiotic family, structurally similar to erythromycin. The pharmacokinetic profile is more favorable than erythromycin, and it is dosed twice daily. Clarithromycin is well distributed in tissues, including the eye. Clarithromycin inhibits bacterial protein synthesis by preventing peptidyl transferase attachment to a growing peptide chain [222].

12.14.2 Role in Lymphoma

Clarithromycin, known for its ability to treat chronic infections and its antineoplastic properties [222–233], has been employed in treating patients with relapsed or refractory ocular adnexal EMZL. A prospective study was conducted using clarithromycin to treat EMZL in patients with various involvement sites, including the conjunctiva, orbits, stomach, kidney, bone marrow, lymph nodes, and breast. In the study by Govi et al. ($n = 13$), a baseline assessment included testing for infectious agents. Results showed the presence of *Helicobacter pylori* in one patient, *Chlamydophila psittaci* in four, and hepatitis C virus in two [234].

In a different study involving 23 patients, testing for various infectious etiologies was also performed. This study found that seven patients had previously eradicated *Helicobacter pylori* and *Chlamydophila psittaci* infections 2 years before enrollment, with no current infections detected at the trial's start. This suggests that clarithromycin's effectiveness may be due to non-antimicrobial mechanisms. The treatment regimens included oral clarithromycin (500 mg twice daily) for 6 months [215, 216] or 2 grams daily in 2-week cycles over 3 months [216]. In terms of effectiveness, one study reported that 22% of patients achieved a complete response and 25% a partial response, but half did not respond to the treatment. After 24 months, relapse rates were observed to be between 30% and 50% [215, 216].

12.14.3 Dosage

In one of the studies, clarithromycin (500 mg) is taken orally, twice daily, for 6 months [234]. In the other study, clarithromycin (2 g) is taken daily for 14-day cycles with 1 week off and repeated for 3 months [235].

12.14.4 Side Effects

Few side effects have been reported with clarithromycin. The most common side effects are nausea, diarrhea, and abnormal taste [236].

12.15 Doxycycline

12.15.1 Pharmacology

Doxycycline is a member of the tetracycline antibiotic family. It works by binding to the 30s ribosomal subunit and blocking the binding of aminoacyl-tRNA to the ribosomal complex, thus interfering with protein synthesis and interrupting proper cell function [237].

12.15.2 Role in Lymphoma

As mentioned above, due to the association between chronic antigen stimulation and lymphoma, doxycycline has been used with the aim of eradicating bacterial infection to induce regression of the lymphoma. Some studies suggest that the use of doxycycline in patients with *Chlamydophila psittaci* DNA-positive infections can be beneficial, and, interestingly, it has a positive impact on tumor regression in *Chlamydophila psittaci* DNA-negative patients as well. This parallels the finding that H. pylori-negative gastric MALT lymphoma also may respond to antibiotic therapy [238, 239]. It has been used as a part of primary treatment or in patients with relapse of lymphoma.

In two large prospective studies [240, 241], a total of 117 patients with EMZL were treated with oral doxycycline 100 mg twice daily in 1–2 cycles. In the study by Han et al., doxycycline was given as a first-line treatment to patients with newly diagnosed ocular adnexal EMZL without previous chemotherapy or radiotherapy($n = 90$). No testing of *Chlamydophila psittaci* DNA was performed. The tumors were localized in the conjunctiva (82%), orbit (13%), eyelid (3%), and lacrimal gland (2%). At the time of analysis, 24 patients (27%) achieved complete or partial response, and 34 (38%) remained with stable disease. The patients with partial response or progressive disease after doxycycline received salvage treatment (chemotherapy and/or radiotherapy) achieving progression-free survival (PFS) of 100% at the last follow-up date [240]. In the other study, 27 patients, 15 newly diagnosed and 12 with relapsed disease, were enrolled and tested for *Chlamydophila psittaci* DNA. Patients with positive and negative test were included in the trial. If *Helicobacter pylori* was identified, it was treated with erythromycin 500 mg twice a day, omeprazole 20 mg twice a day, and tinidazole 500 mg twice a day. In the eligible patients, doxycycline was administered as 100 mg twice a day for 3 weeks. The patient population at enrollment presented with lymphoma in conjunctiva (45%), lacrimal gland or orbit (55%), and bilateral orbit (27%). Chlamydophila psittaci was positive in 11 patients (41%) and negative in 16 patients (59%). At a median follow-up of 14 months, six patients (22%) experienced a complete response, and 7 patients (26%) achieved a partial response. Response to the treatment was observed in patients with a positive *Chlamydophila psittaci* DNA test (7 of 11 patients), and in patients with a negative test (6 of 16 patients). Seven patients had failure to the treatment but a correlation to disease location, *Chlamydophila psittaci* DNA test, or previous treatment was not found, suggesting false-negative tests for *Chlamydophila*, potential associations of lymphoma development with another doxycycline-sensitive bacteria or a result from non-antimicrobial properties of the doxycycline. PFS at 2 years was 74% [241]. Looking at the combined results of the two studies, out of the 117 patients, 10 (8%) patients achieved complete response, and 27 (23%) had partial response. When discontinued, relapse rates were approximately 25% over 14–40 months [240, 241].

In a more recent retrospective study, PFS was analyzed in 67 patients who were treated with oral doxycycline as their primary treatment of EMZL (MALT) lymphoma [242]. All patients received either one or two cycles of oral doxycycline at 100 mg twice a day for 3 weeks. The two cycles were given to patients with a residual mass or ocular discomfort who did not respond to the first cycle with 3 weeks off between cycles. Patients with progression were changed to second-line treatments. After the initial cycle, 25 (37.3%) patients achieved complete response and 8 (11.9%) partial response, 30 (44.8%) had stable disease, and 4 (6%) patients had progression. PFS rates were of 70% at 3 years, 65% at 5 years, and 62% at 10 years; no further progression was observed after 6 years [242].

12.15.3 Dose

Doxycycline, 100 mg, administered twice a day for 3 weeks in cycles [240–242].

12.15.4 Side Effects

The most common side effects of doxycycline are nausea, vomiting, and skin rash [243].

12.16 Pigmented Conjunctival Lesions

12.16.1 Introduction

Pigmented lesions of the ocular surface include conjunctival nevus, complexion-associated melanosis, conjunctival primary acquired melanosis (PAM) with and without atypia, and conjunctival malignant melanoma (CMM) [244], all arising from the conjunctival melanocytes residing in the basal layer of the epithelium. PAM with atypia is the most common progenitor of CMM and appears clinically as a flat and variably brown conjunctival lesion [244, 245] (Fig. 12.5). CMM can arise also from conjunctival nevus and de novo [244]. CMM typically presents as a unilateral, pigmented, immobile, vascular lesion with heterogeneous pigmentation. It is commonly seen on the bulbar conjunctiva with associated feeder vessels but can appear anywhere on the bulbar or palpebral conjunctiva. CMM can also present as an amelanotic lesion or with variable pigmentation and vascularity [246–250]. While the traditional treatment of PAM with atypia is surgical excision [251], in recent years, topical chemotherapy, cryotherapy, and immunotherapy have been used as adjuvant treatment [252–255] (see Chaps. 6 and 7).

12.16.2 Treatment

Complete surgical excision is the mainstay of treatment for conjunctival melanoma. Due to the high rate of local recurrence and potential metastasis [135, 256, 257], surgical excision should always be combined with adjuvant therapy such as cryotherapy, chemotherapy, immunotherapy, and brachytherapy [251, 252, 256, 258]. Chemotherapy is used for diffuse disease (i.e., PAM with atypia and diffuse PAM surrounding CMM). In terms of topical therapy, MMC has been the most studied therapy

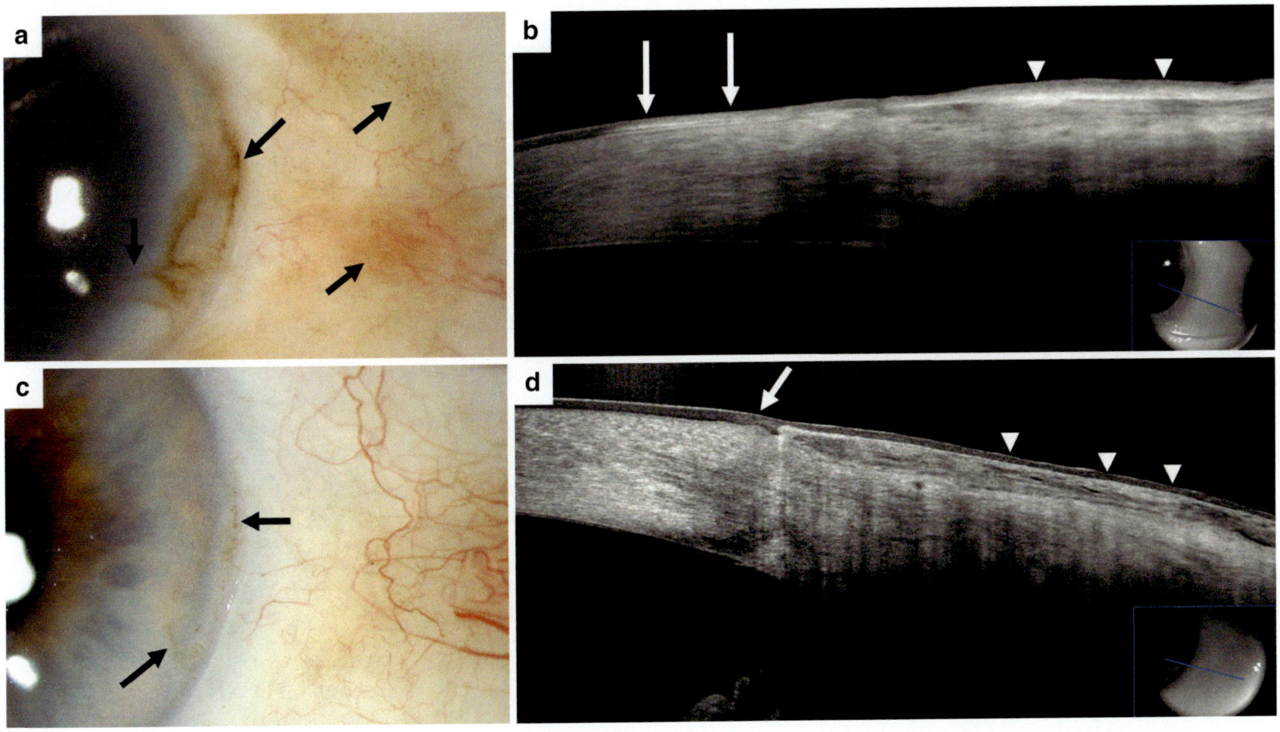

Fig. 12.5 Slit-lamp photography and HR-OCT imaging of a right eye with primary acquired melanosis treated with MMC as neoadjuvant before excision. (**a**) Slit lamp photograph of the right eye demonstrates diffuse areas of melanosis in the nasal conjunctiva and peripheral cornea (arrows). (**b**) HR-OCT image of nasal conjunctiva and cornea demonstrates hyperreflective epithelium in cornea (arrows) most prominent in the basal epithelium. The adjacent involved conjunctival epithelium similarly has hyperreflectivity in the basal epithelium but also with mild thickening and hyperreflectivity (arrowheads). The lower right inset represents the anatomical location of the OCT raster section. (**c**) Slit lamp photography of right eye demonstrates a reduction in areas of melanosis with subtle remaining melanotic areas in the peripheral cornea after 6 cycles of 0.04% mitomycin C given four times a day for 1 week on with 3 weeks off. The patient had an excision of the remaining areas not eliminated by the MMC. (**d**) HR-OCT image of nasal conjunctiva and cornea demonstrates reduction of hyperreflectivity in corneal and conjunctival epithelium and normalization of conjunctival epithelial thickness (arrowheads). Note area of mild hyperreflectivity in peripheral corneal epithelium (arrow) corresponding to the residual limbal pigmentation. The lower right inset represents anatomical location of OCT raster section. As the MMC resolved the pigmentation, she did not undergo surgical excision. She has been observed

and is the primary topical therapy when adjuvants are needed for PAM [259, 260]. IFN-α2b has been used in small series and when MMC was not tolerated [261–263]. These two drugs are used often also in treating PAM with atypia after diagnostic biopsy and have been used also in combination [253, 259–261, 263, 264].

12.17 Mitomycin C (MMC)

12.17.1 Pharmacology

Described above in the section on OSSN.

12.17.2 Role in Pigmented Conjunctival Lesions

Topical MMC can be used as an adjuvant and neoadjuvant to excision [261, 265]. MMC is not used as a primary therapy in conjunctival malignant melanoma as the results are poor [266]. Whereas in PAM, a short regimen can be used to chemoreduce the tumor prior to excision. It has also been used for extensive and unresectable PAM as a primary treatment with some success. In three large retrospective studies [259, 260, 267], a total of 26 patients were treated primarily with MMC for PAM. The regimen consisted of topical MMC 0.02–0.04%, four times a day for 28 days. Of the 26, 12 (46%) had complete response, and 12 (46%) showed partial response. One patient had no response to the MMC. Follow-up ranges were 4–144 months, and relapse rates were approximately 27% [259, 260, 267]. As a postoperative adjuvant, MMC has been used to aid in the treatment of CMM and PAM with atypia, but its use may be limited because of its known side effects [253, 261, 263].

12.17.3 Dosage

When used as adjuvant and neoadjuvant, MMC is typically administered at 0.02–0.04% four times a day for 7–28 days [259, 260]. MMC can be administered intraoperatively as well [268].

12.17.4 Side Effects

Described above in the section on OSSN.

12.18 Interferon Alpha-2b

12.18.1 Pharmacology

Described above in the OSSN section.

12.18.2 Role in Pigmented Conjunctival Lesions

IFNα-2b is not commonly used in the treatment of pigmented conjunctival lesions as evidence is limited. However, due to its enhancement of the MHC class 1 surface antigen expression, there is biologic plausibility that it may have a positive immune response signaling for the removal of tumor cells [269]. It can be administered topically and as subconjunctival/perilesional injections [266]. The data for topical IFNα-2b for PAM is limited [262]. In four retrospective studies [264, 270–272], a total of 25 patients with PAM/MMC were treated with 1 million IU four to five times a day for 6–36 weeks. Of the 25 patients treated, 7 (28%) had eventual complete response to treatment, and 13 (52%) showed partial response. Approximately 20% did not respond to the IFNα-2b treatment. The follow-up of the previous studies was short (range, 4–17 months) [264, 270–272]. IFNα-2b is currently not available in the United States.

12.18.3 Dosage

The dose of topical IFNα-2b is 1 million IU/mL one drop four or five times a day, for 3–6 months [264, 266, 270–274].

12.18.4 Side Effects

Described above in the section on OSSN (Fig. 12.6).

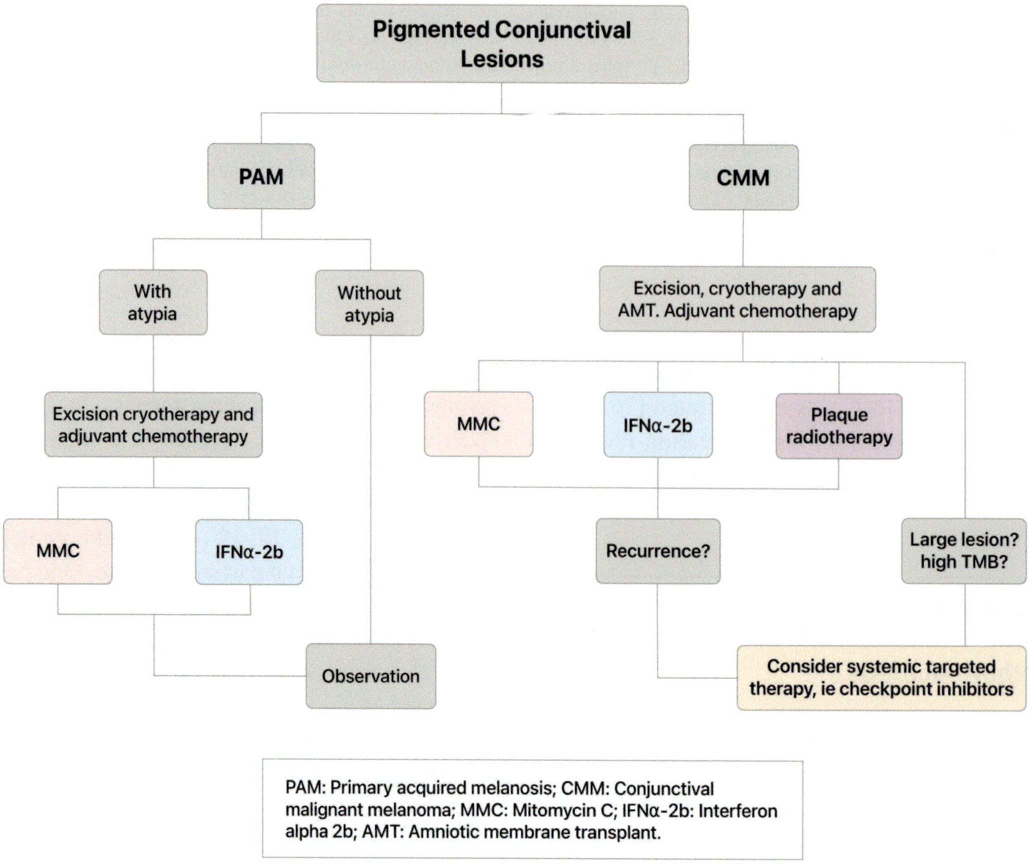

Fig. 12.6 Algorithm for management of pigmented conjunctival lesions

12.19 Checkpoint Inhibitors and Other Targeted Therapies

12.19.1 Pharmacology

Targeted therapies directed toward various mechanisms related to CMM development have been used; this includes those targeted to mutations such as BRAF, MEK, and those blocking immunoregulatory mechanisms such as PD-1, PD-L1, and CTLA-4 (checkpoint inhibitors, described above in the OSSN section).

For instance, anti-PD1 medications such as nivolumab and pembrolizumab, or anti-PD-L1 medications such as avelumab and atezolizumab, are useful in CMM because these cancer cells activate various immune checkpoint pathways to suppress the natural immune response (i.e., expression of PD-L1 molecules) [131, 134]. By blocking these mechanisms, a more appropriate response from the immune system to the malignant cells is generated. In addition to PD-1 and PD-L1 inhibitors, other medications such as vemurafenib and dabrafenib can be used in CMM. These are two monoclonal antibodies directed to interrupt mechanisms where a BRAF mutation exists, which occurs in a high percentage of melanoma cases and leads to promotion of tumoral growth [132, 135, 275, 276]. Other mutation-targeted therapies include the MEK1/MEK2 mutation inhibitors like trametinib and cobimetinib, which have been used in combination with BRAF inhibitors for being part of the same pathway [135, 138, 275].

12.19.2 Role in Pigmented Conjunctival Lesions

These therapies represent "game changers" in the treatment of unresectable and metastatic cancers of several types, especially cutaneous melanoma which is similar in many biological and molecular aspects to conjunctival melanoma [277]. In skin melanoma, particularly in advanced disease (stage III and stage IV), several studies have shown an increase in survival rates using checkpoint inhibitors such as ipilimumab and pembrolizumab as adjuvants for treatment when compared with no treatment or surgical resection alone [278–280], and new studies have shown a longer event-free survivals when used as neoadjuvants followed by adjuvant therapy than those who received the medication as adjuvant alone [281–284].

The expression of PD-1 and PD-L1 has been identified in CMM (Fig. 12.7). In particular, PD-L1 expression (present in about 19% of CMM) is correlated with distant metastases and worse survival [134, 138, 285–290]. Medications like nivolumab and pembrolizumab, anti-PD-1, which have been combined with anti-CTLA-4 like ipilimumab have been successfully used in patients with advanced disease (metastases to several organs or multifocal recurrence) leading to favorable outcomes [289, 291–297].

For instance, when used for unresectable or metastatic conjunctival melanoma in small series, some complete regression or stabilization of the disease has been documented [289, 291–297]. A case by the group of Torres et al. describes a patient with an unresectable recurrent CMM who was treated with vemurafenib, resulting in complete remission [294]. Savig et al. reported a case series of five patients with metastatic CMM where three patients showed no evidence of disease after treatment with checkpoint inhibitors [291]. Another case report detailed a patient who had undergone surgical excision for cutaneous melanoma 5 years prior and later presented with multiple metastases in the chest wall, abdomen, and skin. She then presented with a new dark spot on the temporal conjunctiva of the left eye. The patient was initiated on treatment with nivolumab and ipilimumab. After 3 weeks of systemic treatment, she was seen by an ophthalmologist, and surgical excision was chosen for the conjunctival lesion. Histopathology revealed the presence of melanophages and the absence of viable melanoma cells (Melan-A and SOX10 negative). These findings indicated necrosis and complete regression of the metastasis following treatment with checkpoint inhibitors [298].

In addition to the cases of metastatic CMM treated with checkpoint inhibitors, it is important to consider the current therapeutic strategies for cases of advanced CMM without systemic involvement. This approach for advanced CMM includes exenteration, which continues to be a part of the recommended and standard treatment. However, the significant drawbacks of the exenteration are its highly morbid and disfiguring nature, along with its inability to always prevent metastasis [299]. These limitations of exenteration could be potentially improved by using checkpoint inhibitors as neoadjuvants, as described before in cutaneous melanoma (Fig. 12.7) [281–284].

In addition to their potential use as neoadjuvants, recent studies have begun to explore the efficacy of checkpoint inhibitors as an alternative treatment strategy for those patients unwilling to undergo the recommended orbital exenteration, demonstrating scenarios of complete and partial tumor regression, without signs of recurrence during the subsequent follow-up period [289, 293, 300]. A study by Kini et al. featured a patient with conjunctival melanoma who had previously been treated with excision and cryotherapy. When local recurrence emerged, the patient declined the advised orbital exenteration and was offered pembrolizumab as an alternative, ultimately achieving a complete response [293].

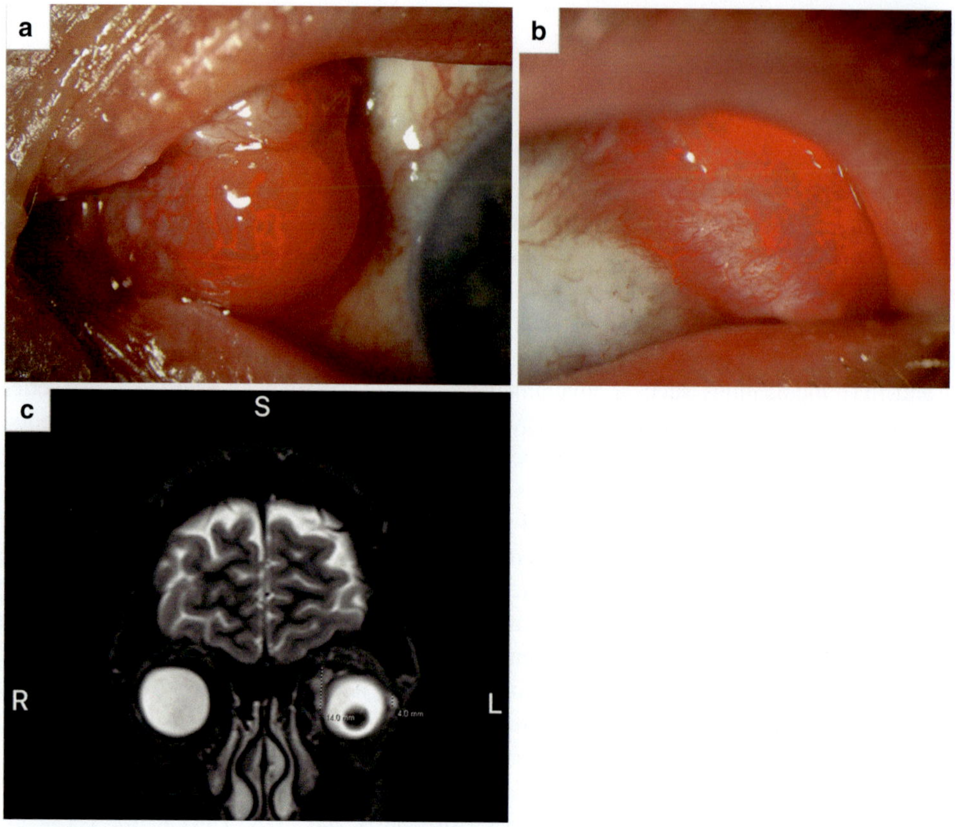

Fig. 12.7 Slit-lamp photography and orbit MRI of a patient with advanced recurrent amelanotic melanoma of the conjunctiva of the left eye (Stage 4: liver and nose metastases) before exenteration and treatment with ipilimumab and nivolumab. (**a**) Slit lamp photograph of the left eye demonstrates a large amelanotic melanoma in nasal conjunctiva involving the area of the caruncle. (**b**) Slit lamp photograph of the same left eye demonstrates a second mass in the temporal conjunctiva. (**c**) Orbital MRI imaging (coronal section) demonstrates the presence of mass at the superior medial left globe (19 mm × 0.8 mm × 14 mm, transverse by anteroposterior by craniocaudal) which mildly deforms the superior medial left eye, and another mass along the anterior superior lateral globe (4 mm × 3 mm × 4 mm, transverse by anteroposterior by craniocaudal) lateral and inferior to the lacrimal gland. Treatment with checkpoint inhibitors was initiated with pembrolizumab but to no effect. This patient ultimately underwent exenteration given orbital extension and no systemic involvement. Unfortunately, 2 months later he developed liver and nasal metastases. After the metastases appeared, he was treated with nivolumab which fortunately led to the resolution of the metastatic lesions and has been tumor-free for 5 years at last follow-up

Similarly, Finger et al. reported a case series of five patients in which three of them with locally advanced disease declined the suggested orbital exenteration and were then treated with checkpoint inhibitors as an alternative to surgery, resulting in favorable outcomes that ranged from partial to complete tumor regression [289].

The literature on the use of checkpoint inhibitors for primary CMM is still scarce, primarily comprising case reports and series. These preliminary results are promising, but the effectiveness of these novel agents across different stages of conjunctival melanoma still requires a large-scale and comprehensive evaluation. For example, six recent case series and case reports with a total of 16 patients (10 females and 6 males, between 28 and 94 years old) were treated for conjunctival melanoma with checkpoint inhibitors. These were patients who declined surgical excision, had extensive disease, or already had metastasis. During follow-up periods ranging from 1 to 48 months, 75% of the patients (n = 13) showed no evidence of disease after treatment, 12.5% (n = 2) experienced partial regression, and 6.25% (n = 1) initially had a recurrence but subsequently achieved a complete response after switching to another checkpoint inhibitor [289, 291–295].

Apart from the checkpoint inhibitors, the study of targeted therapies for CMM includes other biomarkers and specific mutations, including those previously studied for other type of malignancies. Notably, KIT mutations are associated with adverse prognostic features such as higher tumor mitotic index and increased tumor thickness; these mutations could be addressed with targeted medications as imatinib, regorafenib, ripretinib, and sunitinib. Additionally, for BRAF and MEK mutations, therapies, such as vemurafenib, dabrafenib and trametinib, have recently shown favorable response in patients with CMM where these mutations have been detected [132, 135, 275, 294], even in patients with advanced metastatic disease [275, 301–303].

Some other markers and mutations are still being studied to uncover new associations [135], potentially including a higher risk of metastasis and recurrence, as well as other characteristics of tumor spread. These advancements and the availability of molecular information represent an enormous potential to study and develop new targeted therapies that might be useful in conjunctival melanoma. For instance, NRAS mutants were associated with a greater 2-year rate of metastasis (28% vs 14%) and death (16% vs 4%) compared to NRAS wild-type tumors. ATRX mutants were associated with a lower 2-year rate of metastasis than ATRX wild-type tumors (0% vs 24%). Mutant TERT was associated with shorter metastasis-free survival [135]. Targeted medications are expected to become available as the correlation of these markers and clinical progression and prognosis is observed.

Future large-scale clinical trials focusing on conjunctival melanoma are needed to establish whether these emerging therapies can offer outcomes and prognoses comparable to or better than those of extensive surgical interventions like exenteration. There is a need to identify the patient populations for which they are most suitable, and their use as adjuvants and neoadjuvants merits continued study as it has been done with cutaneous melanoma [281–284, 304, 305].

12.19.3 Dosage

Ipilimumab: In unresectable or metastatic melanoma 3 mg/kg every 3 weeks for a maximum of 4 doses with or without combination with nivolumab. As adjuvant treatment of melanoma, 10 mg/kg every 3 weeks for 4 doses followed by 10 mg/kg every 12 weeks for up to 3 years (Product Information: YERVOY® intravenous injection, ipilimumab intravenous injection. Bristol-Myers Squibb Company (per manufacturer), Princeton, NJ, 2018.).

Nivolumab: As adjuvant treatment of melanoma or in unresectable or metastatic melanoma, 240 mg intravenously every 2 weeks or 480 mg intravenously every 4 weeks is administered until disease recurrence or unacceptable toxicity occurs when used as monotherapy. When used in combination with ipilimumab, 1 mg/kg of nivolumab intravenously over 30 min followed by 3 mg/kg of ipilimumab intravenously on the same day, every 3 weeks for 4 doses, then give the dose of nivolumab as monotherapy (Product Information: OPDIVO® intravenous injection, nivolumab intravenous injection. Bristol-Myers Squibb Company (per manufacturer), Princeton, NJ, 2018.).

Pembrolizumab: As adjuvant treatment of melanoma or in unresectable or metastatic melanoma, 200 mg is administered intravenously over 30 min every 3 weeks or 400 mg intravenously over 30 min every 6 weeks until disease progression or for up to 12 months when there is no evidence of recurrence (Product Information: KEYTRUDA® intravenous injection, pembrolizumab intravenous injection. Merck Sharp & Dohme Corp (per FDA), Whitehouse Station, NJ, 2020).

Vemurafenib: In unresectable or metastatic melanoma BRAF V600E mutation positive, 960 mg orally every 12 h is administered until disease progression or unacceptable toxicity occurs (Product Information: ZELBORAF® oral tablets, vemurafenib oral tablets. Genentech USA, Inc. (per FDA), South San Francisco, CA, 2014).

12.19.4 Side Effects

Described above in the section on OSSN.

12.19.5 Funding Sources

NIH Center Core Grant P30EY014801, The RPB Unrestricted Award and Career Development Awards, Dr. Ronald and Alicia Lepke Grant, The Lee and Claire Hager Grant, The Grant and Diana Stanton-Thornbrough, The Robert Baer Family Grant, The Emilyn Page and Mark Feldberg Grant, The Robert Farr Family Grant, The Jose Ferreira de Melo Grant, Mr. and Mrs. Irwin Friedman Grant, The Roberto and Antonia Menendez Family Grant, The Calvin and Flavia Oak Foundation, The Dr. Tim and Cammy Ioannides Grant, The Stephen Takach Grant, The Richard and Kathy Lesser Grant, The Ragheb Family Grant, The Honorable A. Jay Cristol Grant, The Michele and Ted Kaplan Grant, The Zvi Levin Grant, The Carol Soffer Grant, and the Richard Azar Family Grant (institutional grants).

References

1. Pe'er J. Ocular surface squamous neoplasia. Ophthalmol Clin N Am. 2005;18(1):1–13. vii
2. Murillo JC, Galor A, Wu MC, Kye NK, Wong J, Ahmed IO, et al. Intracorneal and intraocular invasion of ocular surface squamous neoplasia after intraocular surgery: report of two cases and review of the literature. Ocul Oncol Pathol. 2017;3(1):66–72.
3. McClellan AJ, McClellan AL, Pezon CF, Karp CL, Feuer W, Galor A. Epidemiology of ocular surface squamous neoplasia in a veterans affairs population. Cornea. 2013;32(10):1354–8.
4. Gichuhi S, Sagoo MS, Weiss HA, Burton MJ. Epidemiology of ocular surface squamous neoplasia in Africa. Trop Med Int Health. 2013;18(12):1424–43.
5. Nanji AA, Mercado C, Galor A, Dubovy S, Karp CL. Updates in ocular surface tumor diagnostics. Int Ophthalmol Clin. 2017;57(3):47–62.
6. Sayed-Ahmed IO, Palioura S, Galor A, Karp CL. Diagnosis and medical management of ocular surface squamous neoplasia. Expert Rev Ophthalmol. 2017;12(1):11–9.

7. Sepulveda R, Pe'er J, Midena E, Seregard S, Dua HS, Singh AD. Topical chemotherapy for ocular surface squamous neoplasia: current status. Br J Ophthalmol. 2010;94(5):532–5.
8. Adler E, Turner JR, Stone DU. Ocular surface squamous neoplasia: a survey of changes in the standard of care from 2003 to 2012. Cornea. 2013;32(12):1558–61.
9. Pe'er J. Ocular surface squamous neoplasia: evidence for topical chemotherapy. Int Ophthalmol Clin. 2015;55(1):9–21.
10. Parker WB, Cheng YC. Metabolism and mechanism of action of 5-fluorouracil. Pharmacol Ther. 1990;48(3):381–95.
11. Xie P, Mo JL, Liu JH, Li X, Tan LM, Zhang W, et al. Pharmacogenomics of 5-fluorouracil in colorectal cancer: review and update. Cell Oncol (Dordr). 2020;43(6):989–1001.
12. Longley DB, Harkin DP, Johnston PG. 5-Fluorouracil: mechanisms of action and clinical strategies. Nat Rev Cancer. 2003;3(5):330–8.
13. Joag MG, Sise A, Murillo JC, Sayed-Ahmed IO, Wong JR, Mercado C, et al. Topical 5-fluorouracil 1% as primary treatment for ocular surface squamous neoplasia. Ophthalmology. 2016;123(7):1442–8.
14. Parrozzani R, Lazzarini D, Alemany-Rubio E, Urban F, Midena E. Topical 1% 5-fluorouracil in ocular surface squamous neoplasia: a long-term safety study. Br J Ophthalmol. 2011;95(3):355–9.
15. Midena E, Angeli CD, Valenti M, de Belvis V, Boccato P. Treatment of conjunctival squamous cell carcinoma with topical 5-fluorouracil. Br J Ophthalmol. 2000;84(3):268–72.
16. Venkateswaran N, Mercado C, Galor A, Karp CL. Comparison of topical 5-fluorouracil and interferon alfa-2b as primary treatment modalities for ocular surface squamous neoplasia. Am J Ophthalmol. 2019;199:216–22.
17. Yeatts RP, Engelbrecht NE, Curry CD, Ford JG, Walter KA. 5-Fluorouracil for the treatment of intraepithelial neoplasia of the conjunctiva and cornea. Ophthalmology. 2000;107(12):2190–5.
18. Monroy D, Serrano A, Galor A, Karp CL. Medical treatment for ocular surface squamous neoplasia. Eye (Lond). 2023;37(5):885–93.
19. Wylegala A, Sripawadkul W, Zein M, Alvarez OP, Al Bayyat G, Galor A, Karp CL. Topical 1% 5-fluorouracil eye drops as primary treatment for ocular surface squamous neoplasia: long-term follow-up study. Ocul Surf. 2023;27:67–74.
20. de Keizer RJ, de Wolff-Rouendaal D, van Delft JL. Topical application of 5-fluorouracil in premalignant lesions of cornea, conjunctiva and eyelid. Doc Ophthalmol. 1986;64(1):31–42.
21. Arits AH, Mosterd K, Essers BA, Spoorenberg E, Sommer A, De Rooij MJ, et al. Photodynamic therapy versus topical imiquimod versus topical fluorouracil for treatment of superficial basal-cell carcinoma: a single blind, non-inferiority, randomised controlled trial. Lancet Oncol. 2013;14(7):647–54.
22. Jansen MHE, Mosterd K, Arits A, Roozeboom MH, Sommer A, Essers BAB, et al. Five-year results of a randomized controlled trial comparing effectiveness of photodynamic therapy, topical imiquimod, and topical 5-fluorouracil in patients with superficial basal cell carcinoma. J Invest Dermatol. 2018;138(3):527–33.
23. Neale H, Michelon M, Jacob S, Pinkston M, Ukaegbu R, Zamor W, et al. Topical 5% 5-fluorouracil versus procedural modalities for squamous cell carcinoma in situ and superficial basal cell carcinoma: a retrospective cohort analysis. J Am Acad Dermatol. 2022;87(2):423–5.
24. Gross K, Kircik L, Kricorian G. 5% 5-Fluorouracil cream for the treatment of small superficial Basal cell carcinoma: efficacy, tolerability, cosmetic outcome, and patient satisfaction. Dermatologic Surg. 2007;33(4):433–9. discussion 40
25. Yeatts RP, Ford JG, Stanton CA, Reed JW. Topical 5-fluorouracil in treating epithelial neoplasia of the conjunctiva and cornea. Ophthalmology. 1995;102(9):1338–44.
26. Al-Barrag A, Al-Shaer M, Al-Matary N, Al-Hamdani M. 5-Fluorouracil for the treatment of intraepithelial neoplasia and squamous cell carcinoma of the conjunctiva, and cornea. Clin Ophthalmol. 2010;4:801–8.
27. Singh S, Trakos N, Ali MJ. Effect of topical 5-fluorouracil on lacrimal drainage system: histopathological evidence from animal experiments and potential clinical implications. Ophthalmic Plast Reconstr Surg. 2023;39(3):288–92.
28. Parrozzani R, Frizziero L, Trainiti S, Testi I, Miglionico G, Pilotto E, et al. Topical 1% 5-fluoruracil as a sole treatment of corneoconjunctival ocular surface squamous neoplasia: long-term study. Br J Ophthalmol. 2017;101(8):1094–9.
29. Chevaliez S, Pawlotsky JM. Interferon-based therapy of hepatitis C. Adv Drug Deliv Rev. 2007;59(12):1222–41.
30. Pestka S, Krause CD, Walter MR. Interferons, interferon-like cytokines, and their receptors. Immunol Rev. 2004;202:8–32.
31. Houglum JE. Interferon: mechanisms of action and clinical value. Clin Pharm. 1983;2(1):20–8.
32. Randall RE, Goodbourn S. Interferons and viruses: an interplay between induction, signalling, antiviral responses and virus countermeasures. J Gen Virol. 2008;89(Pt 1):1–47.
33. Ferrantini M, Capone I, Belardelli F. Interferon-alpha and cancer: mechanisms of action and new perspectives of clinical use. Biochimie. 2007;89(6–7):884–93.
34. Zaman R, Islam RA, Chowdhury EH. Evolving therapeutic proteins to precisely kill cancer cells. J Control Release. 2022;351:779–804.
35. Shah SU, Kaliki S, Kim HJ, Lally SE, Shields JA, Shields CL. Topical interferon alfa-2b for management of ocular surface squamous neoplasia in 23 cases: outcomes based on American Joint Committee on Cancer classification. Arch Ophthalmol. 2012;130(2):159–64.
36. Karp CL, Galor A, Chhabra S, Barnes SD, Alfonso EC. Subconjunctival/perilesional recombinant interferon alpha2b for ocular surface squamous neoplasia: a 10-year review. Ophthalmology. 2010;117(12):2241–6.
37. Vann RR, Karp CL. Perilesional and topical interferon alfa-2b for conjunctival and corneal neoplasia. Ophthalmology. 1999;106(1):91–7.
38. Tsatsos M, Karp CL. Modern management of ocular surface squamous neoplasia. Expert Rev Ophthalmol. 2013;8(3):287–95.
39. Sripawadkul W, Reyes-Capo D, Zein M, Wylegala A, Albayyat G, Galor A, Karp CL. Long term study of topical interferon alpha-2b eye drops as primary treatment of ocular surface squamous neoplasia. Ocul Surf. 2023;28:108–14.
40. Karp CL, Moore JK, Rosa RH Jr. Treatment of conjunctival and corneal intraepithelial neoplasia with topical interferon alpha-2b. Ophthalmology. 2001;108(6):1093–8.
41. Kusumesh R, Ambastha A, Sinha B, Kumar R. Topical interferon alpha-2b as a single therapy for primary ocular surface squamous neoplasia. Asia Pac J Ophthalmol (Phila). 2015;4(5):279–82.
42. Shields CL, Constantinescu AB, Paulose SA, Yaghy A, Dalvin LA, Shields JA, Lally SE. Primary treatment of ocular surface squamous neoplasia with topical interferon alpha-2b: comparative analysis of outcomes based on original tumor configuration. Indian J Ophthalmol. 2021;69(3):563–7.
43. Kaliki S, Sharma A, Vempuluru VS. Interferon alfa-2b for pigmented ocular surface squamous neoplasia: a report of 8 lesions. Cornea. 2021;40(2):142–6.
44. Boehm MD, Huang AJ. Treatment of recurrent corneal and conjunctival intraepithelial neoplasia with topical interferon alfa 2b. Ophthalmology. 2004;111(9):1755–61.
45. Yeoh CHY, Lee JJR, Lim BXH, Sundar G, Mehta JS, Chan ASY, et al. The management of Ocular Surface Squamous Neoplasia (OSSN). Int J Mol Sci. 2022;24(1)

46. Kim HJ, Shields CL, Shah SU, Kaliki S, Lally SE. Giant ocular surface squamous neoplasia managed with interferon alpha-2b as immunotherapy or immunoreduction. Ophthalmology. 2012;119(5):938–44.
47. Galvis V, Moreno NJ, Tello A, Carreno NI. Topical interferon alpha-2b for a giant ocular surface squamous neoplasia: 7 years of follow-up after complete remission. BMJ Case Rep. 2021;14(2)
48. Shields CL, Paulose SA, Yaghy A, Dalvin LA, Constantinescu AB, Lally SE, Shields JA. Ocular surface squamous neoplasia managed with primary interferon alpha2b: a comparative analysis of 212 tumors in smokers versus nonsmokers. Cornea. 2021;40(11):1387–94.
49. Kim SE, Salvi SM. Immunoreduction of ocular surface tumours with intralesional interferon alpha-2a. Eye (Lond). 2018;32(2):460–2.
50. Rishi P, Shields CL. Intralesional and topical interferon therapy following incomplete primary excision of ocular surface squamous neoplasia. Indian J Ophthalmol. 2016;64(6):460–1.
51. Karp CL, Galor A, Lee Y, Yoo SH. Pegylated interferon alpha 2b for treatment of ocular surface squamous neoplasia: a pilot study. Ocul Immunol Inflamm. 2010;18(4):254–60.
52. Park J, Han J, Chung TY, Lim DH, Choi CY. Pegylated interferon alpha 2a for the treatment of ocular surface squamous neoplasia. Cornea. 2022;41(10):1271–5.
53. Nuruddin M, Roy SR, Hoque F. Pegylated interferon-alpha-2a for the treatment of ocular surface squamous neoplasia. Oman J Ophthalmol. 2022;15(1):81–4.
54. Kaliki S, Singh S, Iram S, Tripuraneni D. Recombinant interferon alpha 2b for ocular surface squamous neoplasia: an efficient and cost-effective treatment modality in Asian Indian patients. Indian J Ophthalmol. 2016;64(10):702–9.
55. Galor A, Karp CL, Chhabra S, Barnes S, Alfonso EC. Topical interferon alpha 2b eye-drops for treatment of ocular surface squamous neoplasia: a dose comparison study. Br J Ophthalmol. 2010;94(5):551–4.
56. Lewczuk N, Zdebik A, Boguslawska J. Interferon alpha 2a and 2b in ophthalmology: a review. J Interf Cytokine Res. 2019;39(5):259–72.
57. Aldave AJ, Nguyen A. Ocular surface toxicity associated with topical interferon alpha-2b. Br J Ophthalmol. 2007;91(8):1087–8.
58. Verweij J, Pinedo HM. Mitomycin C: mechanism of action, usefulness and limitations. Anti-Cancer Drugs. 1990;1(1):5–13.
59. Singh P. Mitomycin-C use in ophthalmology. IOSR J Pharma (IOSRPHR). 2013;3(1):12–4.
60. Frucht-Pery J, Sugar J, Baum J, Sutphin JE, Pe'er J, Savir H, et al. Mitomycin C treatment for conjunctival-corneal intraepithelial neoplasia: a multicenter experience. Ophthalmology. 1997;104(12):2085–93.
61. Shields CL, Naseripour M, Shields JA. Topical mitomycin C for extensive, recurrent conjunctival-corneal squamous cell carcinoma. Am J Ophthalmol. 2002;133(5):601–6.
62. Blasi MA, Maceroni M, Sammarco MG, Pagliara MM. Mitomycin C or interferon as adjuvant therapy to surgery for ocular surface squamous neoplasia: comparative study. Eur J Ophthalmol. 2018;28(2):204–9.
63. Siganos CS, Kozobolis VP, Christodoulakis EV. The intraoperative use of mitomycin-C in excision of ocular surface neoplasia with or without limbal autograft transplantation. Cornea. 2002;21(1):12–6.
64. Prabhasawat P, Tarinvorakup P, Tesavibul N, Uiprasertkul M, Kosrirukvongs P, Booranapong W, Srivannaboon S. Topical 0.002% mitomycin C for the treatment of conjunctival-corneal intraepithelial neoplasia and squamous cell carcinoma. Cornea. 2005;24(4):443–8.
65. Ballalai PL, Erwenne CM, Martins MC, Lowen MS, Barros JN. Long-term results of topical mitomycin C 0.02% for primary and recurrent conjunctival-corneal intraepithelial neoplasia. Ophthalmic. Plast Reconstr Surg. 2009;25(4):296–9.
66. Alvarez OP, Zein M, Galor A, Karp CL. Management of ocular surface squamous neoplasia: Bowman Club Lecture 2021. BMJ Open Ophthalmol. 2021;6(1):e000842.
67. Quebbeman EJ, Hoffman NE, Ausman RK, Hamid AA. Stability of mitomycin admixtures. Am J Hosp Pharm. 1985;42(8):1750–4.
68. Chen C, Louis D, Dodd T, Muecke J. Mitomycin C as an adjunct in the treatment of localised ocular surface squamous neoplasia. Br J Ophthalmol. 2004;88(1):17–8.
69. Frucht-Pery J, Rozenman Y, Pe'er J. Topical mitomycin-C for partially excised conjunctival squamous cell carcinoma. Ophthalmology. 2002;109(3):548–52.
70. Höllhumer R, Williams S, Michelow P. Ocular surface squamous neoplasia: management and outcomes. Eye (Lond). 2021;35(6):1562–73.
71. Cohen VML, O'Day RF. Management issues in conjunctival tumours: ocular surface squamous neoplasia. Ophthalmol Ther. 2020;9(1):181–90.
72. Khong JJ, Muecke J. Complications of mitomycin C therapy in 100 eyes with ocular surface neoplasia. Br J Ophthalmol. 2006;90(7):819–22.
73. Mearza AA, Aslanides IM. Uses and complications of mitomycin C in ophthalmology. Expert Opin Drug Saf. 2007;6(1):27–32.
74. Russell HC, Chadha V, Lockington D, Kemp EG. Topical mitomycin C chemotherapy in the management of ocular surface neoplasia: a 10-year review of treatment outcomes and complications. Br J Ophthalmol. 2010;94(10):1316–21.
75. Abraham LM, Selva D, Casson R, Leibovitch I. Mitomycin: clinical applications in ophthalmic practice. Drugs. 2006;66(3):321–40.
76. Lichtinger A, Pe'er J, Frucht-Pery J, Solomon A. Limbal stem cell deficiency after topical mitomycin C therapy for primary acquired melanosis with atypia. Ophthalmology. 2010;117(3):431–7.
77. Tunc M, Erbilen E. Topical cyclosporine-a combined with mitomycin C for conjunctival and corneal squamous cell carcinoma. Am J Ophthalmol. 2006;142(4):673–5.
78. Billing K, Karagiannis A, Selva D. Punctal-canalicular stenosis associated with mitomycin-C for corneal epithelial dysplasia. Am J Ophthalmol. 2003;136(4):746–7.
79. Bushue N, Wan YJ. Retinoid pathway and cancer therapeutics. Adv Drug Deliv Rev. 2010;62(13):1285–98.
80. Klaassen I, Braakhuis BJ. Anticancer activity and mechanism of action of retinoids in oral and pharyngeal cancer. Oral Oncol. 2002;38(6):532–42.
81. Freemantle SJ, Spinella MJ, Dmitrovsky E. Retinoids in cancer therapy and chemoprevention: promise meets resistance. Oncogene. 2003;22(47):7305–15.
82. Tallman MS, Andersen JW, Schiffer CA, Appelbaum FR, Feusner JH, Ogden A, et al. All-trans-retinoic acid in acute promyelocytic leukemia. N Engl J Med. 1997;337(15):1021–8.
83. Nagai Y, Ambinder AJ. The promise of retinoids in the treatment of cancer: neither burnt out nor fading away. Cancers (Basel). 2023;15(14)
84. Herbort CP, Zografos L, Zwingli M, Schoeneich M. Topical retinoic acid in dysplastic and metaplastic keratinization of corneoconjunctival epithelium. Graefes Arch Clin Exp Ophthalmol. 1988;226(1):22–6.
85. Krilis M, Tsang H, Coroneo M. Treatment of conjunctival and corneal epithelial neoplasia with retinoic acid and topical interferon alfa-2b: long-term follow-up. Ophthalmology. 2012;119(10):1969–73.
86. Skippen B, Tsang HH, Assaad NN, Coroneo MT. Rapid response of refractory ocular surface dysplasia to combination treatment with topical all-trans retinoic acid and interferon alfa-2b. Arch Ophthalmol. 2010;128(10):1368–9.

87. Moore DM, Kalvakolanu DV, Lippman SM, Kavanagh JJ, Hong WK, Borden EC, et al. Retinoic acid and interferon in human cancer: mechanistic and clinical studies. Semin Hematol. 1994;31(4 Suppl 5):31–7.
88. French LE, Shapiro M, Junkins-Hopkins JM, Vittorio CC, Rook AH. Regression of multifocal, skin-restricted, CD30-positive large T-cell lymphoma with interferon alfa and bexarotene therapy. J Am Acad Dermatol. 2001;45(6):914–8.
89. McGinnis KS, Junkins-Hopkins JM, Crawford G, Shapiro M, Rook AH, Vittorio CC. Low-dose oral bexarotene in combination with low-dose interferon alfa in the treatment of cutaneous T-cell lymphoma: clinical synergism and possible immunologic mechanisms. J Am Acad Dermatol. 2004;50(3):375–9.
90. Peck GL, Olsen TG, Yoder FW, Strauss JS, Downing DT, Pandya M, et al. Prolonged remissions of cystic and conglobate acne with 13-cis-retinoic acid. N Engl J Med. 1979;300(7):329–33.
91. Weinstock MA, Bingham SF, Digiovanna JJ, Rizzo AE, Marcolivio K, Hall R, et al. Tretinoin and the prevention of keratinocyte carcinoma (Basal and squamous cell carcinoma of the skin): a veterans affairs randomized chemoprevention trial. J Invest Dermatol. 2012;132(6):1583–90.
92. Zhang C, Duvic M. Retinoids: therapeutic applications and mechanisms of action in cutaneous T-cell lymphoma. Dermatol Ther. 2003;16(4):322–30.
93. Tang JY, Chiou AS, Mackay-Wiggan JM, Aszterbaum M, Chanana AM, Lee W, et al. Tazarotene: randomized, double-blind, vehicle-controlled, and open-label concurrent trials for basal cell carcinoma prevention and therapy in patients with basal cell nevus syndrome. Cancer Prev Res (Phila). 2014;7(3):292–9.
94. Abbott RA, Whittaker SJ, Morris SL, Russell-Jones R, Hung T, Bashir SJ, Scarisbrick JJ. Bexarotene therapy for mycosis fungoides and Sezary syndrome. Br J Dermatol. 2009;160(6):1299–307.
95. Chen L, Wang J, Hu X, Xu X. Meta-analysis of all-trans retinoic acid-linked arsenic trioxide treatment for acute promyelocytic leukemia. Hematology. 2014;19(4):202–7.
96. Uray IP, Dmitrovsky E, Brown PH. Retinoids and rexinoids in cancer prevention: from laboratory to clinic. Semin Oncol. 2016;43(1):49–64.
97. Lippman SM, Batsakis JG, Toth BB, Weber RS, Lee JJ, Martin JW, et al. Comparison of low-dose isotretinoin with beta carotene to prevent oral carcinogenesis. N Engl J Med. 1993;328(1):15–20.
98. Hong WK, Endicott J, Itri LM, Doos W, Batsakis JG, Bell R, et al. 13-cis-retinoic acid in the treatment of oral leukoplakia. N Engl J Med. 1986;315(24):1501–5.
99. Bolla M, Lefur R, Ton Van J, Domenge C, Badet JM, Koskas Y, Laplanche A. Prevention of second primary tumours with etretinate in squamous cell carcinoma of the oral cavity and oropharynx. Results of a multicentric double-blind randomised study. Eur J Cancer. 1994;30A(6):767–72.
100. Orfanos CE, Zouboulis CC, Almond-Roesler B, Geilen CC. Current use and future potential role of retinoids in dermatology. Drugs. 1997;53(3):358–88.
101. Harlev E, Nevo E, Lansky EP, Ofir R, Bishayee A. Anticancer potential of aloes: antioxidant, antiproliferative, and immunostimulatory attributes. Planta Med. 2012;78(9):843–52.
102. Pecere T, Ponterio E, Di Iorio E, Carli M, Fassan M, Santoro L, et al. On the mechanism of tumor cell entry of aloe-emodin, a natural compound endowed with anticancer activity. Int J Cancer. 2021;149(5):1129–36.
103. Jeon W, Jeon YK, Nam MJ. Apoptosis by aloe-emodin is mediated through down-regulation of calpain-2 and ubiquitin-protein ligase E3A in human hepatoma Huh-7 cells. Cell Biol Int. 2012;36(2):163–7.
104. Yagi A, Nakamori J, Yamada T, Iwase H, Tanaka T, Kaneo Y, et al. In vivo metabolism of aloemannan. Planta Med. 1999;65(5):417–20.
105. Damani MR, Shah AR, Karp CL, Orlin SE. Treatment of ocular surface squamous neoplasia with topical Aloe vera drops. Cornea. 2015;34(1):87–9.
106. Snoeck R, Sakuma T, De Clercq E, Rosenberg I, Holy A. (S)-1-(3-hydroxy-2-phosphonylmethoxypropyl)cytosine, a potent and selective inhibitor of human cytomegalovirus replication. Antimicrob Agents Chemother. 1988;32(12):1839–44.
107. Zabawski EJ Jr, Cockerell CJ. Topical and intralesional cidofovir: a review of pharmacology and therapeutic effects. J Am Acad Dermatol. 1998;39(5 Pt 1):741–5.
108. Snoeck R, Wellens W, Desloovere C, Van Ranst M, Naesens L, De Clercq E, Feenstra L. Treatment of severe laryngeal papillomatosis with intralesional injections of cidofovir [(S)-1-(3-hydroxy-2-phosphonylmethoxypropyl)cytosine]. J Med Virol. 1998;54(3):219–25.
109. Woods M, Chow S, Heng B, Glenn W, Whitaker N, Waring D, et al. Detecting human papillomavirus in ocular surface diseases. Invest Ophthalmol Vis Sci. 2013;54(13):8069–78.
110. Ip MH, Robert George CR, Naing Z, Perlman EM, Rawlinson W, Coroneo MT. Topical Cidofovir for treatment-refractory ocular surface squamous neoplasia. Ophthalmology. 2018;125(4):617–9.
111. Sherman MD, Feldman KA, Farahmand SM, Margolis TP. Treatment of conjunctival squamous cell carcinoma with topical cidofovir. Am J Ophthalmol. 2002;134(3):432–3.
112. Hurt CN, Nedjai B, Alvarez-Mendoza C, Powell N, Tristram A, Jones S. Combined HPV 16 E2 and L1 methylation predict response to treatment with cidofovir and imiquimod in patients with vulval intraepithelial neoplasia. Cancer Biomark. 2022;35(2):143–53.
113. Burgos J, Campany D, Garcia J, Landolfi S, Falco V, Curran A. Effectiveness of topical cidofovir for treatment of refractory anal high-grade squamous intraepithelial lesion. AIDS. 2023;37(9):1425–9.
114. Solarz P, Bodnar M, Czech J, Mackiewicz-Nartowicz H, Sinkiewicz A, Szylberg L, et al. Assessment of immunomodulation and regulation of cell cycle in epithelium and stroma after Cidofovir injection in patients with recurrent respiratory papillomatosis-pilot study. J Med Virol. 2023;95(1):e28303.
115. Ip MH, Coroneo MT. Treatment of previously refractory ocular surface squamous neoplasia with topical Cidofovir. JAMA Ophthalmol. 2017;135(5):500–2.
116. Kim LA, D'Amore PA. A brief history of anti-VEGF for the treatment of ocular angiogenesis. Am J Pathol. 2012;181(2):376–9.
117. Leung DW, Cachianes G, Kuang WJ, Goeddel DV, Ferrara N. Vascular endothelial growth factor is a secreted angiogenic mitogen. Science. 1989;246(4935):1306–9.
118. Friedman HS, Prados MD, Wen PY, Mikkelsen T, Schiff D, Abrey LE, et al. Bevacizumab alone and in combination with irinotecan in recurrent glioblastoma. J Clin Oncol. 2009;27(28):4733–40.
119. Kabbinavar FF, Hambleton J, Mass RD, Hurwitz HI, Bergsland E, Sarkar S. Combined analysis of efficacy: the addition of bevacizumab to fluorouracil/leucovorin improves survival for patients with metastatic colorectal cancer. J Clin Oncol. 2005;23(16):3706–12.
120. Li Z, Guo F, Han Y, Wang J, Xu B. Efficacy and safety of bevacizumab in pretreated metastatic breast cancer: a systematic review and meta-analysis. Oncol Res Treat. 2022;45(10):608–17.
121. Furugaki K, Fukumura J, Iwai T, Yorozu K, Kurasawa M, Yanagisawa M, et al. Impact of bevacizumab in combination with erlotinib on EGFR-mutated non-small cell lung cancer xenograft models with T790M mutation or MET amplification. Int J Cancer. 2016;138(4):1024–32.
122. Yin L, Li W, Chen X, Wang R, Zhang T, Meng J, et al. HOOK1 inhibits the progression of renal cell carcinoma via

TGF-beta and TNFSF13B/VEGF-A axis. Adv Sci (Weinh). 2023;10(17):e2206955.
123. Ma J, Sawai H, Ochi N, Matsuo Y, Xu D, Yasuda A, et al. PTEN regulates angiogenesis through PI3K/Akt/VEGF signaling pathway in human pancreatic cancer cells. Mol Cell Biochem. 2009;331(1–2):161–71.
124. Nagy JA, Dvorak AM, Dvorak HF. VEGF-A and the induction of pathological angiogenesis. Annu Rev Pathol. 2007;2:251–75.
125. Ozcan AA, Ciloglu E, Esen E, Simdivar GH. Use of topical bevacizumab for conjunctival intraepithelial neoplasia. Cornea. 2014;33(11):1205–9.
126. Asena L, Dursun AD. Topical bevacizumab for the treatment of ocular surface squamous neoplasia. J Ocul Pharmacol Ther. 2015;31(8):487–90.
127. Lee CY, Chen HC, Meir YJ, Ma DH, Wu WC. Subconjunctival injection of bevacizumab for recurrent conjunctival papilloma: a case report. Can J Ophthalmol. 2017;52(5):e156–e9.
128. Finger PT, Chin KJ. Refractory squamous cell carcinoma of the conjunctiva treated with subconjunctival ranibizumab (Lucentis): a two-year study. Ophthalmic Plast Reconstr Surg. 2012;28(2):85–9.
129. Paul S, Stone DU. Intralesional bevacizumab use for invasive ocular surface squamous neoplasia. J Ocul Pharmacol Ther. 2012;28(6):647–9.
130. Faramarzi A, Feizi S. Subconjunctival bevacizumab injection for ocular surface squamous neoplasia. Cornea. 2013;32(7):998–1001.
131. Dunn GP, Bruce AT, Ikeda H, Old LJ, Schreiber RD. Cancer immunoediting: from immunosurveillance to tumor escape. Nat Immunol. 2002;3(11):991–8.
132. Bollag G, Tsai J, Zhang J, Zhang C, Ibrahim P, Nolop K, Hirth P. Vemurafenib: the first drug approved for BRAF-mutant cancer. Nat Rev Drug Discov. 2012;11(11):873–86.
133. Barone A, Hazarika M, Theoret MR, Mishra-Kalyani P, Chen H, He K, et al. FDA approval summary: pembrolizumab for the treatment of patients with unresectable or metastatic melanoma. Clin Cancer Res. 2017;23(19):5661–5.
134. Cao J, Brouwer NJ, Richards KE, Marinkovic M, van Duinen S, Hurkmans D, et al. PD-L1/PD-1 expression and tumor-infiltrating lymphocytes in conjunctival melanoma. Oncotarget. 2017;8(33):54722–34.
135. Zeiger JS, Lally SE, Dalvin LA, Shields CL. Advances in conjunctival melanoma: clinical features, diagnostic modalities, staging, genetic markers, and management. Can J Ophthalmol. 2023;59:209.
136. Pedoeem A, Azoulay-Alfaguter I, Strazza M, Silverman GJ, Mor A. Programmed death-1 pathway in cancer and autoimmunity. Clin Immunol. 2014;153(1):145–52.
137. Keir ME, Francisco LM, Sharpe AH. PD-1 and its ligands in T-cell immunity. Curr Opin Immunol. 2007;19(3):309–14.
138. Larkin J, Chiarion-Sileni V, Gonzalez R, Grob JJ, Cowey CL, Lao CD, et al. Combined nivolumab and ipilimumab or monotherapy in untreated melanoma. N Engl J Med. 2015;373(1):23–34.
139. Weber JS, Hamid O, Chasalow SD, Wu DY, Parker SM, Galbraith S, et al. Ipilimumab increases activated T cells and enhances humoral immunity in patients with advanced melanoma. J Immunother. 2012;35(1):89–97.
140. Hooiveld-Noeken JS, Eggen AC, Racz E, de Vries EGE, Reyners AKL, Jalving M. Towards less mutilating treatments in patients with advanced non-melanoma skin cancers by earlier use of immune checkpoint inhibitors. Crit Rev Oncol Hematol. 2022;180:103855.
141. Gross ND, Miller DM, Khushalani NI, Divi V, Ruiz ES, Lipson EJ, et al. Neoadjuvant cemiplimab and surgery for stage II-IV cutaneous squamous-cell carcinoma: follow-up and survival outcomes of a single-arm, multicentre, phase 2 study. Lancet Oncol. 2023;24(11):1196–205.
142. Ferrarotto R, Amit M, Nagarajan P, Rubin ML, Yuan Y, Bell D, et al. Pilot phase II trial of neoadjuvant immunotherapy in locoregionally advanced, resectable cutaneous squamous cell carcinoma of the head and neck. Clin Cancer Res. 2021;27(16):4557–65.
143. Migden MR, Rischin D, Schmults CD, Guminski A, Hauschild A, Lewis KD, et al. PD-1 blockade with cemiplimab in advanced cutaneous squamous-cell carcinoma. N Engl J Med. 2018;379(4):341–51.
144. Wolkow N, Jakobiec FA, Afrogheh AH, Eagle RC Jr, Pai SI, Faquin WC. Programmed cell death 1 ligand 1 and programmed cell death 1 ligand 2 are expressed in conjunctival invasive squamous cell carcinoma: therapeutic implications. Am J Ophthalmol. 2019;200:226–41.
145. Nagarajan P, El-Hadad C, Gruschkus SK, Ning J, Hudgens CW, Sagiv O, et al. PD-L1/PD1 expression, composition of tumor-associated immune infiltrate, and HPV status in conjunctival squamous cell carcinoma. Invest Ophthalmol Vis Sci. 2019;60(6):2388–98.
146. Sun C, Mezzadra R, Schumacher TN. Regulation and function of the PD-L1 checkpoint. Immunity. 2018;48(3):434–52.
147. Pai SI, Zandberg DP, Strome SE. The role of antagonists of the PD-1:PD-L1/PD-L2 axis in head and neck cancer treatment. Oral Oncol. 2016;61:152–8.
148. Pai SI, Faquin WC. Programmed cell death ligand 1 as a biomarker in head and neck cancer. Cancer Cytopathol. 2017;125(7):529–33.
149. Demirci H, Elner VM, Demirci FY, Robinson DR, Chinnaiyan A, Schlachter D, et al. Immunotherapy for conjunctival squamous cell carcinoma with orbital extension. Ophthalmology. 2021;128(5):801–4.
150. Esmaeli B. Immune checkpoint inhibitor therapy for orbital and ocular adnexal squamous cell carcinomas: International Society of Ocular Oncology President's Lecture, 2022. Invest Ophthalmol Vis Sci. 2023;64(7):29.
151. Goodman AM, Kato S, Bazhenova L, Patel SP, Frampton GM, Miller V, et al. Tumor mutational burden as an independent predictor of response to immunotherapy in diverse cancers. Mol Cancer Ther. 2017;16(11):2598–608.
152. Addeo A, Friedlaender A, Banna GL, Weiss GJ. TMB or not TMB as a biomarker: that is the question. Crit Rev Oncol Hematol. 2021;163:103374.
153. Hoffmann M, Schardt J, Ionescu C, Wolf-Schnurrbusch UE, Wagner F, Dettmer MS, et al. Long lasting response to anti-PD-1 therapy of recurrent conjunctival squamous cell carcinoma—a case report and systematic review of the literature. Curr Prob Cancer-C R. 2021;4:100088.
154. Shen YC, Upadhyayula R, Cevallos S, Messick RJ, Hsia T, Leese MP, et al. Targeted NF1 cancer therapeutics with multiple modes of action: small molecule hormone-like agents resembling the natural anticancer metabolite, 2-methoxyoestradiol. Br J Cancer. 2015;113(8):1158–67.
155. Populo H, Soares P, Rocha AS, Silva P, Lopes JM. Evaluation of the mTOR pathway in ocular (uvea and conjunctiva) melanoma. Melanoma Res. 2010;20(2):107–17.
156. van Ipenburg JA, Naus NC, Dubbink HJ, van Ginderdeuren R, Missotten GS, Paridaens D, Verdijk RM. Prognostic value of TERT promoter mutations in conjunctival melanomas in addition to clinicopathological features. Br J Ophthalmol. 2021;105(10):1454–61.
157. Lewis CM, Glisson BS, Feng L, Wan F, Tang X, Wistuba II, et al. A phase II study of gefitinib for aggressive cutaneous squamous cell carcinoma of the head and neck. Clin Cancer Res. 2012;18(5):1435–46.
158. Maubec E, Petrow P, Scheer-Senyarich I, Duvillard P, Lacroix L, Gelly J, et al. Phase II study of cetuximab as first-line single-drug therapy in patients with unresectable squamous cell carcinoma of the skin. J Clin Oncol. 2011;29(25):3419–26.

159. de Lima PO, Joseph S, Panizza B, Simpson F. Epidermal growth factor receptor's function in cutaneous squamous cell carcinoma and its role as a therapeutic target in the age of immunotherapies. Curr Treat Options in Oncol. 2020;21(1):9.
160. Khayyati Kohnehshahri M, Sarkesh A, Mohamed Khosroshahi L, HajiEsmailPoor Z, Aghebati-Maleki A, Yousefi M, Aghebati-Maleki L. Current status of skin cancers with a focus on immunology and immunotherapy. Cancer Cell Int. 2023;23(1):174.
161. Wollina U, Tchernev G, Lotti T. Chimeric monoclonal antibody cetuximab targeting epidermal growth factor-receptor in advanced non-melanoma skin cancer. Open Access Maced J Med Sci. 2018;6(1):152–5.
162. Bitton K, Michot JM, Barreau E, Lambotte O, Haigh O, Marabelle A, et al. Prevalence and clinical patterns of ocular complications associated with anti-PD-1/PD-L1 anticancer immunotherapy. Am J Ophthalmol. 2019;202:109–17.
163. Park RB, Jain S, Han H, Park J. Ocular surface disease associated with immune checkpoint inhibitor therapy. Ocul Surf. 2021;20:115–29.
164. Alba-Linero C, Alba E. Ocular side effects of checkpoint inhibitors. Surv Ophthalmol. 2021;66(6):951–9.
165. Hartmann EM, Ott G, Rosenwald A. Molecular biology and genetics of lymphomas. Hematol Oncol Clin North Am. 2008;22(5):807–23. vii
166. Tanenbaum RE, Galor A, Dubovy SR, Karp CL. Classification, diagnosis, and management of conjunctival lymphoma. Eye Vis (Lond). 2019;6:22.
167. McGrath LA, Ryan DA, Warrier SK, Coupland SE, Glasson WJ. Conjunctival lymphoma. Eye (Lond). 2023;37(5):837–48.
168. Kirkegaard MM, Coupland SE, Prause JU, Heegaard S. Malignant lymphoma of the conjunctiva. Surv Ophthalmol. 2015;60(5):444–58.
169. Wotherspoon AC, Ortiz-Hidalgo C, Falzon MR, Isaacson PG. Helicobacter pylori-associated gastritis and primary B-cell gastric lymphoma. Lancet. 1991;338(8776):1175–6.
170. Nakamura S, Aoyagi K, Furuse M, Suekane H, Matsumoto T, Yao T, et al. B-cell monoclonality precedes the development of gastric MALT lymphoma in Helicobacter pylori-associated chronic gastritis. Am J Pathol. 1998;152(5):1271–9.
171. Aigelsreiter A, Gerlza T, Deutsch AJ, Leitner E, Beham-Schmid C, Beham A, et al. Chlamydia psittaci infection in nongastrointestinal extranodal MALT lymphomas and their precursor lesions. Am J Clin Pathol. 2011;135(1):70–5.
172. Mesnard B, De Vroey B, Maunoury V, Lecuit M. Immunoproliferative small intestinal disease associated with Campylobacter jejuni. Dig Liver Dis. 2012;44(9):799–800.
173. Leopizzi M, Mundo L, Messina E, Campolo F, Lazzi S, Angeloni A, et al. Epstein-Barr virus encoded EBNA2 downregulates ICOSL by inducing miR-24 in B-cell lymphoma. Blood. 2023;
174. Lyons SF, Liebowitz DN. The roles of human viruses in the pathogenesis of lymphoma. Semin Oncol. 1998;25(4):461–75.
175. Zhang W, Du F, Wang L, Bai T, Zhou X, Mei H. Hepatitis virus-associated non-Hodgkin lymphoma: pathogenesis and treatment strategies. J Clin Transl Hepatol. 2023;11(5):1256–66.
176. Sassone M, Ponzoni M, Ferreri AJ. Ocular adnexal marginal zone lymphoma: clinical presentation, pathogenesis, diagnosis, prognosis, and treatment. Best Pract Res Clin Haematol. 2017;30(1–2):118–30.
177. Shields CL, Shields JA, Carvalho C, Rundle P, Smith AF. Conjunctival lymphoid tumors: clinical analysis of 117 cases and relationship to systemic lymphoma. Ophthalmology. 2001;108(5):979–84.
178. Lee J, Yoon JS, Kim JS, Koom WS, Cho J, Suh CO. Long-term outcome, relapse patterns, and toxicity after radiotherapy for orbital mucosa-associated lymphoid tissue lymphoma: implications for radiotherapy optimization. Jpn J Clin Oncol. 2019;49(7):664–70.
179. Lee GI, Oh D, Kim WS, Kim SJ, Ko YH, Woo KI, et al. Low-dose radiation therapy for primary conjunctival marginal zone B-cell lymphoma. Cancer Res Treat. 2018;50(2):575–81.
180. Pereira-Da Silva MV, Di Nicola ML, Altomare F, Xu W, Tsang R, Laperriere N, Krema H. Radiation therapy for primary orbital and ocular adnexal lymphoma. Clin Transl Radiat Oncol. 2023;38:15–20.
181. Fasola CE, Jones JC, Huang DD, Le QT, Hoppe RT, Donaldson SS. Low-dose radiation therapy (2 Gy x 2) in the treatment of orbital lymphoma. Int J Radiat Oncol Biol Phys. 2013;86(5):930–5.
182. Pinnix CC, Dabaja BS, Milgrom SA, Smith GL, Abou Z, Nastoupil L, et al. Ultra-low-dose radiotherapy for definitive management of ocular adnexal B-cell lymphoma. Head Neck. 2017;39(6):1095–100.
183. de Castro B, Peixeiro RP, Mariz JM, Oliveira A. Ultra-low dose radiotherapy in the management of low-grade orbital lymphomas. Rep Pract Oncol Radiother. 2022;27(3):467–73.
184. Cerrato M, Orlandi E, Vella A, Bartoncini S, Iorio GC, Bongiovanni D, et al. Efficacy of low-dose radiotherapy (2 Gy x 2) in the treatment of marginal zone and mucosa-associated lymphoid tissue lymphomas. Br J Radiol. 2021;94(1123):20210012.
185. Park J, Yea JW, Oh SA, Kim MK, Son JH, Park JW. Prospective study of 4 Gy radiotherapy for orbital mucosa-associated lymphoid tissue lymphoma (FORMAL). Cancers (Basel). 2022;14(17)
186. Parada-Vasquez RH, Lomas-Guaman VE, Leon-Roldan CR. Conjunctival lymphoma in right eye: case report. Arch Soc Esp Oftalmol. 2017;92(2):78–81.
187. Ben Simon GJ, Cheung N, McKelvie P, Fox R, McNab AA. Oral chlorambucil for extranodal, marginal zone, B-cell lymphoma of mucosa-associated lymphoid tissue of the orbit. Ophthalmology. 2006;113(7):1209–13.
188. Seker M, Ozdemir B, Bilici A, Ustaalioglu BB, Sonmez B, Yilmaz BE, et al. Bilateral conjunctival MALT lymphoma mimicking chronic conjunctivitis. Onkologie. 2010;33(6):317–20.
189. Shimomura I, Miki Y, Suzuki E, Katsumata M, Hashimoto D, Arai Y, et al. Mucosa-associated lymphoid tissue lymphoma with metachronous involvement of the palpebral conjunctiva and bronchus: a case report. Respir Med Case Rep. 2019;26:101–4.
190. Viani GA, Fendi LI. Adjuvant treatment or primary topical monotherapy for ocular surface squamous neoplasia: a systematic review. Arq Bras Oftalmol. 2017;80(2):131–6.
191. Kim SY, Lee WS, Oh SY, Yang DH, Kim HJ, Park SK, et al. Relapse in patients with limited-stage ocular adnexal lymphoma treated by chemoimmunotherapy: extended follow-up of a phase 2 study. Cancer Med. 2022;11(14):2817–23.
192. Blasi MA, Tiberti AC, Valente P, Laguardia M, Sammarco MG, Balestrazzi A, et al. Intralesional interferon-alpha for conjunctival mucosa-associated lymphoid tissue lymphoma: long-term results. Ophthalmology. 2012;119(3):494–500.
193. Lachapelle KR, Rathee R, Kratky V, Dexter DF. Treatment of conjunctival mucosa-associated lymphoid tissue lymphoma with intralesional injection of interferon alfa-2b. Arch Ophthalmol. 2000;118(2):284–5.
194. Ross JJ, Tu KL, Damato BE. Systemic remission of non-Hodgkin's lymphoma after intralesional interferon alpha-2b to bilateral conjunctival lymphomas. Am J Ophthalmol. 2004;138(4):672–3.
195. Holds J, Buchanan A, Hanson R. Intralesional interferon-alpha for the treatment of bilateral conjunctival mucosa-associated lymphoid tissue lymphoma. Pediatr Blood Cancer. 2012;59(1):176–8.
196. Tsai PS, Colby KA. Treatment of conjunctival lymphomas. Semin Ophthalmol. 2005;20(4):239–46.

197. Zayed M, Sears K, Salvi SM, Rundle PA, Rennie IG, Mudhar HS. Intra-lesional interferon injection for recurrent conjunctival MALT lymphoma. Eye (Lond). 2013;27(5):680–2.
198. Cerny T, Borisch B, Introna M, Johnson P, Rose AL. Mechanism of action of rituximab. Anti-Cancer Drugs. 2002;13(Suppl 2):S3–10.
199. Sein JSA, Karp CL. Diagnosis and treatment of conjunctival lymphoma: American Academy of. Ophthalmology. 2012; Available from: https://www.aao.org/eyenet/article/diagnosis-treatment-of-conjunctival-lymphoma
200. Banchereau J, Rousset F. Human B lymphocytes: phenotype, proliferation, and differentiation. Adv Immunol. 1992;52:125–262.
201. Dreyling M, Ghielmini M, Rule S, Salles G, Vitolo U, Ladetto M, Committee EG. Newly diagnosed and relapsed follicular lymphoma: ESMO Clinical Practice Guidelines for diagnosis, treatment and follow-up. Ann Oncol. 2016;27(suppl 5):v83–90.
202. Tilly H, Gomes da Silva M, Vitolo U, Jack A, Meignan M, Lopez-Guillermo A, et al. Diffuse large B-cell lymphoma (DLBCL): ESMO Clinical Practice Guidelines for diagnosis, treatment and follow-up. Ann Oncol. 2015;26(Suppl 5):v116–25.
203. Eichhorst B, Robak T, Montserrat E, Ghia P, Hillmen P, Hallek M, et al. Chronic lymphocytic leukaemia: ESMO Clinical Practice Guidelines for diagnosis, treatment and follow-up. Ann Oncol. 2015;26(Suppl 5):v78–84.
204. Salles G, Barrett M, Foa R, Maurer J, O'Brien S, Valente N, et al. Rituximab in B-cell hematologic malignancies: a review of 20 years of clinical experience. Adv Ther. 2017;34(10):2232–73.
205. Minard-Colin V, Auperin A, Pillon M, Burke GAA, Barkauskas DA, Wheatley K, et al. Rituximab for high-risk, mature B-cell non-Hodgkin's lymphoma in children. N Engl J Med. 2020;382(23):2207–19.
206. Alvarez-Sanchez AI, Martinez-Losada C. Rituximab monotherapy become an optimal treatment for primary pulmonary malt lymphoma. Leuk Res Rep. 2018;9:21–2.
207. Foran JM, Cunningham D, Coiffier B, Solal-Celigny P, Reyes F, Ghielmini M, et al. Treatment of mantle-cell lymphoma with Rituximab (chimeric monoclonal anti-CD20 antibody): analysis of factors associated with response. Ann Oncol. 2000;11(Suppl 1):117–21.
208. Brown JR, Cymbalista F, Sharman J, Jacobs I, Nava-Parada P, Mato A. The role of rituximab in chronic lymphocytic leukemia treatment and the potential utility of biosimilars. Oncologist. 2018;23(3):288–96.
209. Dotan E, Aggarwal C, Smith MR. Impact of rituximab (Rituxan) on the treatment of B-cell non-Hodgkin's lymphoma. P T. 2010;35(3):148–57.
210. Annibali O, Chiodi F, Sarlo C, Cortes M, Quaranta-Leoni FM, Quattrocchi C, et al. Rituximab as single agent in primary MALT lymphoma of the ocular adnexa. Biomed Res Int. 2015;2015:895105.
211. Tuncer S, Tanyildiz B, Basaran M, Buyukbabani N, Dogan O. Systemic rituximab immunotherapy in the management of primary ocular adnexal lymphoma: single institution experience. Curr Eye Res. 2015;40(8):780–5.
212. Yazicioglu T, Oklar M, Kocabas S, Karadag E, Elibol V, Tezcan ME. A case report of conjunctival extranodal marginal zone lymphoma treated with intralesional rituximab injection therapy. Ocul Immunol Inflamm. 2022;30(6):1329–33.
213. Demirci H, Kauh CY, Rajaii F, Elner VM. Intralesional rituximab for the treatment of recurrent ocular adnexal lymphoma. Ophthalmic Plast Reconstr Surg. 2017;33(3S Suppl 1):S70–1.
214. Ferreri AJ, Govi S, Colucci A, Crocchiolo R, Modorati G. Intralesional rituximab: a new therapeutic approach for patients with conjunctival lymphomas. Ophthalmology. 2011;118(1):24–8.
215. Biotti D, Lerebours F, Bonneville F, Ciron J, Clanet M, Brassat D. Late-onset neutropenia and neurological relapse, during long-term rituximab therapy in myelin oligodendrocyte glycoprotein-antibody spectrum disorder. Mult Scler. 2018;24(12):1645–7.
216. Yi JH, Kim SJ, Ahn HK, Lee SJ, Chang MH, Kim WS. Rituximab-induced acute thrombocytopenia: a case report and review of the literature. Med Oncol. 2009;26(1):45–8.
217. Oellers P, Savar A, Samaniego F, Pro B, Esmaeli B. Second-line 90Yttrium-ibritumomab tiuxetan (Zevalin) in a patient with conjunctival mucosa-associated lymphoid tissue lymphoma refractory to rituximab. Ophthalmic Plast Reconstr Surg. 2012;28(6):e145–6.
218. Esmaeli B, McLaughlin P, Pro B, Samaniego F, Gayed I, Hagemeister F, et al. Prospective trial of targeted radioimmunotherapy with Y-90 ibritumomab tiuxetan (Zevalin) for front-line treatment of early-stage extranodal indolent ocular adnexal lymphoma. Ann Oncol. 2009;20(4):709–14.
219. Witzig TE, White CA, Gordon LI, Wiseman GA, Emmanouilides C, Murray JL, et al. Safety of yttrium-90 ibritumomab tiuxetan radioimmunotherapy for relapsed low-grade, follicular, or transformed non-Hodgkin's lymphoma. J Clin Oncol. 2003;21(7):1263–70.
220. Witzig TE, Flinn IW, Gordon LI, Emmanouilides C, Czuczman MS, Saleh MN, et al. Treatment with ibritumomab tiuxetan radioimmunotherapy in patients with rituximab-refractory follicular non-Hodgkin's lymphoma. J Clin Oncol. 2002;20(15):3262–9.
221. Wiseman GA, White CA, Stabin M, Dunn WL, Erwin W, Dahlbom M, et al. Phase I/II 90Y-Zevalin (yttrium-90 ibritumomab tiuxetan, IDEC-Y2B8) radioimmunotherapy dosimetry results in relapsed or refractory non-Hodgkin's lymphoma. Eur J Nucl Med. 2000;27(7):766–77.
222. Hamada K, Mikasa K, Yunou Y, Kurioka T, Majima T, Narita N, Kita E. Adjuvant effect of clarithromycin on chemotherapy for murine lung cancer. Chemotherapy. 2000;46(1):49–61.
223. Carella AM, Beltrami G, Pica G, Carella A, Catania G. Clarithromycin potentiates tyrosine kinase inhibitor treatment in patients with resistant chronic myeloid leukemia. Leuk Lymphoma. 2012;53(7):1409–11.
224. Hirasawa K, Moriya S, Miyahara K, Kazama H, Hirota A, Takemura J, et al. Macrolide antibiotics exhibit cytotoxic effect under amino acid-depleted culture condition by blocking autophagy flux in head and neck squamous cell carcinoma cell lines. PLoS One. 2016;11(12):e0164529.
225. Komatsu S, Miyazawa K, Moriya S, Takase A, Naito M, Inazu M, et al. Clarithromycin enhances bortezomib-induced cytotoxicity via endoplasmic reticulum stress-mediated CHOP (GADD153) induction and autophagy in breast cancer cells. Int J Oncol. 2012;40(4):1029–39.
226. Mikasa K, Sawaki M, Kita E, Hamada K, Teramoto S, Sakamoto M, et al. Significant survival benefit to patients with advanced non-small-cell lung cancer from treatment with clarithromycin. Chemotherapy. 1997;43(4):288–96.
227. Nakamura M, Kikukawa Y, Takeya M, Mitsuya H, Hata H. Clarithromycin attenuates autophagy in myeloma cells. Int J Oncol. 2010;37(4):815–20.
228. Ohara T, Morishita T, Suzuki H, Masaoka T, Ishii H, Hibi T. Antibiotics directly induce apoptosis in B cell lymphoma cells derived from BALB/c mice. Anticancer Res. 2004;24(6):3723–30.
229. Ohe M, Hashino S. A case of follicular B-cell lymphoma treated using clarithromycin. Korean J Hematol. 2011;46(3):203–6.
230. Ohe M, Hashino S. Successful treatment of angioimmunoblastic T-cell lymphoma with clarithromycin. Blood Res. 2016;51(2):139–42.
231. Pillozzi S, Masselli M, Gasparoli L, D'Amico M, Polletta L, Veltroni M, et al. Macrolide antibiotics exert antileukemic effects by modulating the autophagic flux through inhibition of hERG1 potassium channels. Blood Cancer J. 2016;6(5):e423.

232. Schafranek L, Leclercq TM, White DL, Hughes TP. Clarithromycin enhances dasatinib-induced cell death in chronic myeloid leukemia cells, by inhibition of late stage autophagy. Leuk Lymphoma. 2013;54(1):198–201.
233. Yatsunami J, Turuta N, Wakamatsu K, Hara N, Hayashi S. Clarithromycin is a potent inhibitor of tumor-induced angiogenesis. Res Exp Med (Berl). 1997;197(4):189–97.
234. Govi S, Dognini GP, Licata G, Crocchiolo R, Resti AG, Ponzoni M, Ferreri AJ. Six-month oral clarithromycin regimen is safe and active in extranodal marginal zone B-cell lymphomas: final results of a single-centre phase II trial. Br J Haematol. 2010;150(2):226–9.
235. Ferreri AJ, Sassone M, Kiesewetter B, Govi S, Scarfo L, Donadoni G, Raderer M. High-dose clarithromycin is an active monotherapy for patients with relapsed/refractory extranodal marginal zone lymphoma of mucosa-associated lymphoid tissue (MALT): the HD-K phase II trial. Ann Oncol. 2015;26(8):1760–5.
236. Peters DH, Clissold SP. Clarithromycin. A review of its antimicrobial activity, pharmacokinetic properties and therapeutic potential. Drugs. 1992;44(1):117–64.
237. Griffin MO, Fricovsky E, Ceballos G, Villarreal F. Tetracyclines: a pleitropic family of compounds with promising therapeutic properties. Review of the literature. Am J Physiol Cell Physiol. 2010;299(3):C539–48.
238. Jung K, Kim DH, Seo HI, Gong EJ, Bang CS. Efficacy of eradication therapy in Helicobacter pylori-negative gastric mucosa-associated lymphoid tissue lymphoma: a meta-analysis. Helicobacter. 2021;26(2):e12774.
239. Xie YL, He CY, Wei SQ, Guan WJ, Jiang Z. Clinical efficacy of the modified Helicobacter pylori eradication therapy for Helicobacter pylori-negative gastric mucosa-associated lymphoid tissue lymphoma: a meta analysis. Chin Med J. 2020;133(11):1337–46.
240. Han JJ, Kim TM, Jeon YK, Kim MK, Khwarg SI, Kim CW, et al. Long-term outcomes of first-line treatment with doxycycline in patients with previously untreated ocular adnexal marginal zone B cell lymphoma. Ann Hematol. 2015;94(4):575–81.
241. Ferreri AJ, Ponzoni M, Guidoboni M, Resti AG, Politi LS, Cortelazzo S, et al. Bacteria-eradicating therapy with doxycycline in ocular adnexal MALT lymphoma: a multicenter prospective trial. J Natl Cancer Inst. 2006;98(19):1375–82.
242. Choi SH, Yang MK, Kim TM, Choi HJ. Feasibility of oral doxycycline as first-line therapy for conjunctival mucosa-associated lymphoid tissue lymphoma. Eye (Lond). 2023;
243. Bryant SG, Fisher S, Kluge RM. Increased frequency of doxycycline side effects. Pharmacotherapy. 1987;7(4):125–9.
244. Jakobiec FA, Folberg R, Iwamoto T. Clinicopathologic characteristics of premalignant and malignant melanocytic lesions of the conjunctiva. Ophthalmology. 1989;96(2):147–66.
245. Shields JA, Shields CL, Mashayekhi A, Marr BP, Benavides R, Thangappan A, et al. Primary acquired melanosis of the conjunctiva: experience with 311 eyes. Trans Am Ophthalmol Soc 2007;105:61–71; discussion –2.
246. Kenworthy MK, Kenworthy SJ, De Guzman P, Morlet N. Conjunctival amelanotic melanoma presenting as a multifocal pink lesion. BMJ Case Rep. 2022;15(12)
247. Vishnevskia-Dai V, Davidy T, Zloto O. Amelanotic conjunctival melanoma in a child. Am J Ophthalmol Case Rep. 2023;29:101735.
248. Kovacevic D, Lukanovic-Primc K, Markusic V, Babic MB, Ledic D. Conjunctival amelanotic melanoma—a case report. Coll Antropol. 2011;35(Suppl 2):295–7.
249. Damani MR, O'Brien JM. Amelanotic conjunctival melanoma. JAMA Ophthalmol. 2016;134(1):e153568.
250. Kopsachilis N, Chatzibougias D, Ziakas N, Detorakis E, Tsatsos M. Chronic red eye due to amelanotic conjuctival melanoma masquerading as pyogenic granuloma. More than meets the eye. Clin Exp Optom. 2015;98(3):283–5.
251. Shields CL, Shields JA. Tumors of the conjunctiva and cornea. Surv Ophthalmol. 2004;49(1):3–24.
252. Huerva V, Vilardell F, Cid-Bertomeu P. Cryotherapy after topical interferon alpha 2b to treat conjunctival primary acquired melanosis. Case Rep Ophthalmol. 2023;14(1):111–4.
253. Ghassemi F, Ghadimi H, Nikdel M. Resolution of primary acquired melanosis with atypia after treatment with topical mitomycin C and interferon alfa-2b. J Ophthalmic Vis Res. 2015;10(1):84–6.
254. Kikuchi I, Kase S, Ishijima K, Ishida S. Long-term follow-up of conjunctival melanoma treated with topical interferon alpha-2b eye drops as adjunctive therapy following surgical resection. Graefes Arch Clin Exp Ophthalmol. 2017;255(11):2271–6.
255. Benage MJ, Morrow NC, Janson BJ, Greiner MA. Evaluation of interferon alpha 2b as adjunctive therapy for conjunctival melanoma. Am J Ophthalmol Case Rep. 2019;15:100467.
256. Goemaere J, Lauwers N, de Keizer RO, Verdijk RM, de Keizer RJ. Bone metastasis in a case of primary acquired melanosis with atypia resulting from conjunctiva melanoma. Am J Ophthalmol Case Rep. 2023;29:101730.
257. Calis Karanfil F, Gunduz AK, Gunduz OO, Ozalp Ates FS. Factors affecting recurrence and metastasis in conjunctival melanoma. Int Ophthalmol. 2023;43(11):4203–15.
258. Damato BE, Coupland SE. Ocular melanoma. Saudi J Ophthalmol. 2012;26(2):137–44.
259. Pe'er J, Frucht-Pery J. The treatment of primary acquired melanosis (PAM) with atypia by topical Mitomycin C. Am J Ophthalmol. 2005;139(2):229–34.
260. Finger PT, Czechonska G, Liarikos S. Topical mitomycin C chemotherapy for conjunctival melanoma and PAM with atypia. Br J Ophthalmol. 1998;82(5):476–9.
261. Nuessle S, Auw-Haedrich C, Jiang J, Boehringer D, Reinhard T. Real-life data of adjuvant IFN-alpha2b and MMC in conjunctival melanocytic lesions. Graefes Arch Clin Exp Ophthalmol. 2023;261(4):1159–66.
262. Cid-Bertomeu P, Huerva V. Use of interferon alpha 2b to manage conjunctival primary acquired melanosis and conjunctival melanoma. Surv Ophthalmol. 2022;67(5):1391–404.
263. Chaparro Tapias TA, Diaz Diaz AL, Secondi R, Coy Villamil H, Sanchez Espana JC. Resolution of conjunctival melanoma with topical interferon alpha 2b in a patient with mitomycin C intolerance. Arch Soc Esp Oftalmol (Engl Ed). 2018;93(11):558–61.
264. Huerva V, Traveset AE, Vilardell F. Topical interferon alpha-2b for diffuse conjunctival primary acquired melanosis with atypia. Ocul Immunol Inflamm. 2017;25(2):284–6.
265. Mazzini C, Pieretti G, Vicini G, Nicolosi C, Virgili G, Giansanti F. Extensive conjunctival melanoma successfully treated with surgical resection and pre- and postoperative topical mitomycin C. Eur J Ophthalmol. 2021;31(6):NP71-NP4:NP71.
266. Wong JR, Nanji AA, Galor A, Karp CL. Management of conjunctival malignant melanoma: a review and update. Expert Rev Ophthalmol. 2014;9(3):185–204.
267. Kurli M, Finger PT. Topical mitomycin chemotherapy for conjunctival malignant melanoma and primary acquired melanosis with atypia: 12 years' experience. Graefes Arch Clin Exp Ophthalmol. 2005;243(11):1108–14.
268. Chalasani R, Giblin M, Conway RM. Role of topical chemotherapy for primary acquired melanosis and malignant melanoma of the conjunctiva and cornea: review of the evidence and recommendations for treatment. Clin Experiment Ophthalmol. 2006;34(7):708–14.

269. Bender C, Hassel JC, Enk A. Immunotherapy of melanoma. Oncol Res Treat. 2016;39(6):369–76.
270. Finger PT, Sedeek RW, Chin KJ. Topical interferon alfa in the treatment of conjunctival melanoma and primary acquired melanosis complex. Am J Ophthalmol. 2008;145(1):124–9.
271. Garip A, Schaumberger MM, Wolf A, Herold TR, Miller CV, Klingenstein A, et al. Evaluation of a short-term topical interferon alpha-2b treatment for histologically proven melanoma and primary acquired melanosis with atypia. Orbit. 2016;35(1):29–34.
272. Herold TR, Hintschich C. Interferon alpha for the treatment of melanocytic conjunctival lesions. Graefes Arch Clin Exp Ophthalmol. 2010;248(1):111–5.
273. Oellers P, Karp CL. Management of pigmented conjunctival lesions. Ocul Surf. 2012;10(4):251–63.
274. Bratton EM, Knutsen-Larson S, Durairaj VD, Gregory DG, Mellette JR. Combination topical therapy for conjunctival primary acquired melanosis with atypia and periocular lentigo maligna. Cornea. 2015;34(1):90–3.
275. Kim JM, Weiss S, Sinard JH, Pointdujour-Lim R. Dabrafenib and trametinib for BRAF-mutated conjunctival melanoma. Ocul Oncol Pathol. 2020;6(1):35–8.
276. Gkiala A, Palioura S. Conjunctival melanoma: update on genetics, epigenetics and targeted molecular and immune-based therapies. Clin Ophthalmol. 2020;14:3137–52.
277. Rossi E, Schinzari G, Maiorano BA, Pagliara MM, Di Stefani A, Bria E, et al. Conjunctival melanoma: genetic and epigenetic insights of a distinct type of melanoma. Int J Mol Sci. 2019;20(21)
278. Weber J, Mandala M, Del Vecchio M, Gogas HJ, Arance AM, Cowey CL, et al. Adjuvant nivolumab versus ipilimumab in resected stage III or IV melanoma. N Engl J Med. 2017;377(19):1824–35.
279. Eggermont AMM, Blank CU, Mandala M, Long GV, Atkinson V, Dalle S, et al. Adjuvant pembrolizumab versus placebo in resected stage III melanoma. N Engl J Med. 2018;378(19):1789–801.
280. Grossmann KF, Othus M, Patel SP, Tarhini AA, Sondak VK, Knopp MV, et al. Adjuvant pembrolizumab versus IFNalpha2b or ipilimumab in resected high-risk melanoma. Cancer Discov. 2022;12(3):644–53.
281. Patel SP, Othus M, Chen Y, Wright GP Jr, Yost KJ, Hyngstrom JR, et al. Neoadjuvant-adjuvant or adjuvant-only pembrolizumab in advanced melanoma. N Engl J Med. 2023;388(9):813–23.
282. Amaria RN, Prieto PA, Tetzlaff MT, Reuben A, Andrews MC, Ross MI, et al. Neoadjuvant plus adjuvant dabrafenib and trametinib versus standard of care in patients with high-risk, surgically resectable melanoma: a single-centre, open-label, randomised, phase 2 trial. Lancet Oncol. 2018;19(2):181–93.
283. Holder AM, Wargo JA, Ross MI. Timing is everything: neoadjuvant versus adjuvant immunotherapy in patients with resectable metastatic melanoma. Ann Surg Oncol. 2023;30(12):6953–7.
284. Versluis JM, Menzies AM, Sikorska K, Rozeman EA, Saw RPM, van Houdt WJ, et al. Survival update of neoadjuvant ipilimumab plus nivolumab in macroscopic stage III melanoma in the OpACIN and OpACIN-neo trials. Ann Oncol. 2023;34(4):420–30.
285. Abaza A, Sid Idris F, Anis Shaikh H, Vahora I, Moparthi KP, Al Rushaidi MT, et al. Programmed cell death protein 1 (PD-1) and programmed cell death ligand 1 (PD-L1) immunotherapy: a promising breakthrough in cancer therapeutics. Cureus. 2023;15(9):e44582.
286. Shields CL, Lally SE, Orloff M. Controlling conjunctival melanoma-to infinity and beyond. JAMA Ophthalmol. 2020;138(6):608–9.
287. Muller AJ, Scherle PA. Targeting the mechanisms of tumoral immune tolerance with small-molecule inhibitors. Nat Rev Cancer. 2006;6(8):613–25.
288. Santella RM, Hsieh LL, Perera F. Immunologic quantification of carcinogen-DNA adducts. Basic Life Sci. 1986;38:509–17.
289. Finger PT, Pavlick AC. Checkpoint inhibition immunotherapy for advanced local and systemic conjunctival melanoma: a clinical case series. J Immunother Cancer. 2019;7(1):83.
290. Dalvin LA, Shields CL, Orloff M, Sato T, Shields JA. Checkpoint inhibitor immune therapy: systemic indications and ophthalmic side effects. Retina. 2018;38(6):1063–78.
291. Sagiv O, Thakar SD, Kandl TJ, Ford J, Sniegowski MC, Hwu WJ, Esmaeli B. Immunotherapy with programmed cell death 1 inhibitors for 5 patients with conjunctival melanoma. JAMA Ophthalmol. 2018;136(11):1236–41.
292. Hong BY, Ford JR, Glitza IC, Torres Cabala CA, Tetzlaff M, Prieto VG, et al. Immune checkpoint inhibitor therapy as an eye-preserving treatment for locally advanced conjunctival melanoma. Ophthalmic Plast Reconstr Surg. 2021;37(1):e9–e13.
293. Kini A, Fu R, Compton C, Miller DM, Ramasubramanian A. Pembrolizumab for recurrent conjunctival melanoma. JAMA Ophthalmol. 2017;135(8):891–2.
294. Pinto Torres S, Andre T, Gouveia E, Costa L, Passos MJ. Systemic treatment of metastatic conjunctival melanoma. Case Rep Oncol Med. 2017;2017:4623964.
295. Chaves LJ, Huth B, Augsburger JJ, Correa ZM. Eye-sparing treatment for diffuse invasive conjunctival melanoma. Ocul Oncol Pathol. 2018;4(4):261–6.
296. Ford J, Thuro BA, Thakar S, Hwu WJ, Richani K, Esmaeli B. Immune checkpoint inhibitors for treatment of metastatic melanoma of the orbit and ocular adnexa. Ophthalmic Plast Reconstr Surg. 2017;33(4):e82–e5.
297. Sa HS, Daniel C, Esmaeli B. Update on immune checkpoint inhibitors for conjunctival melanoma. J Ophthalmic Vis Res. 2022;17(3):405–12.
298. DeSimone JD, Lally SE, Shields CL. Conjunctival metastasis from cutaneous melanoma demonstrating complete regression following checkpoint inhibitor therapy. JAMA Ophthalmol. 2022;140(1):e214786.
299. Paridaens AD, Minassian DC, McCartney AC, Hungerford JL. Prognostic factors in primary malignant melanoma of the conjunctiva: a clinicopathological study of 256 cases. Br J Ophthalmol. 1994;78(4):252–9.
300. Matsuo T, Yamasaki O, Tanaka T, Katsui K, Waki T. Proton beam therapy followed by pembrolizumab for giant ocular surface conjunctival malignant melanoma: a case report. Mol Clin Oncol. 2022;16(1):12.
301. Dagi Glass LR, Lawrence DP, Jakobiec FA, Freitag SK. Conjunctival melanoma responsive to combined systemic BRAF/MEK inhibitors. Ophthalmic Plast Reconstr Surg. 2017;33(5):e114–e6.
302. Kiyohara T, Tanimura H, Miyamoto M, Shijimaya T, Nagano N, Nakamaru S, et al. Two cases of BRAF-mutated, bulbar conjunctival melanoma, and review of the published literature. Clin Exp Dermatol. 2020;45(2):207–11.
303. Rossi E, Maiorano BA, Pagliara MM, Sammarco MG, Dosa T, Martini M, et al. Dabrafenib and trametinib in BRAF mutant metastatic conjunctival melanoma. Front Oncol. 2019;9:232.
304. Bushara O, Tidwell J, Wester JR, Miura J. The current state of neoadjuvant therapy in resectable advanced stage melanoma. Cancers (Basel). 2023;15(13)
305. Blankenstein SA, Rohaan MW, Klop WMC, van der Hiel B, van de Wiel BA, Lahaye MJ, et al. Neoadjuvant cytoreductive treatment with BRAF/MEK inhibition of prior unresectable regionally advanced melanoma to allow complete surgical resection, REDUCTOR: a prospective, single-arm, open-label phase II trial. Ann Surg. 2021;274(2):383–9.

Conjunctival Tumors: Surgical Techniques

13

Arun D. Singh

13.1 Introduction

A variety of tumors affect the conjunctiva and cornea, ranging from benign growths to malignant neoplasms. Several types of conjunctival neoplasms originate from or involve the limbus region and extend into the cornea. Therefore, surgical techniques involve excision of both corneal and conjunctival tissues. Several aspects of the tumor such as location, depth of involvement, and suspected diagnosis influence the surgical intent (incisional, map, or excisional), extent of surgical margins, choice of instruments, and use of adjuvant procedures. Various techniques of wound closure can be selected based on wound size, depth, and location (Table 13.1).

Table 13.1 Considerations for conjunctival surgery

Clinical diagnosis	Benign	Malignant (low grade)	Malignant (high grade)		
Intent	Incisional	Map	Excisional		
Location	Cornea				
	Limbus				
	Conjunctiva	Bulbar	Tarsal	Forniceal	Plica
	Caruncle				
Depth	Conjunctiva				
	Sclera	Superficial (<50%)	Deep sclera (>50%)		
Extent	Localized	Diffuse			
Planned margins	1 mm	2 mm	4 mm		
Instruments	Scissors	Punch	Blade	Cautery needle	
Adjuvant	Cryotherapy	Alcohol	Chemotherapy	Brachytherapy	
Graft	Autograft	Amniotic membrane	Sclera/pericardium		
Closure	None	Suture	Glue		
Cover	Patch	Bandage contact les	Kontour lens	K Pro	

A. D. Singh (✉)
Department of Ophthalmic Oncology, Cole Eye Institute, Cleveland Clinic, Cleveland, OH, USA
e-mail: SINGHA@ccf.org

© The Author(s), under exclusive license to Springer Nature Switzerland AG 2024
J. Pe'er et al. (eds.), *Clinical Ophthalmic Oncology*, https://doi.org/10.1007/978-3-031-72443-5_13

13.2 Presurgical Evaluation

A detailed slit lamp examination is not only vital to correctly diagnose conjunctival and corneal tumors but also critical for planning the appropriate surgery. It is also important to evaluate the upper and lower palpebral conjunctivae to look for extension of lesions (Fig. 13.1) and to palpate the preauricular and submandibular areas for enlarged lymph nodes. Corneal involvement must be accurately documented since it is difficult to appreciate under the diffuse lighting of an operating microscope. Rose Bengal stain can be used to help delineate abnormal epithelium. A drawing or photograph clearly depicting the extent of involvement, which can be readily seen during surgery, is helpful for obtaining adequate surgical margins. Free movement of the abnormal conjunctiva, as tested by gentle pushing with a cotton-tipped applicator, indicates the sparing of the sclera.

Anterior segment optical coherence tomography (OCT) (Fig. 13.2) and ultrasound biomicroscopy can greatly aid in the preoperative evaluation of surface extension (OCT) and depth (UBM) of conjunctival lesions [1].

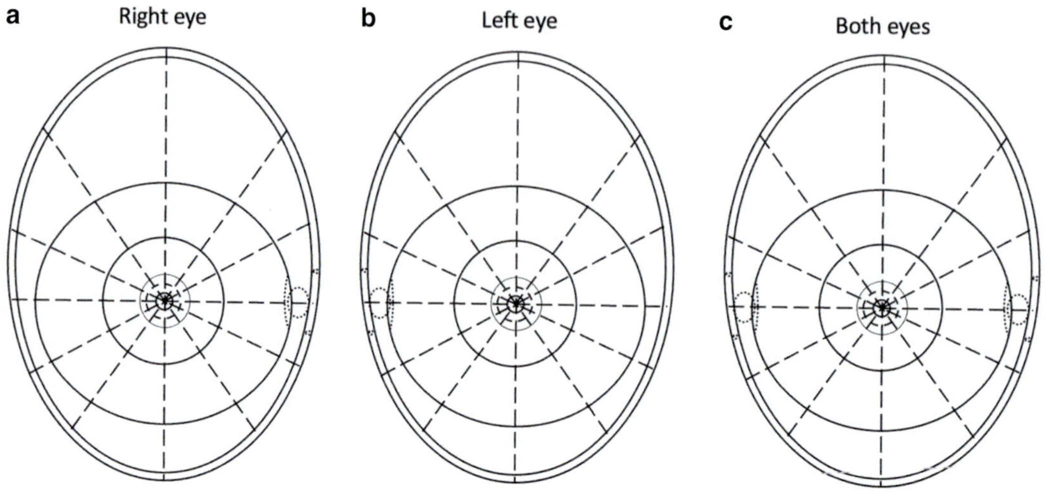

Fig. 13.1 A system for clinically mapping conjunctival tumor location and extent. Right eye (**a**), left eye (**b**) and for both eyes (**c**). Courtesy Prof. Bertil Damato, London, UK

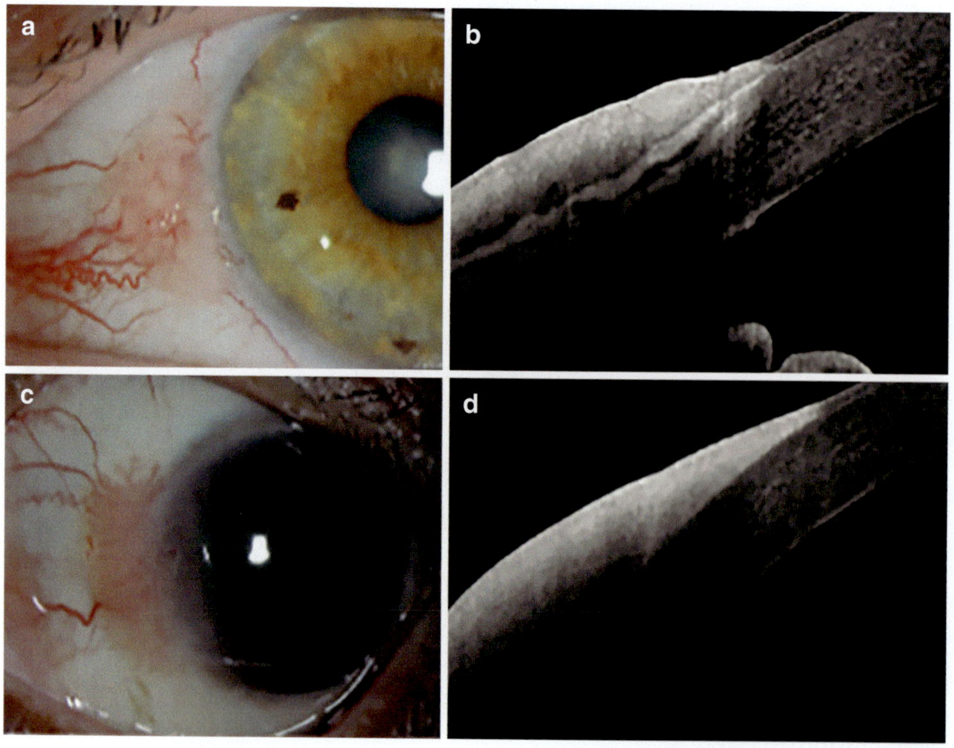

Fig. 13.2 Gelatinous CIN on nasal bulbar limbus with intralesional and surrounding vascularity (**a**) with corresponding AS-OCT showing abrupt epithelial thickening and hyper-reflectivity (**b**). Gelatinous CIN with greater corneal involvement with intralesional and surrounding vascularity (**c**). AS-OCT with abrupt thickening of epithelium, hyper-reflective thickened epithelium, and a distinct boarder below lesion (**d**)

13.3 Anesthesia

Local anesthesia can be used for most procedures, depending on patient cooperation. Subconjunctival injection of 1% lidocaine with epinephrine to elevate the lesion from the underlying sclera [2]. Most authors recommend retrobulbar anesthesia with sedation to avoid disruption of conjunctival architecture and to control the pain associated with conjunctival manipulation and cryotherapy [3]. General anesthesia may be required in exceptional cases.

13.4 General Surgical Principles

Surgical intent can vary from incisional biopsy for diffuse lesion to total removal of tissues (conjunctiva, cornea, sclera) that are affected by the neoplasm (excisional). All but the most extensive conjunctival lesions can be approached by excisional biopsy to achieve this goal. Map biopsy may be performed in cases suspected of pagetoid spread of sebaceous carcinoma [4, 5] or primary acquired melanosis [6].

13.5 General Surgical Technique

In general, the surgical technique depends on the location and the type of tumor. The surgical procedure can be divided into four sequential steps: conjunctival excision, corneal excision (if corneal involvement is present), supplemental cryotherapy (if needed), and ocular surface reconstruction.

13.5.1 Conjunctival Excision

The removal technique for the conjunctival portion of a neoplasm depends on the type of lesion and its depth of invasion.

13.5.1.1 Simple Incisional Biopsy

A simple incisional biopsy should be considered in cases where medical therapy is the planned primary therapy for an ocular surface squamous neoplasia. This procedure can be performed at the slit lamp under topical anesthesia or under sedation in the operating room. Forceps are used to grasp nearby uninvolved tissue, and scissors are then used to remove a sufficient tumor sample. Given the certainty of positive margins, specimen orientation is not needed. The sample is positioned on a small piece of paper and placed in formalin to allow for pathologic review. A Beaver blade can then be used to separate and remove abnormal corneal epithelium, which should also be sent to the pathologist. While this technique is a good option in cases of suspected CIN, it should be avoided in cases of suspected melanoma as complete excisional biopsy is preferred in the latter malignancy.

13.5.1.2 Simple Conjunctival Excision

Benign lesions that do not penetrate the Tenon, or sclera can be removed by a simple excisional biopsy. The surrounding conjunctiva is grasped with non-toothed forceps and excised along with a 1 mm margin of clinically non-affected tissue using scissors. The depth of incision can be limited only to the full thickness sparing the underlying Tenon's fascia or may extend up to the sclera (including Tenon's fascia) (Fig. 13.3). It is important not to touch the affected conjunctiva and use different instruments for affected and non-affected conjunctiva so as not to iatrogenically plant tumor cells on the unaffected tissue.

13.5.1.3 Complex Conjunctival Excision

For potentially malignant tumors, a more extensive excision is suggested with a wider margin of excision of clinically non-affected tissue (3–4 mm) and lamellar sclerectomy if scleral involvement is present. The area to be resected is first outlined with a surgical marker, with care to include 2 mm of unaffected conjunctival tissue for low-grade malignant tumors such as CIN or squamous cell carcinoma [7].

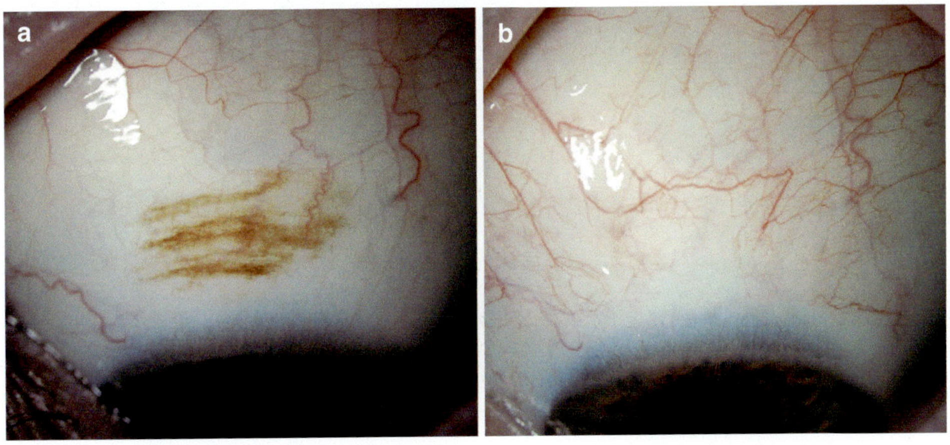

Fig. 13.3 Simple conjunctival excision for PAM. The depth of incision was limited to the full thickness of the conjunctiva sparing the underlying Tenon's fascia (**a**). The wound (8 × 6 mm) was left to heal by secondary intention (with approximation—avoiding sutures or glue). Note full surface epithelialization at 4 weeks (**b**)

However, in suspected cases of melanoma, 4 mm margin is advisable. Using a no-touch technique, the conjunctiva and Tenon's fascia are then incised with scissors to expose the underlying sclera (Fig. 13.4a). Once the conjunctival margins have been released, tumor removal should be completed by cutting flush with the corneal margin. Bipolar cautery is applied to the episcleral vessels to achieve hemostasis. In cases where scleral involvement is suspected, a partial sclerectomy should be performed with a fresh no. 57 Beaver blade by fashioning a semicircular groove, approximately 20% of scleral depth and 2 mm posterior to the tumor margin (Fig. 13.4b). A thin scleral flap can then be dissected with a crescent blade anteriorly up to the limbus (Fig. 13.4c). If the scleral dissection reaches about 50% involvement, wound closure can be supplemented with a donor scleral patch graft (Fig. 13.5). Deeper scleral dissection is not advisable.

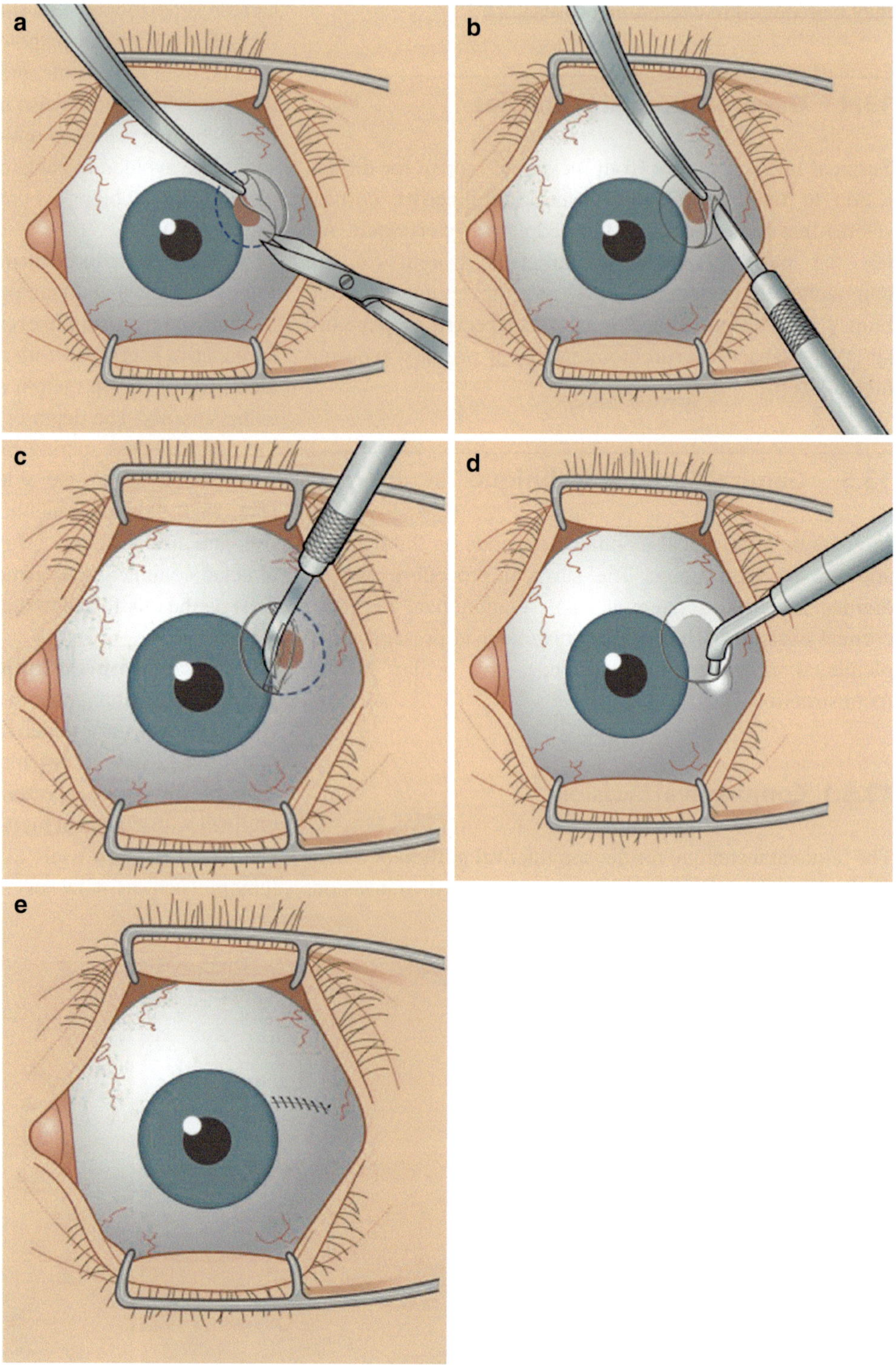

Fig. 13.4 Complex conjunctival excision. Large conjunctival lesion being excised with a 4-mm margin of unaffected conjunctiva. (**a**) Conjunctival flap being fashioned. (**b**) Partial-thickness scleral incision with a no. 57 Beaver blade. (**c**) Lamellar scleral dissection with a crescent blade. (**d**) Cryotherapy to the edges of the conjunctival wound. (**e**) Closure of the wound

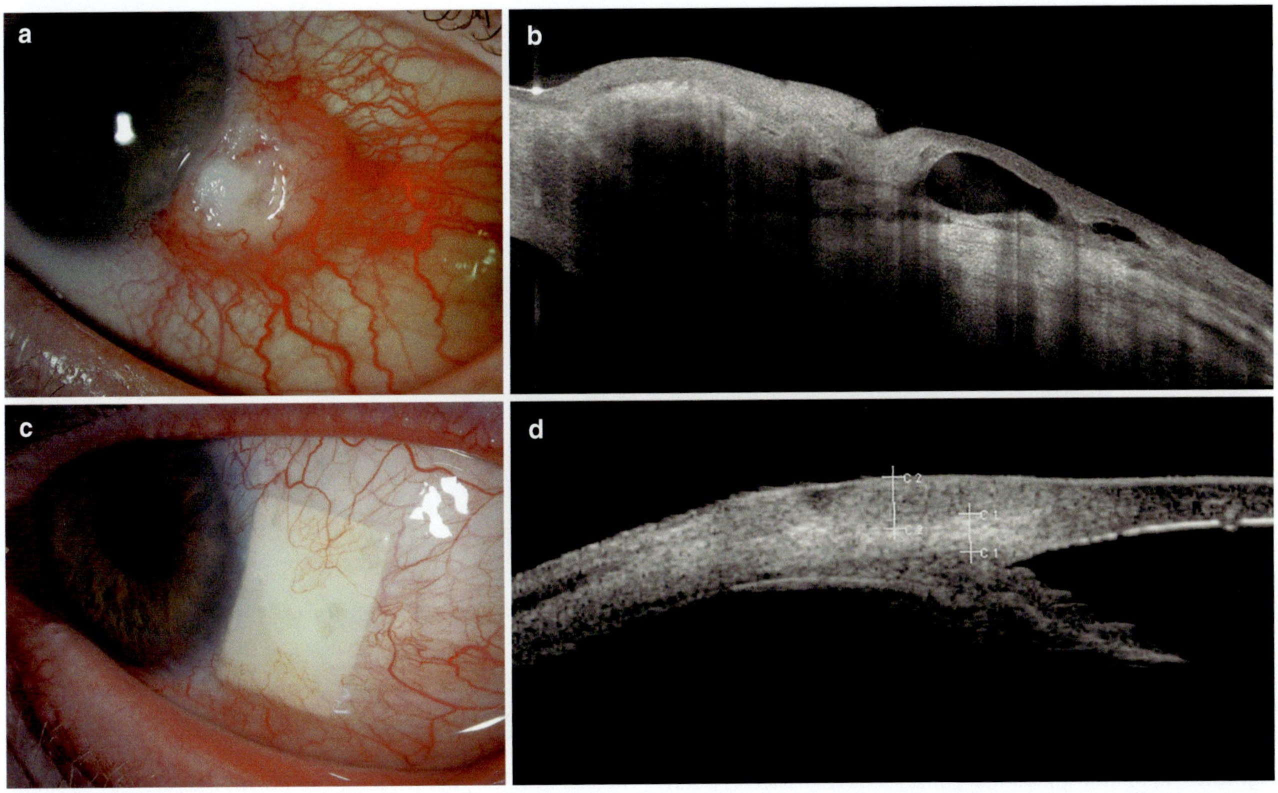

Fig. 13.5 Nodulo-ulcerative squamous cell carcinoma (7 × 6 mm) centered at 4 o'clock (**a**). Preoperative AS OCT suggestive of scleral invasion (**b**). A traction suture was applied, and the globe rotated superonasally. The cornea was protected by viscoelastic and absolute alcohol applied to the involved corneal epithelium and adjacent strip of 1 mm healthy epithelium. The corneal epithelium was incised and reflected off the Bowman's membrane toward the limbus. The conjunctival incision was outlined with cautery (2 mm beyond the visible margin). As the conjunctiva was dissected from sclera, adhesion to the underlying sclera was observed. Therefore, partial-thickness scleral dissection was performed to reflect the conjunctival and the scleral component toward the limbus. Finally, the limbal dissection was performed removing the conjunctival, corneal, and scleral component as a single piece (Taco technique). From the base of the tumor, a rectangular (6 × 4 mm) partial-thickness scleral flap (10% in thickness) was excised and submitted for histopathology as deep margin. At this point, the sclera appeared to be less than 50% in thickness; therefore, it was elected to reinforce it with a donor scleral patch graft that was also 6 × 4 mm in size (**c**). It was tied into position with 8-0 vicryl sutures. The conjunctiva could be mobilized and closed with interrupted 8-0 vicryl sutures after applying double freeze-thaw cryotherapy to the conjunctival margins. Postoperative appearance of the wound site with intact and scleral graft that is flush with the surface (**d**, UBM)

Instead, such cases can be preferentially treated with postoperative adjuvant brachytherapy (Fig. 13.6) [8, 9]. For tumors extending more than 5 mm posterior to the limbus, it is helpful to hook and isolate the appropriate rectus muscle with a suture to provide traction, to allow for better exposure and to avoid inadvertent injury to the muscle.

13.5.2 Corneal Excision

As corneal involvement by a conjunctival tumor tends to be superficial, the corneal excision is usually limited to the removal of the corneal epithelium (corneal epitheliectomy). Care must be taken not to disrupt Bowman's layer as it is thought to serve as a natural ocular barrier to invasion. Deeper invasion of the cornea, if present, necessitates lamellar keratectomy. Prior to scraping off the affected epithelium with no. 57 Beaver blade, absolute alcohol is applied for 1 min with a Weck-cell applicator to the involved corneal epithelium and a 1-mm margin of clinically non-affected tissue. The corneal epithelium is removed in one piece, placed on a filter paper, and submitted to pathology. In the presence of concomitant conjunctival involvement, authors prefer to perform conjunctival resection of the tumor followed by corneal dissection and finally removal of both components in toto by undertaking limbal dissection (Taco technique) (Fig. 13.7).

13.5.3 Adjuvant Procedures

13.5.3.1 Cryotherapy

Nitrous oxide probe is used as a supplemental treatment of malignant lesions to decrease recurrence rates (31% versus 16% at 5 years) [10]. The probe is placed on the underside of the conjunctival edge, lifting the conjunctiva

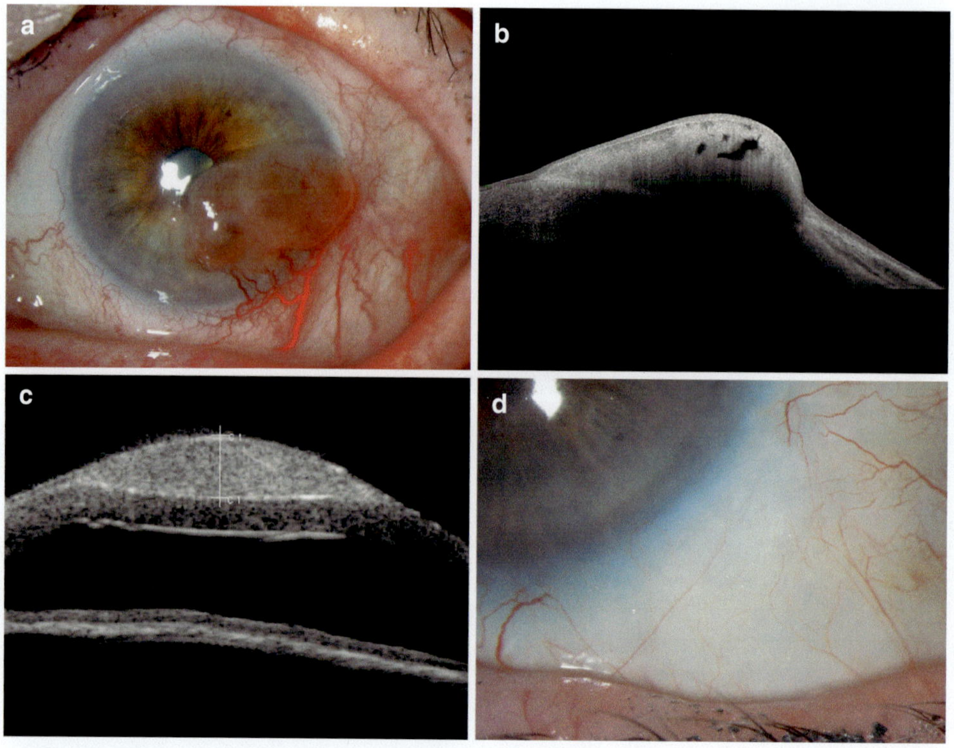

Fig. 13.6 An 81 year woman with primary acquired melanosis (PAM) with multifocal of melanoma. The temporal bulbar melanoma was less conspicuous (5 × 3 × 1 mm) than the corneal melanoma (7.5 × 5.6 × 1.1 mm) with feeder vessels (**a**). Anterior segment OCT (**b**) and UBM did not suggest extension into corneal stroma (**c**). Both conjunctival and corneal melanoma were excised as a single tumor combined with alcohol corneal epitheliectomy, cryotherapy to the conjunctival margins, and map biopsies. Total excision was 12 × 7 mm in size that was repaired with Tenon closure and postoperative use of 16 mm Kontur bandage soft lens (Kontur Kontact Lens, Co., Inc. Hercules, CA, USA). Histopathology confirmed invasive melanoma with negative corneal and conjunctival epithelial, but deep margin was positive. Map biopsies were negative for PAM elsewhere. Allowing for 4 weeks of healing, episcleral/corneal plaque brachytherapy was performed with plaque being centered over the area of corneal stromal involvement. 45 Gy was delivered over 72 h using an I-125 source using EP 917 plaque. Patient remained free from local recurrence and metastasis at 2.5-year follow-up visit with visual acuity of 20/40 (**d**) and only slight corneal stromal opacity and corneal thinning

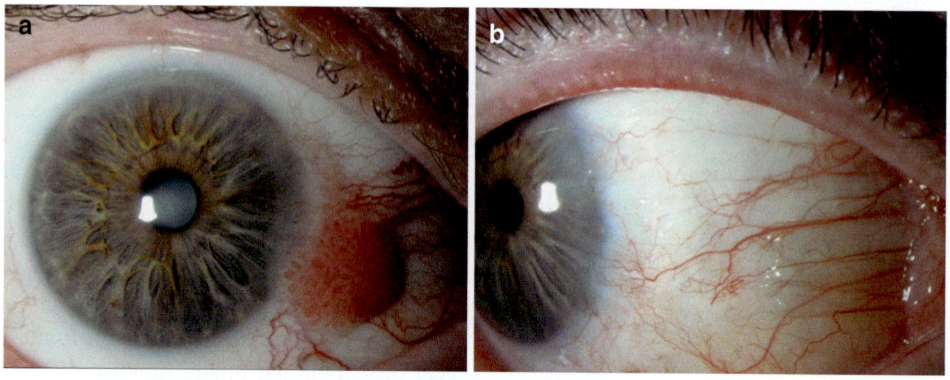

Fig. 13.7 Ocular surface squamous neoplasia prior and post-surgical excision with 2 mm margins. Papillomatous conjunctival intraepithelial neoplasia with corneal involvement (**a**) and post-operative results (**b**). (Reproduced with permission from Bowen et al. [7])

to avoid damage to the sclera, and applied to the tissue for 3–10 s (Fig. 13.4d) [11]. The tissue is allowed to thaw spontaneously and is refrozen in a similar manner for a "double freeze-thaw" cycle. The probe is applied to the margin to overlap with the previously treated area, and the process is repeated until all margins have been treated. The affected limbus is then similarly treated with a double freeze-thaw cycle.

13.5.3.2 Absolute Alcohol

Prior to scraping off the affected epithelium with no. 57 Beaver blade, absolute alcohol is applied for 1 min with a Weck-cell applicator to the involved corneal epithelium and a 1-mm margin of clinically non-affected tissue. The purpose of alcohol application is to denature the cells, thereby minimizing the risk of seeding cancer cells. Alcohol is applied to the dry cornea so as to limit spillage [12].

13.5.3.3 Topical Chemotherapy

Intraoperative adjuvant 0.02% mitomycin-C (MMC) may delay epithelial healing [13].

13.5.3.4 Brachytherapy

Adjuvant brachytherapy applied 2–4 weeks after surgery for conjunctival melanoma excised with 2 mm margin and dissected to bare sclera has been advocated, despite local recurrence rate of 22% 13/58 cases) [9].

13.6 Ocular Surface Reconstruction

To prevent the possibility of planting tumor cells on unaffected tissue, it is important to use a different set of instruments for reconstructing the ocular surface than those that were used for lesion removal.

13.6.1 Healing by Secondary Intention

Conjunctival dissection that is Tenon sparing can be allowed to heal with secondary intention without the need for sutures or graft (Fig. 13.8). Excision of tumors located in plica, fornices, and caruncle are generally allowed to heal by secondary intention.

13.6.2 Primary Closure

Conjunctival defects that are 12 mm or less in diameter can be easily closed by the primary close after undermining the conjunctival on the bulbar surface and trimming it at the limbal attachment (Fig. 13.9).

13.6.3 Grafts

For larger conjunctival defects or those with prior surgery, the conjunctival defect can be closed either by conjunctival autograft obtained from the superolateral bulbar region or amniotic membrane. The preferred technique involves cutting an amniotic membrane to the appropriate size, placing it (substrate side down) over the defect area, and tucking the margins under the healthy conjunctivae. Fibrin glue is then utilized to secure the membrane to the underlying sclera. The thicker component (fibrinogen) is first introduced under the graft with a 27-gauge cannula and gently spread so that a thin layer of uniform thickness is achieved. The thinner compo-

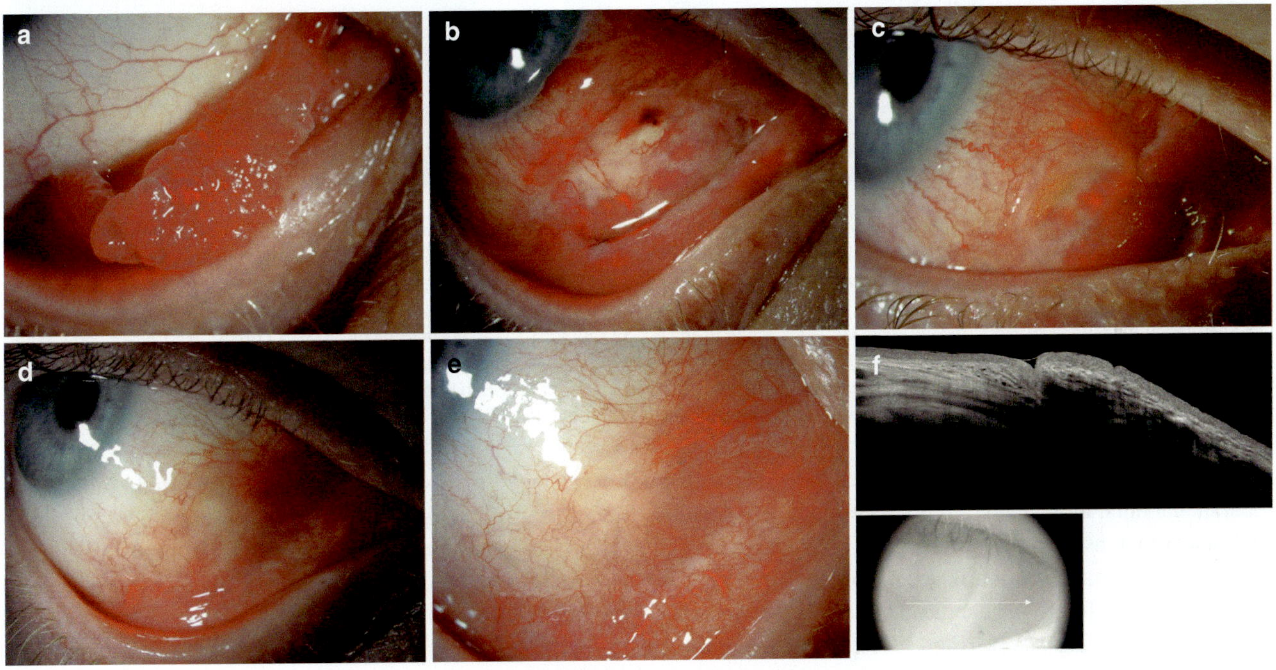

Fig. 13.8 Healing by secondary intention. In the inferior nasal bulbar conjunctiva region, a single 20 × 10 mm papillomatous lesion had narrow base without deep stromal extension (**a**). Inferior bulbar conjunctiva was infiltrated with 2% lidocaine with epinephrine and conjunctiva lifted away from the underlying Tenons. Using monopolar cautery needle, conjunctiva was incised 2 mm beyond the visible margin cauterizing the vessels and providing a clean incision sparing the underlying Tenon. The wound was approximately 18 × 12 mm in size. Double freeze-thaw cryotherapy was applied to the margin. Since the Tenons were intact, the wound was left to granulate by secondary intention. Steroid antibiotic ointment and eye patch were applied. Appearance 2 days (**b**), 2 weeks (**c**), 6 weeks (**d**), and 12 weeks (**e**) after surgery showing gradual epithelialization of the underlying Tenon as confirmed by OCT (**f**)

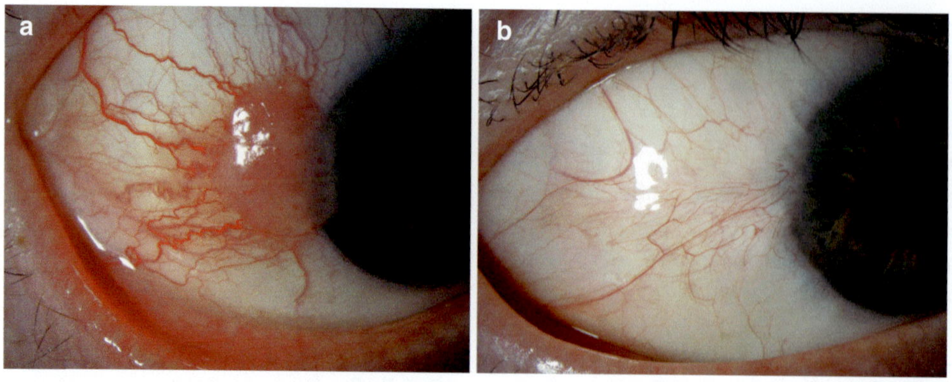

Fig. 13.9 Healing by primary closure. CIN lesion (5.7 × 5.0 mm) with limbal involvement from 8:30 to 10:00 position and 1.5 mm extension into the cornea (**a**). The corneal component was excised first following alcohol epitheliectomy, reflecting it toward the limbus. Conjunctival excision was then performed with 2 mm margin. The conjunctiva and underlying Tenons were incised and dissected up to the level of the sclera. Using hockey-stick blade, the tumor was dissected off the sclera toward the limbus. There appeared to be no deeper extension. Finally, the limbal dissection was performed (Taco technique). Once the plane of the distal dissection was identified, a crescent blade was used to remove the conjunctival and corneal component together as a single piece. This was submitted on filter paper for histopathology. Double freeze thaw cryotherapy was applied to the conjunctival margins. The wound was 10 mm vertical and 8 mm in horizontal dimension. The conjunctiva could be mobilized easily for primary closure using 8-0 vicryl sutures. Postoperative appearance with pseudopterygium like appearance due to conjunctivalization of the corneal limbal dissection site (**b**, 3 months)

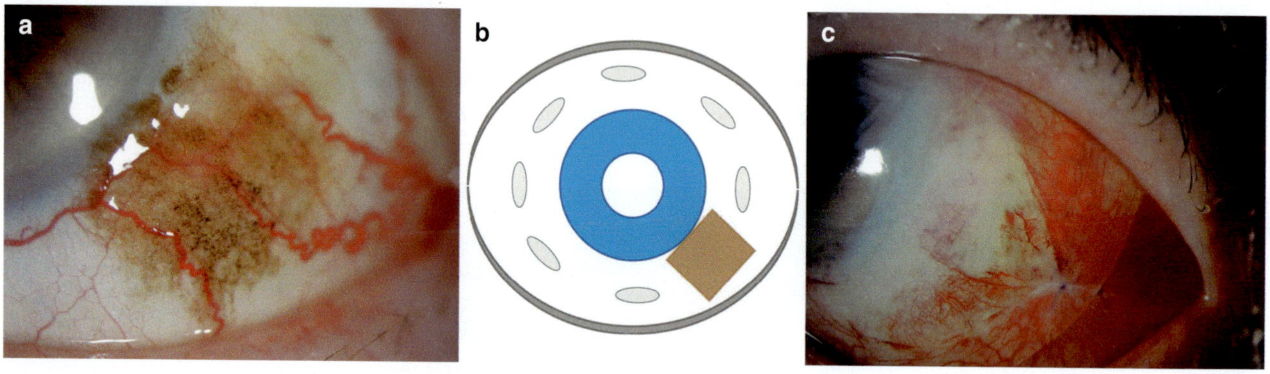

Fig. 13.10 Healing by amniotic graft. Conjunctival primary acquire melanosis (6.0 × 6.0 mm) lesion at the limbus from 3:30 to 5 o'clock (**a**). 2 mm outside the visible margin of the conjunctival lesion was marked with fine tip pen and then with cautery. Conjunctival incision was then made with Westcott scissors and a hockey stick blade used to reflect the lesion off the sclera. Double freeze-thaw cryotherapy was applied to the conjunctival margins. The wound defect was 10 mm vertical and 11 mm in horizontal dimensions. Two 8-0 vicryl sutures were placed to partially close the conjunctival wound. The remaining size was 7 × 10 mm. Next, freeze-dried amniotic membrane was cut to fit over the remaining defect (7 × 10 mm) and tissue glue used as adhesive. Next conjunctival map biopsies were obtained from 12 O'clock, 1:30 O'clock, 3 O'clock, 6 O'clock, 7:30 O'clock, 9 O'clock, and 10:30 O'clock (**b**). There was a total of 8 biopsies which were placed on filter paper and sent to pathology. A 22 mm Kontur lens was placed (**c**, postoperative day #10)

nent (thrombin) is then introduced under the graft with a separate cannula, and, again, a thin layer is applied. A muscle hook is then used to smooth the graft and remove excess glue. Once the graft position is acceptable, a 2-min wait is usually sufficient for good adherence to develop between the graft and underlying sclera (Fig. 13.4e). Use of amniotic membrane helps to decrease inflammation and to facilitate epithelialization (Fig. 13.10) [14, 15]. Recent reports suggest the use of sutureless cryopreserved amniotic membrane transplantation (ProKera® (Bio-Tissue, Inc., Miami, FL, USA) [16]. In cases that require extensive limbal dissection, repair can be performed by incorporating simple limbal epithelial transplantation (SLET) to avoid limbal stem failure [17]. Use of any type of graft generally requires a bandage contact lens and topical treatment for a longer time.

13.6.4 Sutures

Use of fibrin glue when compared with 8-0 Vicryl conjunctival sutures is associated with less ocular irritation and inflammation [18].

13.7 Specific Surgical Techniques

13.7.1 Melanocytic Tumors

13.7.1.1 Conjunctival Nevus

Excision of conjunctival nevus is considered for cosmetic reasons, ocular irritation, or parental concern. A simple excisional biopsy is the procedure of choice [3].

13.7.1.2 Primary Acquired Melanosis

Because of the diffuse nature of primary acquired melanosis (PAM), the surgical approach is different from that of an isolated conjunctival lesion. Corneal epitheliectomy is performed if corneal involvement is documented. Suspicious nodules are excised to evaluate for the possibility of melanoma. Complete removal is possible with small areas of PAM, whereas diffuse areas may be treated with map biopsy combined with double freeze-thaw cycle cryotherapy [6, 19].

The technique of map biopsy involves three components: clinical drawing, biopsy sites, and sample handling. The first component, the clinical drawing, indicates the biopsy sites and to be used for clinic pathologic correlation (Fig. 13.10). The first step is the diagnostic biopsy of the main tumor (excisional or incisional) based on the size and extent of the tumor. The most suspicious lesion is labeled as "diagnostic biopsy—main tumor," followed by the location (e.g., Sample #1 "main tumor" at 3:00). Additional samples ("map biopsy") are taken in a clockwise manner starting at 12:00, provided that was not the location of the main tumor, at intervals of 1.5 clock hours from the previous sample. The number of additional samples is chosen depending on the extension of the clinically affected area in each case. Each map biopsy sample is full thickness conjunctival epithelium about 3 × 1 mm in size. Double freeze-thaw cryotherapy is applied at the diagnostic site and all other clinically affected areas. These small areas can be left to heal without sutures [3]. All samples are placed on filter paper disc with great care to unroll the edges [6].

Map biopsy enhances overall assessment of the anatomic and pathologic extent, impacting subsequent management, particularly the use of adjuvant topical chemotherapy [6]. If severe atypia is documented histopathologically, topical mitomycin-C (MMC) is prescribed [6, 20].

13.7.1.3 Conjunctival Malignant Melanoma

Conjunctival melanomas are managed by wide excision and cryotherapy [12, 21]. Recurrent conjunctival melanoma is managed by repeat excision, cryotherapy, or irradiation. MMC use is limited to melanoma in situ. More extensive recurrences may require exenteration.

13.7.2 Squamous Tumors

13.7.2.1 Squamous Cell Papilloma

If removal is contemplated, combined modality treatment should be used since simple excision often leads to a more extensive recurrence than the original lesion. Cryotherapy, as described above, is the supplemental treatment of choice. Alternatively, a medical approach using interferon alpha 2b drops or injections may be utilized (currently unavailable).

13.7.2.2 Conjunctival Epithelial Neoplasia

Combined modality treatment (excision supplemented with cryotherapy) as described above is advocated given the high rate of recurrence of simple excision. Other variations to the above technique have been described and include application of cryotherapy to the scleral bed as well as the surrounding conjunctivae [11] and performing cryosurgery prior to and after excision [2]. A variant of Mohs' micrographic surgery has been described as an approach to treating CIN [22]. Topical MMC [23] or topical 5-fluorouracil can be used as an adjuvant treatment for patients with incompletely excised lesions (i.e., those with positive surgical margins) [24]. In patients with positive surgical margins, the use of postoperative interferon therapy reduced recurrences to a level similar to the one seen in patients with negative surgical margins (currently unavailable) [10]. Medical modalities can also be considered as a primary treatment, especially in patients with diffuse disease or in those with multiple recurrences after surgery [25].

13.7.3 Substantia Propria Tumors

13.7.3.1 Lymphoid Tumor

An incisional approach is typically reserved for suspected lymphoid tumors. Even so, overlying conjunctival can be spared while dissecting the episcleral lymphoid infiltrate (Fig. 13.11). Tissue must be kept fresh to allow for flow cytometric assessment to differentiate between hyperplasia and malignancy. External beam radiation is typically used to treat low-grade lymphoma. Excision with or without cryotherapeutic ablation of conjunctival lymphoma has limited use as it only debulks the diffuse tumor without complete elimination of malignant tissue. It may have application in a limited number of patients who are unable to receive other treatment modalities, accepting higher chances of recurrence [26].

13.7.3.2 Limbal Dermoid

Limbal dermoids can cause irregular astigmatism, irritation, or unacceptable cosmesis. Given the deep extent of these tumors, one surgical approach is a lamellar sclerectomy and keratectomy. The lesion can be excised manually

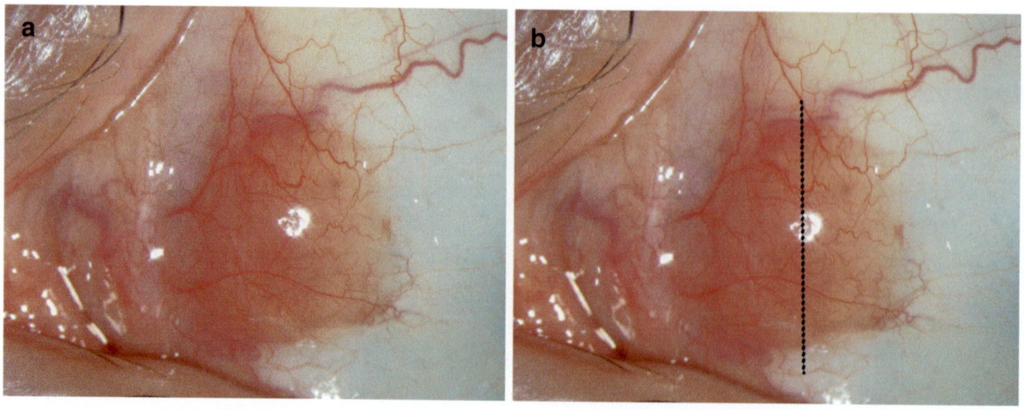

Fig. 13.11 Excision biopsy of lymphoid conjunctival lesion that is pink colored (6.0 × 5.5 mm), slightly mobile, firm, and extending into plica (**a**). About 2 mm from the anterior margin, incision was marked with a fine tip marking pen (**b**). Subconjunctival anesthesia (2% lidocaine with epinephrine) was injected in the subconjunctival space for ballooning the conjunctiva anteriorly. The lesion was excised by monopolar cautery needle within the episcleral plane sparing the medial rectus muscle insertion. Conjunctiva was then reapproximated with interrupted 8-0 Vicryl sutures

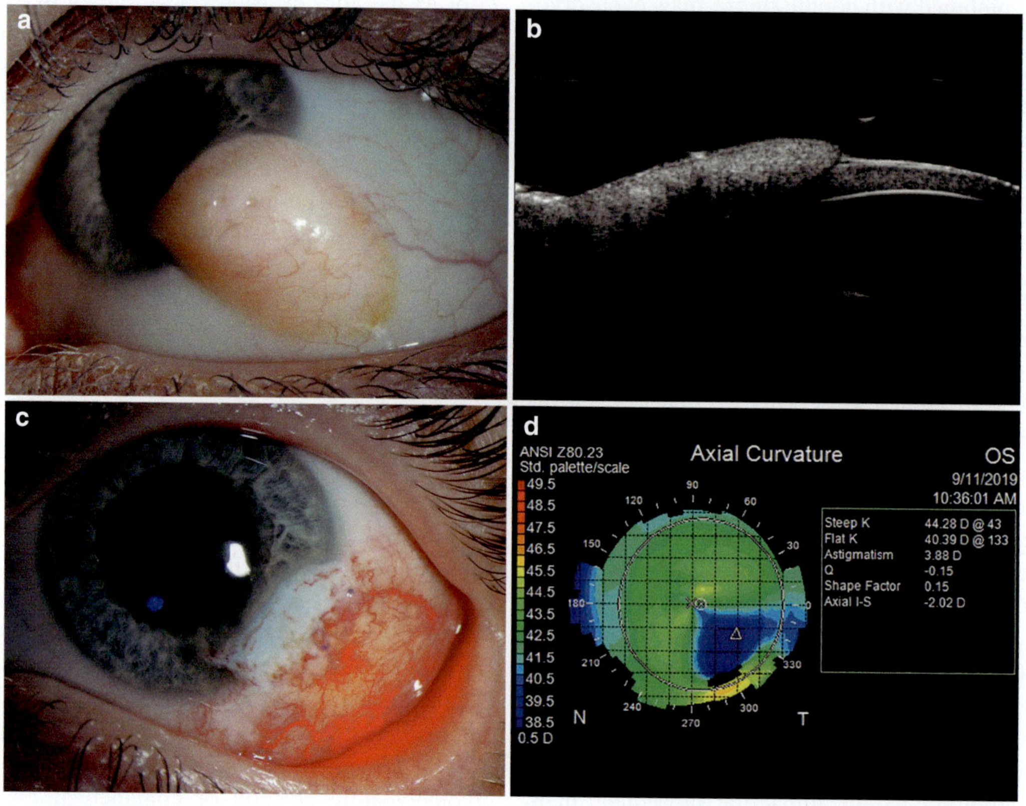

Fig. 13.12 Limbal dermoid (9.0 × 6.0 × 3.0 mm) with 3 mm corneal component at limbus from 3 to 5:30 o'clock (**a**). UBM showing corneoscleral extension (**b**). Using a monopolar cautery needle, the conjunctival incisions were made allowing for the lesion to be mobilized which was then incised down to the sclera. Using careful horizontal motions, the lesion was separated along the plane parallel with the sclera up to the limbus 180°. Next, using a crescent blade, the remaining 180 portion of the dermoid lesion was removed from the cornea without complications or perforation into the anterior chamber. Using 8-0 vicryl suture, the conjunctiva was reapproximated achieving primary closure of the 6 × 12 mm defect. A 14 mm bandage contact lens was then placed on the eye along with steroid antibiotic drops (**c**, postoperative #10 day). Visual acuity at 3 week was 20/25 (same as preop) despite moderate (3.88 D) astigmatism (**d**, corneal topography)

by lifting the conjunctival edge with forceps and locating a plane of normal sclera under the tumor with a blade (Fig. 13.12). Alternatively, a handheld trephine on bare sclera can be used to delineate the boundaries of the lesion. A slightly oversized trephine is then used to remove donor corneoscleral tissue after a lamellar dissection is performed of equal depth. The donor is sewn into the recipient bed with interrupted 10-0 nylon sutures [27]. Another surgical approach involves cutting the lesion flush with the surrounding tissue [28].

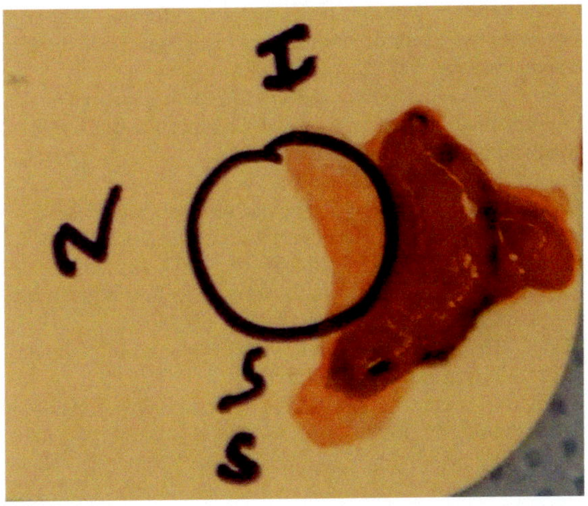

Fig. 13.13 Intraoperative photograph demonstrating the orientation of an ocular surface squamous neoplasia after excisional removal and prior to placement in formalin. (Courtesy of Dr. Carol L. Karp, Bascom Palmer Eye Institute, Miami, Florida)

13.8 Specimen Preparation

Prior discussion with a pathologist is important to identify the proper fixative agent; most commonly, 10% formalin is used. For suspected lymphoid tumors, tissue should be transported fresh in a small amount of saline for flow cytometric analysis. Specimens are prepared by laying the tissue flat, epithelial side up, on sterile paper wetted with a balanced salt solution. Orientation is drawn with a graphite pencil. The tissue can then be sent to pathology for final diagnosis and margin assessment (Fig. 13.13).

13.9 Postsurgical Management

Following surgery, the eye may be simply patched after installation of steroid antibiotic ointment. If the graft is used for closure, it is the author's preference to use a large bandage contact lens (Kontur Kontact Lens, Co. Hercules, CA) for up to 4 weeks to offer protection to the graft from blink-induced surface movement. Following surgery, topical antibiotics are used until reepithelialization is complete. Corticosteroid eye drops are typically used for approximately 1 month, on a tapering schedule. However, the frequency and duration are titrated based on the degree of inflammation in the surgical bed.

13.10 Complications

Although uncommon, complications can occur after surgical resection including infection, bleeding, delayed epithelial healing, pyogenic granuloma formation, Tenon's cyst formation, conjunctival and corneal scarring, restrictive strabismus, and limbal stem cell deficiency. Vigorous cryotherapy to the scleral bed can result in damage to the sclera, iris, and ciliary body. These complications can be minimized by adhering to good surgical techniques.

References

1. Atallah M, Joag M, Galor A, Amescua G, Nanji A, Wang J, et al. Role of high resolution optical coherence tomography in diagnosing ocular surface squamous neoplasia with coexisting ocular surface diseases. Ocul Surf. 2017;15(4):688–95.
2. Peksayar G, Altan-Yaycioglu R, Onal S. Excision and cryosurgery in the treatment of conjunctival malignant epithelial tumours. Eye (Lond). 2003;17(2):228–32.
3. Shields JA, Shields CL, De Potter P. Surgical management of conjunctival tumors. The 1994 Lynn B. McMahan lecture. Arch Ophthalmol. 1997;115(6):808–15.
4. Putterman AM. Conjunctival map biopsy to determine pagetoid spread. Am J Ophthalmol. 1986;102(1):87–90.
5. Kaliki S, Morawala A, Dharap RS, Mohamed A. Pagetoid tumour spread in periocular sebaceous gland carcinoma: a comparative analysis in 130 patients. Eye (Lond). 2021;35(10):2864–70.
6. Soto H, Bowen RC, Raval V, Yeaney G, Singh A. Primary acquired melanosis/melanoma: utility of conjunctival map biopsy. Br J Ophthalmol. 2022;106(5):605–9.
7. Bowen RC, Soto H, Raval V, Bellerive C, Yeaney G, Singh AD. Ocular surface squamous neoplasia: outcomes following primary excision with 2 mm margin and cryotherapy. Eye (Lond). 2021;35(11):3102–9.
8. Walsh-Conway N, Conway RM. Plaque brachytherapy for the management of ocular surface malignancies with corneoscleral invasion. Clin Experiment Ophthalmol. 2009;37(6):577–83.
9. Brouwer NJ, Marinkovic M, Peters FP, Hulshof M, Pieters BR, de Keizer RJW, et al. Management of conjunctival melanoma with local excision and adjuvant brachytherapy. Eye (Lond). 2021;35(2):490–8.
10. Galor A, Karp CL, Oellers P, Kao AA, Abdelaziz A, Feuer W, et al. Predictors of ocular surface squamous neoplasia recurrence after excisional surgery. Ophthalmology. 2012;119(10):1974–81.
11. Fraunfelder FT, Wingfield D. Management of intraepithelial conjunctival tumors and squamous cell carcinomas. Am J Ophthalmol. 1983;95(3):359–63.
12. Hungerford JL. Surgical treatment of ocular melanoma. Melanoma Res. 1993;3(5):305–12.
13. Sarici AM, Arvas S, Pazarli H. Combined excision, cryotherapy, and intraoperative mitomycin C (EXCRIM) for localized intraepithelial and squamous cell carcinoma of the conjunctiva. Graefes Arch Clin Exp Ophthalmol. 2013;251(9):2201–4.
14. Kobayashi A, Takahira M, Yamada A, Segawa Y, Tanahashi T, Shirao Y, et al. Fornix and conjunctiva reconstruction by amniotic membrane in a patient with conjunctival mucosa-associated lymphoid tissue lymphoma. Jpn J Ophthalmol. 2002;46(3):346–8.
15. Chen Z, Yan J, Yang H, Wu Z, Pang Y, Ai S, et al. Amniotic membrane transplantation for conjunctival tumor. Yan Ke Xue Bao. 2003;19(3):165–7, 45.
16. Chiu HI, Tsai CC. Self-retained, sutureless amniotic membrane transplantation for the management of ocular surface diseases. J Clin Med. 2023;12(19)
17. Kaliki S, Mohammad FA, Tahiliani P, Sangwan VS. Concomitant simple limbal epithelial transplantation after surgical excision of ocular surface squamous neoplasia. Am J Ophthalmol. 2017;174:68–75.

18. Lee JH, Kang NY. Comparison of fibrin glue and sutures for conjunctival wound closure in strabismus surgery. Korean J Ophthalmol. 2011 Jun;25(3):178–84.
19. Jakobiec FA, Rini FJ, Fraunfelder FT, Brownstein S. Cryotherapy for conjunctival primary acquired melanosis and malignant melanoma. Experience with 62 cases. Ophthalmology. 1988;95(8):1058–70.
20. Pe'er J, Frucht-Pery J. The treatment of primary acquired melanosis (PAM) with atypia by topical Mitomycin C. Am J Ophthalmol. 2005;139(2):229–34.
21. Jakobiec FA, Brownstein S, Albert W, Schwarz F, Anderson R. The role of cryotherapy in the management of conjunctival melanoma. Ophthalmology. 1982;89(5):502–15.
22. Buus DR, Tse DT, Folberg R, Buuns DR. Microscopically controlled excision of conjunctival squamous cell carcinoma. Am J Ophthalmol. 1994;117(1):97–102.
23. Frucht-Pery J, Rozenman Y, Pe'er J. Topical mitomycin-C for partially excised conjunctival squamous cell carcinoma. Ophthalmology. 2002;109(3):548–52.
24. Alvarez OP, Zein M, Galor A, Karp CL. Management of ocular surface squamous neoplasia: Bowman Club Lecture 2021. BMJ Open Ophthalmol. 2021;6(1):e000842.
25. Kozma K, Dömötör ZR, Csutak A, Szabó L, Hegyi P, Erőss B, et al. Topical pharmacotherapy for ocular surface squamous neoplasia: systematic review and meta-analysis. Sci Rep. 2022;12(1):14221.
26. Fernandez CA, Henry RK, Shields CL, Bilyk JR, Lally SE, Eagle RC, et al. Ocular adnexal lymphoma: a single-institution retrospective study. Saudi J Ophthalmol. 2021;35(3):230–8.
27. Mader TH, Stulting D. Technique for the removal of limbal dermoids. Cornea. 1998 Jan;17(1):66–7.
28. Burillon C, Durand L. Solid dermoids of the limbus and the cornea. Ophthalmologica. 1997;211(6):367–72.

Conjunctival Tumors: Radiation Therapy

14

David Buchberger, Sheen Cherian, and Arun D. Singh

14.1 Introduction

Ophthalmic radiation therapy in several forms has been used with success to treat conjunctival malignancies. As with other ocular tumors, the goal of radiation therapy is to eradicate tumor burden in a manner that maintains visual function and preserves surrounding sensitive ocular tissues. In the following chapter, the indications and outcomes of various modalities of radiation used to treat conjunctival tumors (SCC and melanoma) are discussed. Radiation therapy of ocular adnexal lymphoma is reviewed with orbital tumors (Fig. 14.1) (Chap. 9).

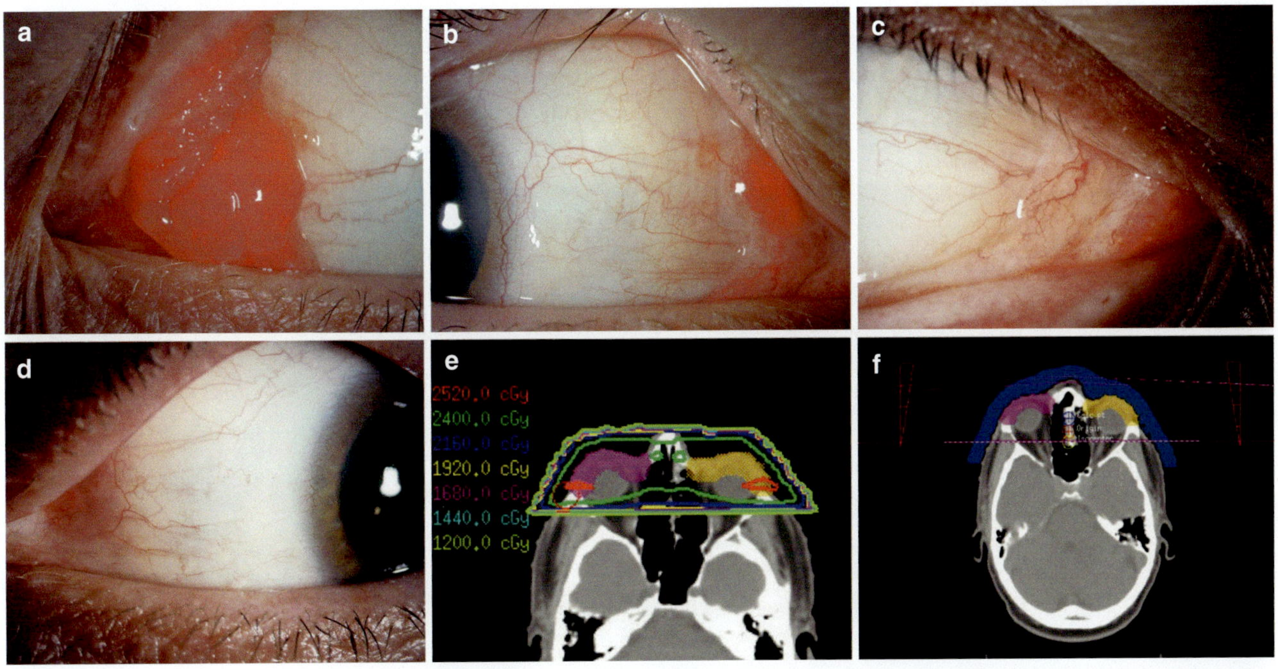

Fig. 14.1 Ocular adnexal lymphoma (EMZL) OU. Response to radiation therapy. Before (**a**, right eye; **b**, left eye) and 3 months (**c**, right eye; **d**, left eye) after 24 Gy (**e**) fractionated radiation therapy delivered using opposed lateral fields (**f**). Note the total regression of the infiltration. Three years later, the patient underwent cataract surgery for radiation-induced cataracts

D. Buchberger · S. Cherian
Department of Radiation Oncology, Cleveland Clinic, Cleveland, OH, USA

A. D. Singh (✉)
Department of Ophthalmic Oncology, Cole Eye Institute, Cleveland Clinic, Cleveland, OH, USA
e-mail: singha@ccf.org

© The Author(s), under exclusive license to Springer Nature Switzerland AG 2024
J. Pe'er et al. (eds.), *Clinical Ophthalmic Oncology*, https://doi.org/10.1007/978-3-031-72443-5_14

14.2 Squamous Cell Carcinoma (SCC)

SCC is the most common neoplasia of the ocular surface. It is a spectrum that ranges from noninvasive intra-epithelial squamous dysplasia to invasive SCC. Surgical excision is traditionally the most frequently employed primary treatment for invasive SCC of the conjunctiva [1, 2]. Adjuvant treatment with cryotherapy is commonly used in conjunction with surgery, and chemotherapy (5-fluorouracil; mitomycin-C) may be used for selected cases such as those with residual conjunctival disease [3].

14.2.1 Indications

Radiation therapy may be indicated in some circumstances, for example, when pathology demonstrates scleral invasion of conjunctival SCC following excision, or in cases of persistently recurrent disease. It may also be used in cases of advanced SCC with intraocular extension or orbital extension or when surgery is not a curative option [4, 5]. Radiation therapy is generally deferred until after the conjunctiva or primary surgical site has healed. Various radiation modalities and treatment regimens have been employed for conjunctival SCC.

14.2.2 Techniques and Results

14.2.2.1 EBRT

EBRT utilizing photons, electrons, and protons alone, or in combination has been used for both curative and palliative treatment for unresponsive and progressive SCC [6–8]. In one series of eight patients with conjunctival SCC who had failed multiple standard treatments and underwent EBRT (dosed in a range of 50–60 Gy in 2.0–2.5 Gy daily fractions), local tumor control and regression were noted in six patients (75%), and recurrences were noted in two. No metastatic spread or tumor-related deaths occurred after a median follow-up of 30.25 months [4]. Case reports in the literature detail successful treatment of conjunctival SCC with EBRT alone for inoperable patients or those with unresectable disease (Fig. 14.2) [9].

For lesions involving the palpebral conjunctiva and fornix, higher radiation doses may be required to achieve local control. For such patients, proton therapy is an option and can be given at a dose of 32 Gy in six fractions followed by a boost to the tumor bed of 14 Gy in 2 fractions [10]. Rarely, intraocular invasion from conjunctival SCC can occur. There are reports of such cases being successfully treated using proton beam therapy employing a total dose of 32 Gy, in 8 Gy divided fractions on 4 consecutive days [11]. A

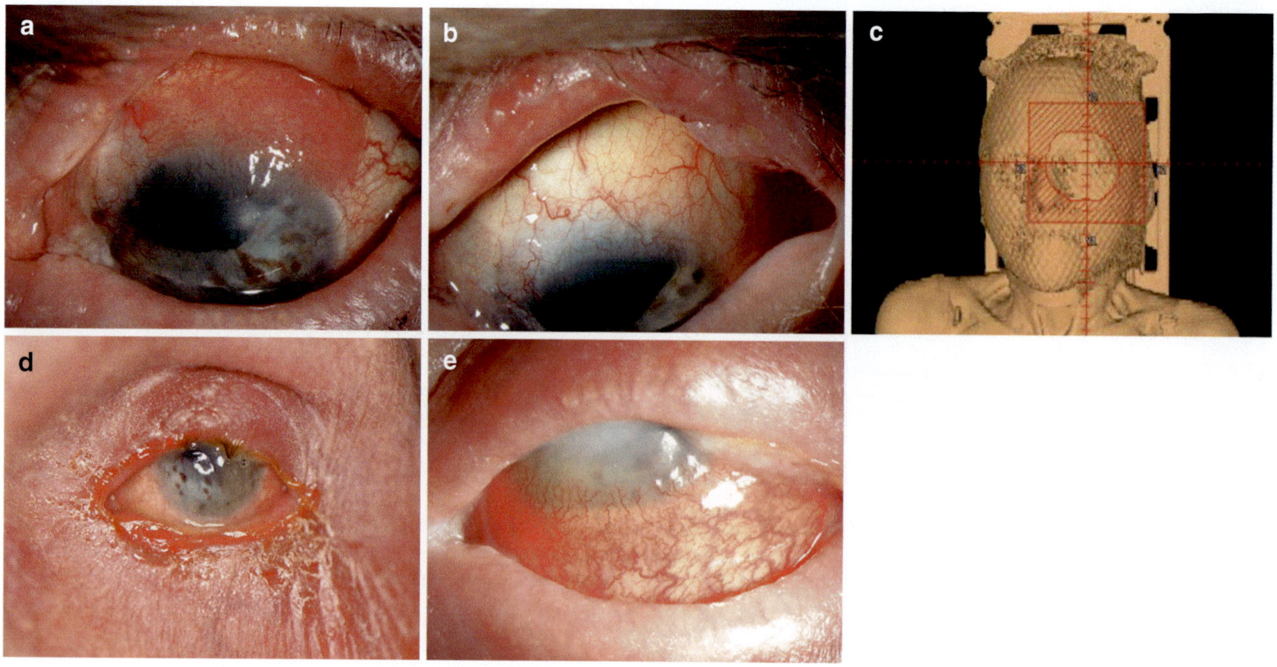

Fig. 14.2 A 94 y/o female presented with redness and crusting OS × 1 week. Examination revealed diffuse squamous cell carcinoma appearing as gelatinous thickening of the superior bulbar and tarsal conjunctiva with corneal extension (**a**). Invasive squamous cell carcinoma was confirmed by punch biopsy of the tarsal conjunctiva. A stepwise conservative plan was implemented. Following 4 cycles of topical 1% 5 fluorouracil (qid × 7 days, repeated every 4 weeks), the bulbar conjunctival involvement was resolved (**b**). Persistent superior tarsal conjunctival involvement was treated with 9 MeV electrons delivered with an En-face technique to a total dose of 40 Gy in 15 fractions (**c**). Following recovery from post-radiation dermatitis and keratitis (**d**), the patient developed a corneal ulcer that required intensive topical therapy. Eight weeks following treatment—there was total regression of residual squamous cell carcinoma (**e**)

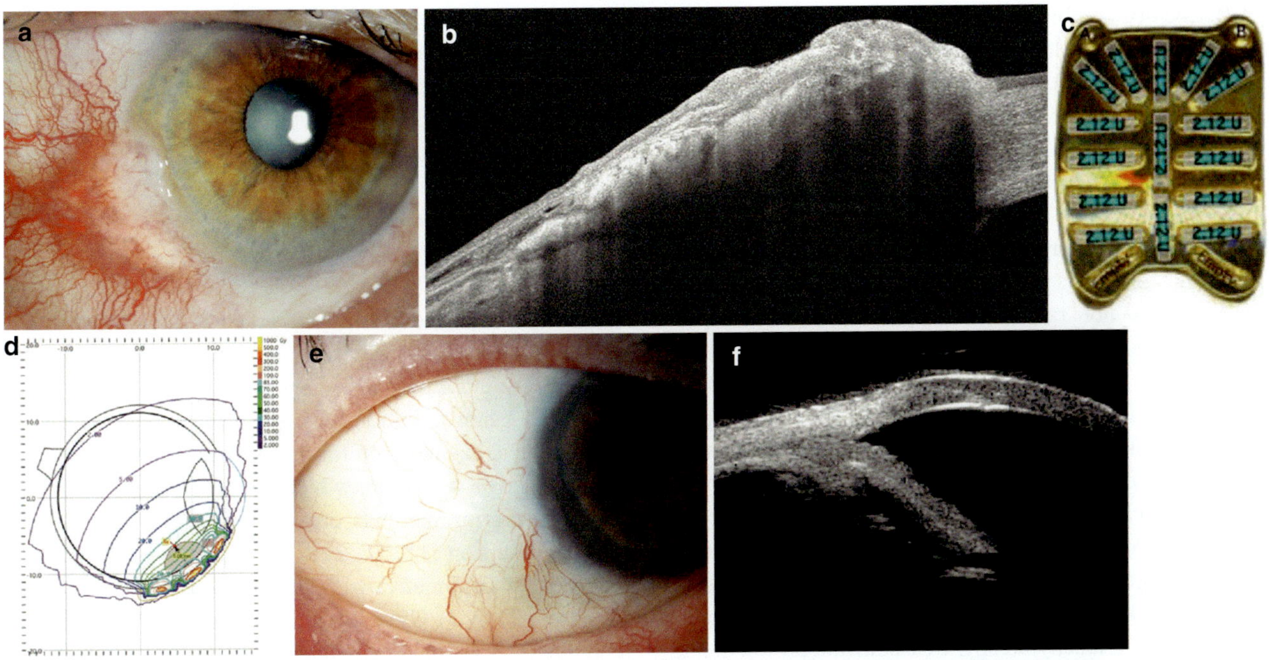

Fig. 14.3 A 65-year-old man with conjunctival invasive squamous cell carcinoma of the right eye (**a**). The tumor was 6 × 6 × 2.0 mm in size and extended at the limbus from 7:30 to 9:30 with corneal involvement of ~2.0 mm (**b**). Excision with 2 mm clear margins, alcohol corneal epitheliectomy, and cryotherapy to conjunctival margins were performed. Near the limbus, the tumor was adherent to the underlying sclera, and the invasive component was transected at the stromal base without an attempt at deep scleral dissection. Histopathology confirmed negative lateral margins and positive deep margins. He was treated with episcleral plaque brachytherapy (**c**) to the depth of 2 mm (**d**, 45 Gy in 72 h). At 4 years follow-up, visual acuity was 20/20 without superficial (**e**) or deep local recurrence (**f**)

recent study from France reviewing outcomes in micro-invasive (<2 mm invasion) and fully invasive SCC of the conjunctiva reported a 2-year local recurrence rate of 12% for invasive SCC treated with surgery and adjuvant proton therapy to a dose of 45 Gy in 8 fractions [12]. This compared favorably to the local recurrence rate of 20% observed in micro-invasive SCC where no patients received adjuvant proton beam therapy [12].

14.2.2.2 Brachytherapy

Brachytherapy, most commonly with strontium-90 (Sr-90), has been used at a dose of 20–180 Gy to the tumor surface [13]. Radiation administration with a handheld Sr-90 applicator delivering 60 Gy to the tumor surface in four fractions once a week or 50 Gy in five daily fractions has also resulted in excellent tumor control [10]. For tumors larger than an available handheld applicator, or those with scleral invasion, iodine-125 (I-125) radioactive plaque can be employed (Fig. 14.3) [10]. One recommended dose for I-125 plaque is 60 Gy at a depth of 2–3 mm [10]. Other investigators have used a treatment dose of 100 Gy to a depth of 1.5–2.5 mm to treat conjunctival SCC following excision for cases with evidence of scleral invasion [14]. After 23.4 months of follow-up, no patients experienced recurrence at the primary treatment site; however, one individual developed a new lesion distant from the initial site of therapy [14]. In treatment centers where ruthenium-106 (Ru-106) is available, the plaque can be applied immediately following excision to deliver a dose of 130 Gy at a depth of 2 mm or after the conjunctiva has healed using a dose of 100 Gy at a depth of 1–2 mm [10, 15]. Another treatment algorithm for Ru-106 is a dose of 320 Gy delivered to the tumor bed. Using this treatment scheme, local control has been achieved (follow-up of 22 months) without major complications from radiation. Recurrence rates following brachytherapy have ranged from 2% to 47%; therefore, brachytherapy alone is typically not recommended as primary therapy [2]. In a recent European series, no local recurrences were reported for 9 patients with SCC of the ocular surface treated with excision followed by Ru-106-based (130 Gy prescribed to a depth of 2 mm with one patient receiving much higher doses in the setting of ciliary body invasion) adjuvant brachytherapy where the range of follow-up was 8.2–52.8 months [16].

14.3 Conjunctival Melanoma

Primary treatment for conjunctival melanoma typically involves complete excision with surgical margins of 3–5 mm when possible [2]. Adjuvant treatments using cryotherapy to the surgical margins and/or tumor bed as well as absolute alcohol epitheliectomy for corneal and limbal involvement are frequently combined with surgery. Other topical therapies are also used in the adjuvant setting such as mitomycin C and interferon [17].

14.3.1 Indications

Radiation therapy may also be used as an adjuvant treatment following primary resection. In general, conjunctival melanoma is not radiosensitive, and therefore radiation should not be used as a sole therapy [18]. Radiation therapy may also be indicated for certain circumstances including deep scleral invasion detected by pathology following primary excision, recurrent disease unresponsive to other therapies, and palliation for extensive disease which is not surgically excisable or in patients who cannot tolerate surgery (Fig. 14.4). A multicenter international retrospective review analyzing outcomes of conjunctival melanoma in 288 patients was published in 2021. In this series, 19% of patients received adjuvant plaque brachytherapy, 14% adjuvant proton therapy, and 5% adjuvant photon-based EBRT [19]. Cumulative rates of local recurrence were 5% at 1 year, 19% at 5 years, and 37% at 10 years with T-stage being predictive of local recurrence likelihood. There was no association with the administration of adjuvant therapy and local recurrence rates [19].

14.3.2 Techniques and Results

14.3.2.1 EBRT

EBRT has been used as adjuvant radiation therapy (total dose of 60 Gy) in tumors with high-risk features such as increased thickness or close margins of resection [6, 17, 20].

Proton beam radiation has also been investigated as an alternative to exenteration for diffuse and multifocal patterns of conjunctival melanoma which are not treatable with standard eye-sparing methods or as adjuvant therapy following primary excision [17, 21, 22]. In one series of 20 patients, areas of the conjunctiva with suspected microscopic disease were treated by 31 Gy in 6 fractions. High-risk regions of the conjunctiva with clinically detectable tumor were treated by an additional boost using a smaller beam size and applying 2

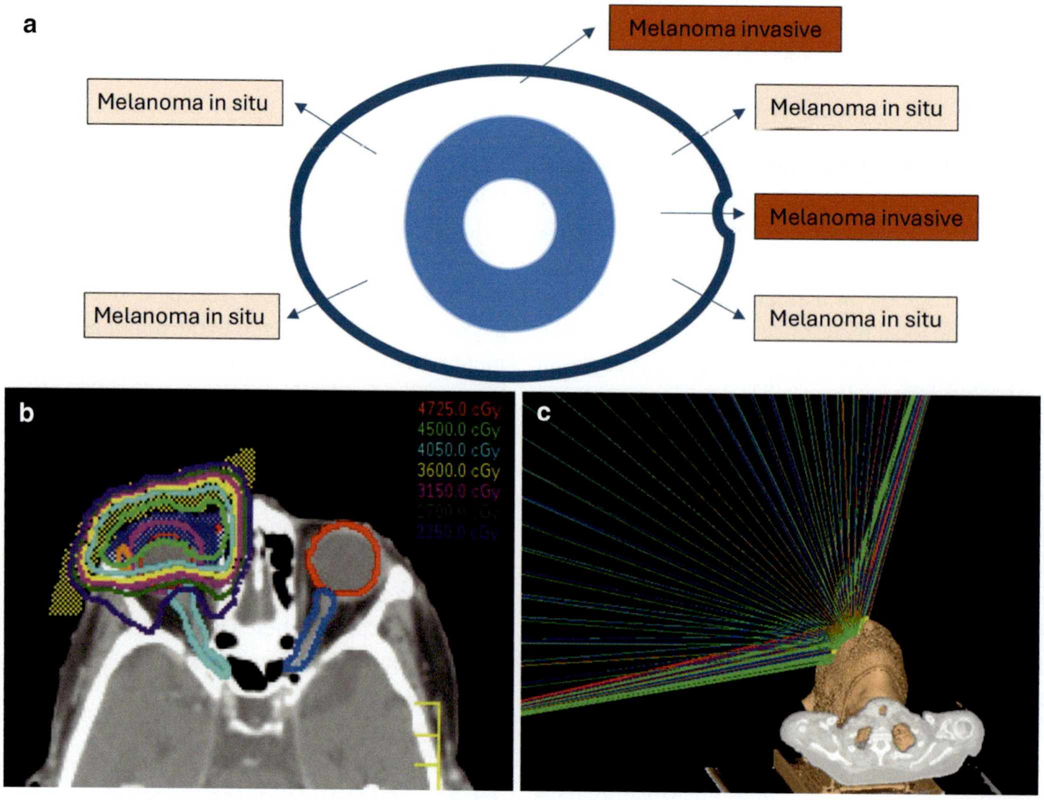

Fig. 14.4 A 96-year-old woman with diffuse invasive amelanotic melanoma extending from the right upper tarsal to bulbar conjunctiva that had been partially excised. Map biopsy revealed a spectrum of melanocytic proliferation ranging from in situ to invasive melanoma in the setting of primary acquired melanosis (**a**). Given the patient's advanced age and the presence of comorbidities, we elected to treat her with radiation therapy. Forty-five Gy in 25 fractions was delivered with a coplanar volumetric modulated arc therapy (VMAT, a form of image-guided and intensity-modulated radiation) utilizing 3 arcs and anterior bolus sparing the posterior structures of the orbit for the treatment of conjunctival melanoma (**b, c**). Follow-up over 2 years showed significant ocular surface changes that included inferior forniceal shortening and symblepharon, nasal conjunctival scarring with keratinization, and stenosis of inferior and superior puncta without local recurrence or pain. She eventually succumbed to brain metastasis

fractions up to 45 Gy. An individually shaped compensator was brought into the beam to modify the range of the protons so that the eye was irradiated at a depth of 2 mm. After a median follow-up of 34 months, recurrent disease occurred in 6 cases (30%); 2 of these were outside the irradiated volume, 3 were within the target volume treated by 31 Gy, and one was in the primary target volume treated by 45 Gy. Exenteration was eventually necessary in two patients (10%). Six patients (30%) developed metastatic disease, and four (20%) deaths occurred suggesting that proton beam therapy should be used with caution in advanced cases of conjunctival melanoma [21]. An additional single institutional experience in France reported a five-year local failure rate of 33% with the use of postoperative proton therapy (45 Gy in 8 fractions) following upfront surgery [22]. In another case, a series of conjunctival melanoma treated with EBRT following excision reported a complete response rate of 63%, with 22% of patients developing metastases in that timeframe [17, 23].

14.3.2.2 Brachytherapy

When brachytherapy is used as adjuvant treatment following excision (Fig. 14.5), one group has advocated for using either Sr-90 or yttrium-90 (Y-90) with a 10 Gy daily dose applied at the tumor surface until a total dose of 150–200 Gy is delivered, depending on the thickness of the neoplasm [18]. In one series of 19 patients treated with I-125 plaque (treatment

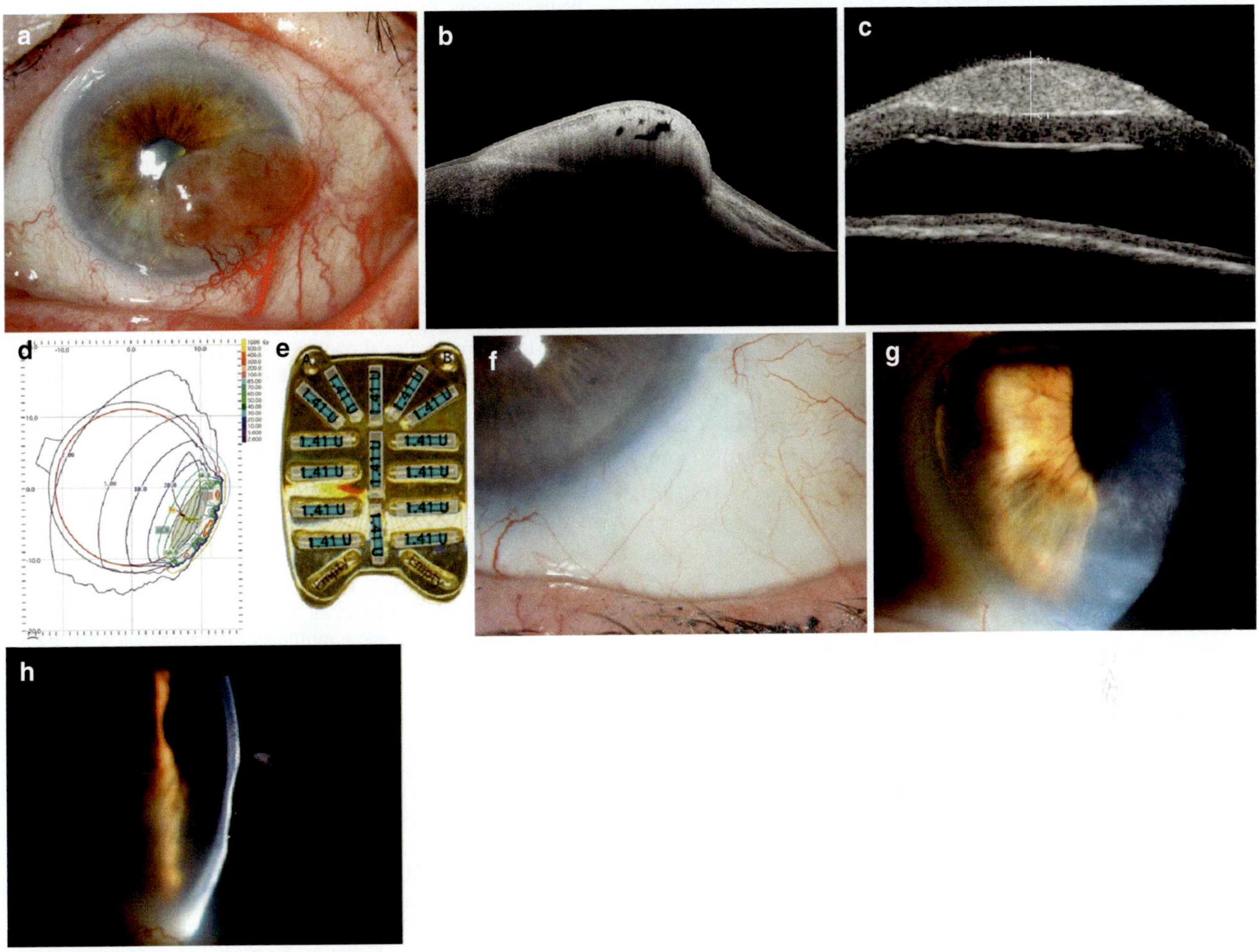

Fig. 14.5 An 81-year-old woman was referred for evaluation of a pyogenic granuloma of the left eye. Examination revealed primary acquired melanosis (PAM) with multifocal melanoma. The temporal bulbar melanoma was less conspicuous (5 × 3 × 1 mm) than the corneal melanoma (7.5 × 5.6 × 1.1 mm) with feeder vessels (**a**). Anterior segment OCT (**b**) and UBM did not suggest extension into corneal stroma (**c**). Both conjunctival and corneal melanoma were excised as a single tumor combined with alcohol corneal epitheliectomy, cryotherapy to the conjunctival margins, and map biopsies. The total excision was 12 × 7 mm in size that was repaired with Tenon closure and postoperative use of 16 mm Contour bandage soft lens (Kontur Kontact Lens, Co., Inc. Hercules, CA, USA). Intraoperatively, there was no involvement of the sclera or the underlying muscle. However, there was evidence of superficial corneal stromal involvement at 6 o'clock position for approximately 3 mm × 3 mm area requiring superficial lamellar keratectomy (approximately 10%). Histopathology confirmed invasive melanoma with negative corneal and conjunctival epithelial, but deep margin was positive. Map biopsies were negative for PAM elsewhere. Allowing for 4 weeks of healing, episcleral/corneal plaque brachytherapy was performed with plaque being centered over the area of corneal stromal involvement. Forty-five Gy was delivered over 72 h (**d**) using an I-125 source using EP 917 plaque (**e**, IsoAid, Port Richey, FL, USA). Patient remained free from local recurrence (**f**) and metastasis at 2.5-year follow-up visit with visual acuity of 20/40 (**f**) and only slight corneal stromal opacity (**g**) and corneal thinning (**h**)

dose of 100 Gy to a depth of 1.5–3.0 mm) following surgical resection, there were no recurrences at the initial treatment site or metastases after a median follow-up of 43.1 months; however, three individuals developed new lesions at a site distant from the primary location [24].

Another analysis of brachytherapy use in the adjuvant treatment of excised conjunctival melanoma showed a complete response rate of 80% with a mean follow-up of 64 months [17, 23]. Additional analyses have reported similar results. In a 58-patient series in which patients had adjuvant treatment with either Sr-90 or Ru-106, the 5-year local recurrence rate was 21% [25]. Common complications included pain, dry eye, symblepharon, ptosis, and cataract formation with excellent vision preservation outcomes [25].

For malignant melanoma affecting the palpebral conjunctiva and fornix, I-125 plaque application following tumor excision has been successfully employed using a dosing schedule of 100 Gy in 4 weekly fractions of 25 Gy [10]. An alternative approach is brachytherapy using I-125 seeds within the eyelid. A perilimbal stainless steel shield attached to the extraocular muscles can be used to protect the cornea and lens. Using this method and a dose of 55–60 Gy delivered over 5 days, one group showed excellent local control in 13 out of 14 patients [26].

14.4 Conclusions

It is important to note that most of the experience using radiation to treat conjunctival tumors is based upon results from small case series. It is therefore difficult to assess overall efficacy and optimal treatment protocols for incorporating radiation into the treatment planning of these tumors. The rare nature of these tumors, varying tumor classification schemes, and confounding prognostic clinical factors such as tumor size and location contribute to the difficulty in analyzing outcomes following radiation. Conjunctival tumors often need well-curated radiation treatment plans and precision radiation delivery techniques, as they are generally surrounded by numerous critical structures; hence, it is imperative they are treated at centers of excellence, by a skilled and experienced multidisciplinary team.

References

1. Cohen VML, O'Day RF. Management issues in conjunctival tumours: ocular surface squamous neoplasia. Ophthalmol Ther. 2020;9(1):181–90.
2. Pe'er J. Ocular surface squamous neoplasia. Ophthalmol Clin N Am. 2005;18(1):1–13. vii
3. Yeoh CHY, Lee JJR, Lim BXH, et al. The management of Ocular Surface Squamous Neoplasia (OSSN). Int J Mol Sci. 2022;24(1)
4. Graue GF, Tena LB, Finger PT. Electron beam radiation for conjunctival squamous carcinoma. Ophthalmic Plast Reconstr Surg. 2011;27(4):277–81.
5. Murthy R, Gupta H, Krishnatry R, Laskar S. Electron beam radiotherapy for the management of recurrent extensive ocular surface squamous neoplasia with orbital extension. Indian J Ophthalmol. 2015;63(8):672–4.
6. Hsu A, Frank SJ, Ballo MT, et al. Postoperative adjuvant external-beam radiation therapy for cancers of the eyelid and conjunctiva. Ophthalmic Plast Reconstr Surg. 2008;24(6):444–9.
7. Caujolle JP, Maschi C, Chauvel P, et al. [Surgery and additional protontherapy for treatment of invasive and recurrent squamous cell carcinomas: technique and preliminary results]. J Fr Ophtalmol. 2009;32(10):707–14.
8. Bowyer JD, Sullivan TJ, Whitehead KJ, et al. The management of perineural spread of squamous cell carcinoma to the ocular adnexae. Ophthalmic Plast Reconstr Surg. 2003;19(4):275–81.
9. Panda BB, Dasmajumdar SK, Sadangi D, Tripathy SR. Radiation therapy in conjunctival squamous cell carcinoma. BMJ Case Rep. 2023;16(7)
10. Stannard C, Sauerwein W, Maree G, Lecuona K. Radiotherapy for ocular tumours. Eye (Lond). 2013;27(2):119–27.
11. Ramonas KM, Conway RM, Daftari IK, et al. Successful treatment of intraocularly invasive conjunctival squamous cell carcinoma with proton beam therapy. Arch Ophthalmol. 2006;124(1):126–8.
12. Santoni A, Thariat J, Maschi C, et al. Management of invasive squamous cell carcinomas of the conjunctiva. Am J Ophthalmol. 2019;200:1–9.
13. Lommatzsch P. Beta-ray treatment of malignant epithelial tumors of the conjunctiva. Am J Ophthalmol. 1976;81(2):198–206.
14. Walsh-Conway N, Conway RM. Plaque brachytherapy for the management of ocular surface malignancies with corneoscleral invasion. Clin Experiment Ophthalmol. 2009;37(6):577–83.
15. Damato B, Coupland SE. An audit of conjunctival melanoma treatment in Liverpool. Eye (Lond). 2009;23(4):801–9.
16. Rahal A, Meller D, Manthey A, et al. Brachytherapy as a curative option for ocular surface squamous neoplasia. Int Ophthalmol. 2023;43(6):1861–5.
17. Grimes JM, Shah NV, Samie FH, et al. Conjunctival melanoma: current treatments and future options. Am J Clin Dermatol. 2020;21(3):371–81.
18. Lommatzsch PK, Lommatzsch RE, Kirsch I, Fuhrmann P. Therapeutic outcome of patients suffering from malignant melanomas of the conjunctiva. Br J Ophthalmol. 1990;74(10):615–9.
19. Jain P, Finger PT, Fili M, et al. Conjunctival melanoma treatment outcomes in 288 patients: a multicentre international data-sharing study. Br J Ophthalmol. 2021;105(10):1358–64.
20. Savar A, Esmaeli B, Ho H, et al. Conjunctival melanoma: local-regional control rates, and impact of high-risk histopathologic features. J Cutan Pathol. 2011;38(1):18–24.
21. Wuestemeyer H, Sauerwein W, Meller D, et al. Proton radiotherapy as an alternative to exenteration in the management of extended conjunctival melanoma. Graefes Arch Clin Exp Ophthalmol. 2006;244(4):438–46.
22. Thariat J, Salleron J, Maschi C, et al. Oncologic and visual outcomes after postoperative proton therapy of localized conjunctival melanomas. Radiat Oncol. 2019;14(1):239.
23. Wong JR, Nanji AA, Galor A, Karp CL. Management of conjunctival malignant melanoma: a review and update. Expert Rev Ophthalmol. 2014;9(3):185–204.
24. Karim R, Conway RM. Conservative resection and adjuvant plaque brachytherapy for early-stage conjunctival melanoma. Clin Experiment Ophthalmol. 2011;39(4):293–8.
25. Brouwer NJ, Marinkovic M, Peters FP, et al. Management of conjunctival melanoma with local excision and adjuvant brachytherapy. Eye (Lond). 2021;35(2):490–8.
26. Stannard CE, Sealy GR, Hering ER, et al. Malignant melanoma of the eyelid and palpebral conjunctiva treated with iodine-125 brachytherapy. Ophthalmology. 2000;107(5):951–8.

Conjunctival and Corneal Complications Following Treatment of an Intraocular Tumor

15

Bertil Damato and Maria Filì

15.1 Introduction

Conjunctival, corneal, and scleral morbidity after treatment for intraocular tumors can cause severe and prolonged discomfort to the patient, as well as cosmetic deficit, visual handicap, and loss of the eye. The type of iatrogenic disease that can develop varies greatly according to the causative therapeutic modality. An understanding of the pathophysiology of these conditions, knowledge of the risk factors, and awareness of the clinical features are essential for prevention, diagnosis, and treatment of these side effects and complications.

15.2 Pathophysiology

The ocular surface comprises the tear film and epithelium. The tear film consists of (a) a superficial layer composed of lipids produced by meibomian glands located in the eyelids, mostly superiorly; (b) an aqueous layer produced by the major lacrimal gland and the accessory lacrimal glands of Krause and Wolfring, which are present mostly in the superior fornix and superior margin of the superior tarsal plate, respectively; and (c) a deep layer of mucin, which is produced by goblet cells, which are most numerous near the inferior and medial fornices. The mucin is tethered to the epithelium by long mucoproteins produced by the superficial epithelial cells, which have microvilli on their outer surface. The epithelium is non-keratinized and consists of columnar and cuboidal squamous cells, which become flattened near the surface, and melanocytes, which are dendritic and located in the basal layer. The epithelial cells rest on Bowman's membrane in the cornea and on a basement membrane in the conjunctiva. In the bulbar conjunctiva, the epithelium overlies the substantia propria, which contains immune cells, arteries, veins, and lymphatics within fibrous tissue. Tenon's capsule is a fibrous tissue layer that is sandwiched between the conjunctiva and the sclera. The corneal epithelial cells are produced by limbal stem cells and migrate toward the central cornea.

15.3 Assessment

The history taking should include questions about photophobia, grittiness, pain, visual symptoms, limited activities, and aggravating factors, such as low humidity and wind. These form the basis of the ocular surface disease index (OSDI) [1].

Tests should be performed in order of increasing invasiveness [2]. The tear film breakup time is measured by touching the bulbar conjunctiva with a moistened fluorescein strip before asking the patient to blink a few times and then to gaze ahead without blinking until the first dry spot in the precorneal tear film is seen with the slit lamp. The extent of corneal and conjunctival staining and the tear film meniscus can be assessed at this time, aided by the fluorescein. Lissamine green and rose Bengal stains are irritating and stimulate reflex tear production so that they should be performed later in the exam, if at all.

Tear production is assessed by placing a Schirmer strip in the lower conjunctival sac without local anesthesia and asking the patient to keep the eyes closed for five minutes, after which the length of the moistened strip is measured. This is done bilaterally to compare the treated eye with the normal eye.

Woo et al. have reported normal tear film breakup time and Schirmer values to be 6.4 ± 2.6 s and 12.3 ± 5.2 mm, respectively [3].

The lid margin should be inspected for blocked meibomian gland orifices, lid margin irregularity, vascular engorge-

B. Damato (✉)
Ocular Oncology Service, St. Erik Eye Hospital, Solna, Sweden

Moorfields Eye Hospital, London, UK
e-mail: bertil.damato@nhs.net

M. Filì
Ocular Oncology Service, St. Erik Eye Hospital, Solna, Sweden

© The Author(s), under exclusive license to Springer Nature Switzerland AG 2024
J. Pe'er et al. (eds.), *Clinical Ophthalmic Oncology*, https://doi.org/10.1007/978-3-031-72443-5_15

ment, and mucocutaneous junction abnormality. By applying digital pressure to the eyelid, meibomian secretion (i.e., "meibum") can be assessed according to whether it is easily expressed and clear or whether it is viscous and cloudy. Studies using a non-contact, infrared system show irradiated meibomian glands to develop dilated and tortuous ducts with loss of acini, which occurs because of radiation damage to the acini and because of squamous metaplasia of these glands with obstruction of the ductules [4].

These procedures are performed in addition to complete ophthalmic examination, which would include visual acuity measurement, tonometry, scleral and anterior chamber examination, and ophthalmoscopy with mydriasis, in addition to any imaging that is indicated by the patient's condition.

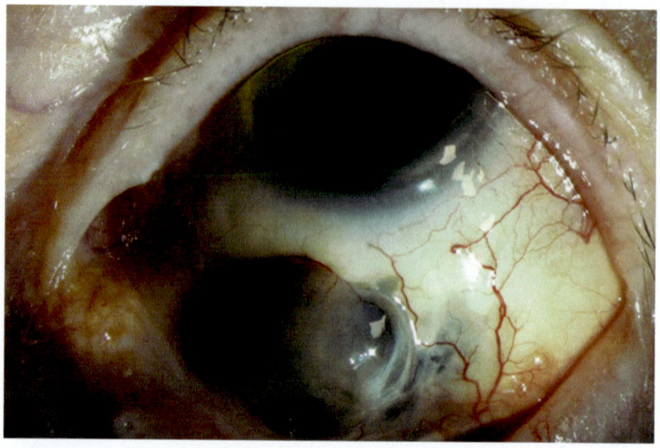

Fig. 15.1 Scleral necrosis and perforation because of conjunctival dehiscence after ruthenium plaque radiotherapy for a ciliochoroidal melanoma. (From: Damato, B. Clinical Atlas of Ocular Oncology. Springer. 2022, with permission)

15.4 Plaque Radiotherapy

In most centers, plaque brachytherapy is the first choice of treatment for uveal melanomas. This is administered with a saucer-shaped, metal applicator containing a radioactive isotope on its inner, concave surface. The isotopes used most widely are iodine-125 and ruthenium-106, which emit gamma and beta radiation, respectively. The plaque is sutured to the sclera overlying the tumor and removed after delivering a minimum dose of 80–100 Gy to the tumor apex. The sclera receives a much higher dose of radiation, especially with thick tumors and especially with ruthenium-106 applicators, because the beta radiation they emit decreases rapidly with distance from the plaque surface.

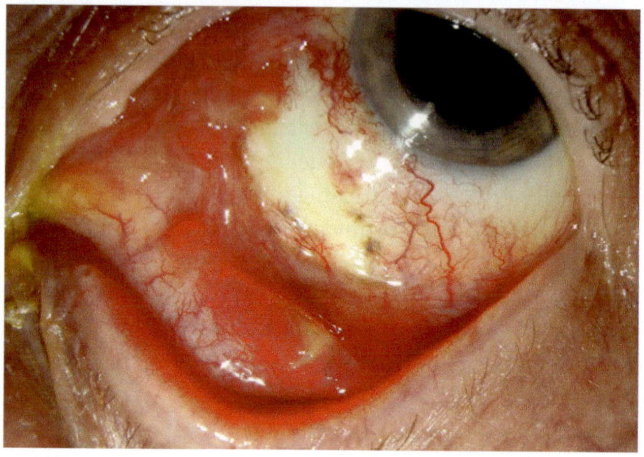

Fig. 15.2 Conjunctival dehiscence after plaque brachytherapy for uveal melanoma

The most serious and common extraocular complication of plaque brachytherapy is scleral necrosis. This may result in scleral transparency if mild, outward bulging of the uveal tissue beneath an intact sclera if moderate, and, in a small proportion of cases, perforation (Fig. 15.1) [5, 6]. This condition may be missed if it develops post-equatorially so that it is not visible subconjunctivally. Risk factors include greater tumor thickness, anterior tumor location, conjunctival wound dehiscence (Fig. 15.2), rectus disinsertion, extraocular tumor spread, and glaucoma.

It may be difficult to differentiate scleral necrosis from extraocular tumor invasion (Fig. 15.3). If the necrosis is adjacent to the irradiated tumor, transpupillary transillumination and ultrasonography would show thin uveal tissue, possibly bulging outward in the area where the sclera is weak or absent. Where tumor is present, the visible changes are more likely to indicate scleral necrosis if the tumor appears to be responding well to the treatment. Biopsy may establish the diagnosis if this is still uncertain despite clinical investigations.

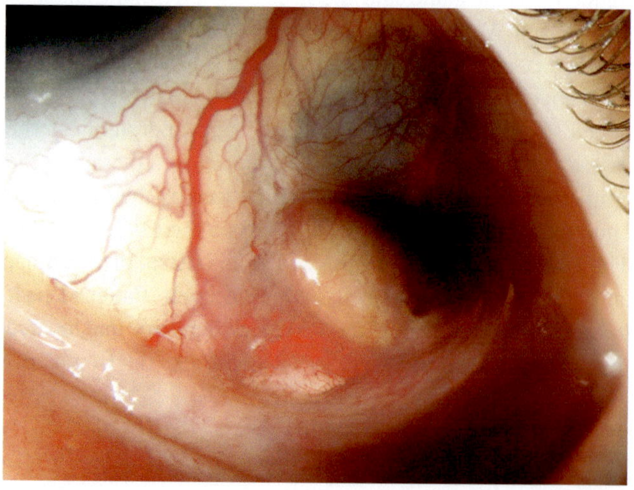

Fig. 15.3 Scleral necrosis and perforation with exposure to a necrotic irradiated choroidal melanoma

The management of scleral necrosis depends on the severity of this condition. No treatment is indicated unless scleral perforation has occurred or is considered imminent, in which case a scleral graft would be indicated. The first author has successfully used lamellar scleral autografts, taken from non-irradiated sclera in the same eye; however, others have used heterologous human sclera, porcine sclera, and other materials. The diameter of the graft should be greater than that of the plaque that caused the necrosis so that sutures can be placed in non-irradiated sclera. Enucleation may be required in some cases.

Plaque brachytherapy is also useful as a treatment for iris melanoma, either as primary or as salvage therapy after iridectomy. The main extraocular complications include dry eye, corneal abrasions and ulcerations, and episcleritis, which usually settle with ocular lubrication and steroid drops [7, 8].

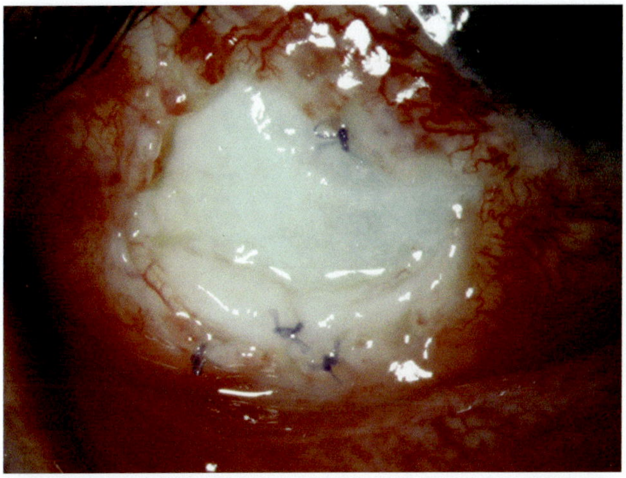

Fig. 15.4 Conjunctival dehiscence after proton beam radiotherapy of a macular choroidal melanoma

15.5 Proton Beam Radiotherapy

Proton beam radiotherapy is being used as a treatment for uveal melanoma in a growing number of centers, either as primary treatment or if plaque radiotherapy is unlikely to succeed, because of tumor size, extent, or location. This treatment involves measurement of tumor dimensions and distance from optic nerve, axial length measurement, and suturing of fiducial tantalum markers at known distances from tumor margins, from each other, and from the limbus. Treatment planning involves the creation of a three-dimensional computer model of the eye and tumor, using these measurements and radiographs showing the tantalum markers. A dose of 50–70 CGE (Cobalt Grey Equivalents) is delivered over 4 or 5 days using a face mask and dental mask to immobilize the patient's head in the correct position. The collimated beam of proton particles produces an ionizing radiation when they stop so that there is a high dose of radiation at the end of the beam (i.e., the "Bragg Peak"), with superficial tissues receiving a relatively low dose of radiation. However, the superficial radiation dose increases when the sharp Bragg peak is transformed into a wide plateau, as is usually required, especially with large tumors. In most patients, therefore, the conjunctiva, sclera, and other structures within the beam receive a high dose of radiation.

Depending on the tumor location and beam diameter, and hence the tissues that are irradiated, ocular side effects of proton beam treatment include: (a) loss of conjunctival healing capacity (Fig. 15.4); (b) conjunctival vascular telangiectasia or avascularity (Figs. 15.5 and 15.6); (c) keratoconjunctivitis sicca, caused by tear film instability (which may improve after several months) [9], dry eye caused by lacrimal gland atrophy; (d) leukoplakia; (e) canalicular occlusion with permanent epiphora (Fig. 15.7); (f) limbal stem-cell failure with keratopathy, especially after total anterior segment irradiation; (g) neurotrophic corneal ulceration [10], possibly with perforation (Fig. 15.8); (h) band keratopathy; (i) superior palpebral conjunctival keratinization, with corneal abrasion and discomfort on blinking, if the mucocutaneous junction of the upper eyelid margin is irradiated [11]; and (j) scleral necrosis and perforation (Fig. 15.9).

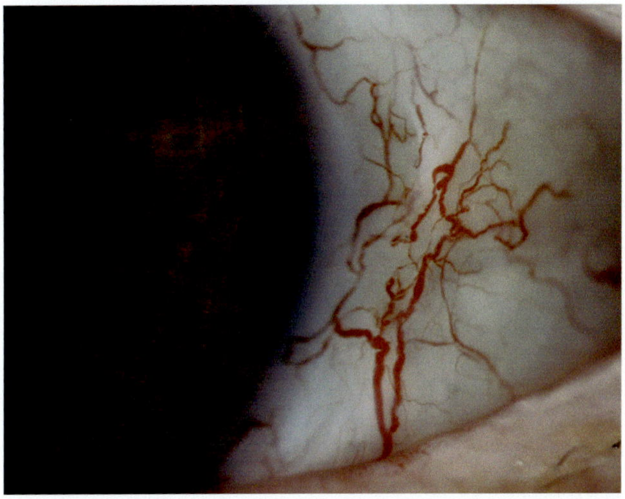

Fig. 15.5 Conjunctival telangiectasia after proton beam radiotherapy for an iridociliary melanoma

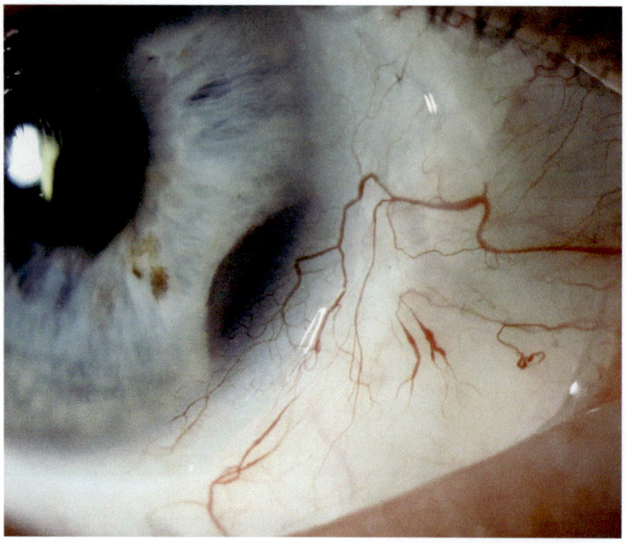

Fig. 15.6 Conjunctival avascularity after proton beam radiotherapy of an iridociliary melanoma

Keratoconjunctivitis sicca is managed with lubricants, punctal plugs, a bandage contact lens, and/or anti-inflammatory drops. Severe limbal stem cell failure may require an amniotic membrane graft or limbal stem cell transplant from the fellow eye; this problem may also be prevented by harvesting limbal stem cells before the radiotherapy and, after storage in culture medium, replacing them after completion of the radiotherapy [12]. Keratinization of the superior palpebral conjunctiva can be avoided by trans-palpebral proton beam radiotherapy (i.e., through the closed eyelid) to avoid irradiating the eyelid margin [11]. Canalicular occlusion may require insertion of a Lester-Jones tube. Scleral necrosis may require grafting, as with plaque brachytherapy.

Dry eye has also been reported after proton beam radiotherapy for diffuse choroidal hemangioma in children, with a total dose of 20 Gy delivered in 10 fractions [13].

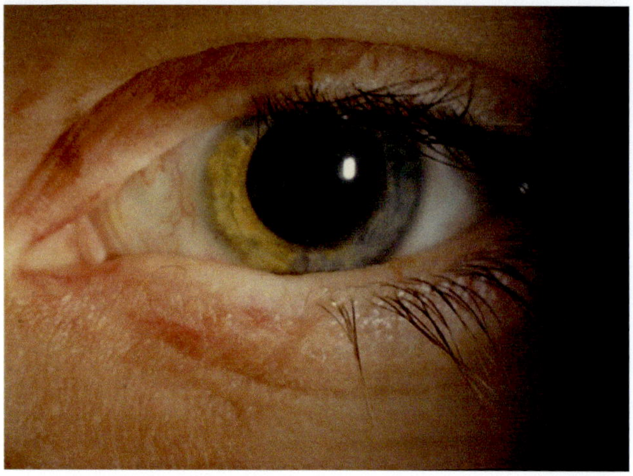

Fig. 15.7 Canalicular occlusion after proton beam radiotherapy for a medial choroidal melanoma

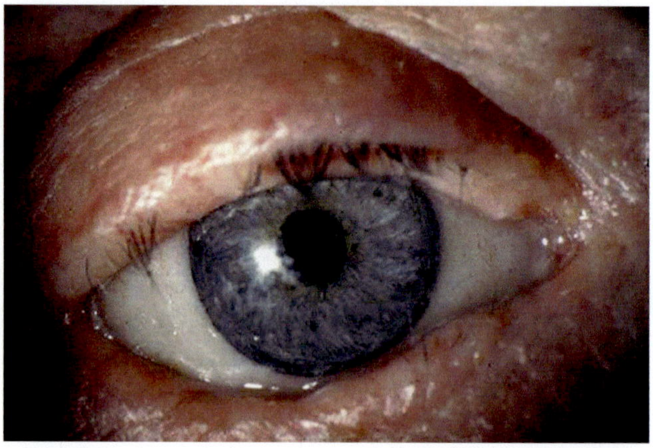

Fig. 15.8 Ocular prosthesis after enucleation for neurotrophic corneal ulceration and perforation following proton beam radiotherapy

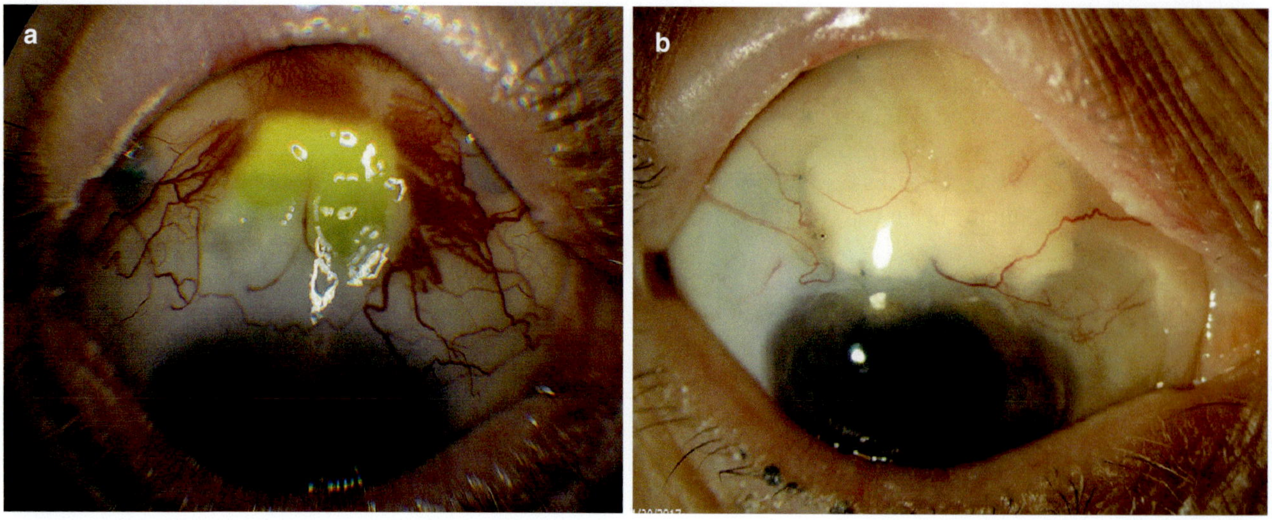

Fig. 15.9 (**a**) Scleral necrosis and perforation after proton beam radiotherapy for a superior choroidal melanoma. (**b**) Appearance after treatment with an autologous lamellar scleral graft

15.6 Stereotactic Radiotherapy

Schmelter et al. reported immediate or delayed keratopathy after robotic CyberKnife radiosurgery for iris melanoma with a good response to lubricating drops [14]. Akbaba et al. reported only mild conjunctivitis in 29% of 24 patients with uveal melanoma treated with linear accelerator-based stereotactic fractionated photon radiotherapy [15].

15.7 External Beam Radiotherapy

Intraocular indications for external beam radiotherapy include uveal metastasis, uveal lymphoma, vitreoretinal lymphoma, and, if photodynamic therapy and proton beam radiotherapy are not possible, choroidal hemangioma. Radiation doses tend to be 30–40 Gy for metastases [16], 28–36 Gy for uveal lymphoma [17], 30–36 Gy for vitreoretinal lymphoma [18], and 20 Gy for choroidal hemangioma [19].

External beam radiotherapy can cause an acute conjunctival reaction (Fig. 15.10). In the long term, all patients who receive radiation doses exceeding 50 Gy develop disordered ocular lubrication, with corneal ulceration in some patients. Such morbidity can also occur with lower radiation doses. Shelukar et al. report dry eye even after administering 4 Gy in two 2-Gy fractions for uveal lymphoma [20].

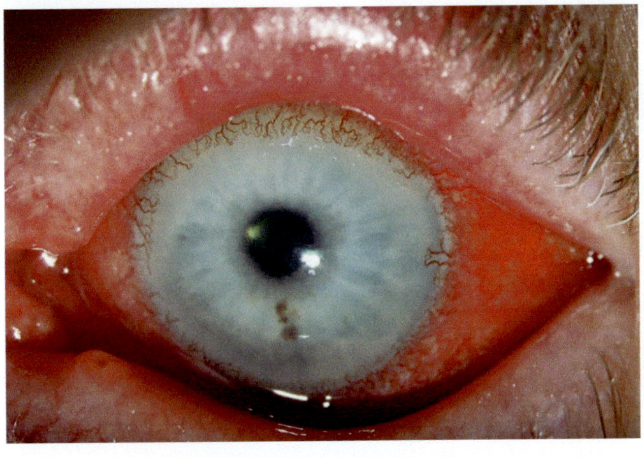

Fig. 15.10 Acute conjunctival reaction after external beam radiotherapy for conjunctival lymphoma

15.8 Chemotherapy

In many centers, vitreoretinal lymphoma is treated with intravitreal methotrexate injections (400 μg/0.05 ml), administered twice a week for 1 month, once a week for the next 2 months, and then once a month for 9 months [21]. Habot-Wilner et al. report that all patients with this regimen develop mild-to-severe superficial punctate keratitis, which resolves after the second month, when the frequency of injections is reduced to monthly [21]. This keratopathy, which can also include filaments, central epithelial defects, and epithelial sheet-like opacity, causes ocular pain, photophobia, tearing, and visual loss. To alleviate this problem, various measures have been proposed, which include applying a cotton bud to the injection site to prevent reflux of the methotrexate; irrigating the eye with saline to wash away any drug that may have spilled onto the cornea; applying a bandage contact lens; prescribing agents such as lubricants, topical antibiotic drops, topical steroids, autologous serum drops, pre-bedtime vitamin A gel, and oral folic acid; and reducing the frequency of methotrexate injections [21–23].

Treatment of advanced retinoblastoma with sub-Tenon's fascia carboplatin injections has largely been abandoned because of irreversible side effects, which include orbital muscle fibrosis, orbital fat atrophy, and conjunctival scarring with shortening of the fornices, which complicated ocular indentation and, therefore, ocular examination and focal treatment of peripheral tumors [24, 25].

15.9 Surgery

With any surgical procedure, disruption of tear flow by limbal conjunctival swelling can cause corneal dellen (Fig. 15.11) [26]. This problem can be prevented and, if necessary, treated by prescribing antibiotics and/or steroids as ointment instead of drops in the immediate postoperative period until the conjunctival swelling resolves.

With proton beam radiotherapy, fiducial tantalum markers can erode the overlying conjunctiva placed anteriorly and within the irradiated field, with scleral exposure resulting in necrosis and possibly perforation (Fig. 15.12). Such conjunctival ulceration can be avoided by placing the markers away from the radiation field and by removing them if they

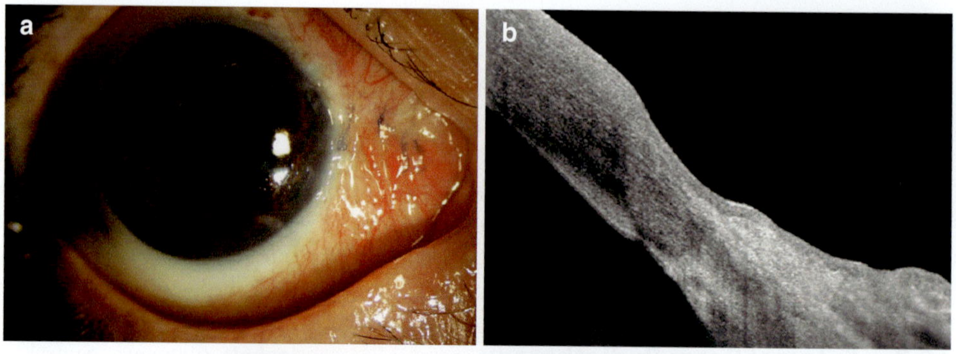

Fig. 15.11 Corneal dellen after medial ocular surgery. (**a**) Color photograph and (**b**) optical coherence tomography scan

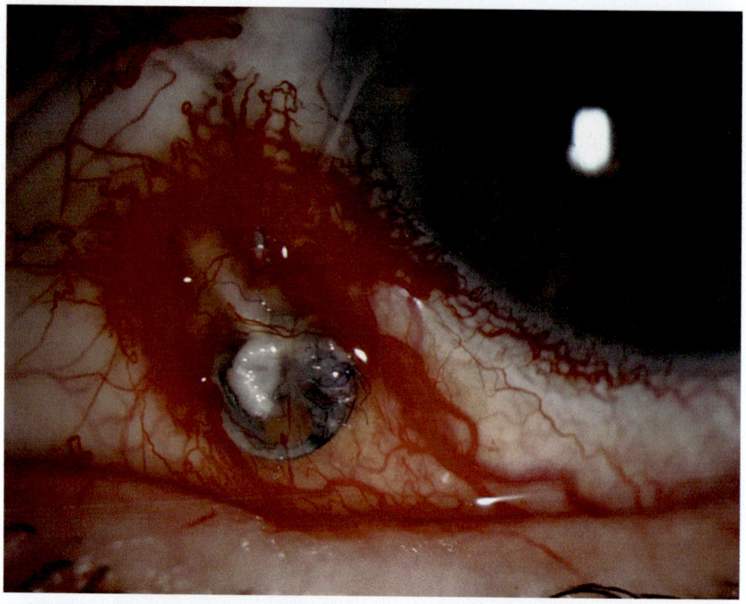

Fig. 15.12 Exposure of tantalum marker after proton beam radiotherapy for choroidal melanoma

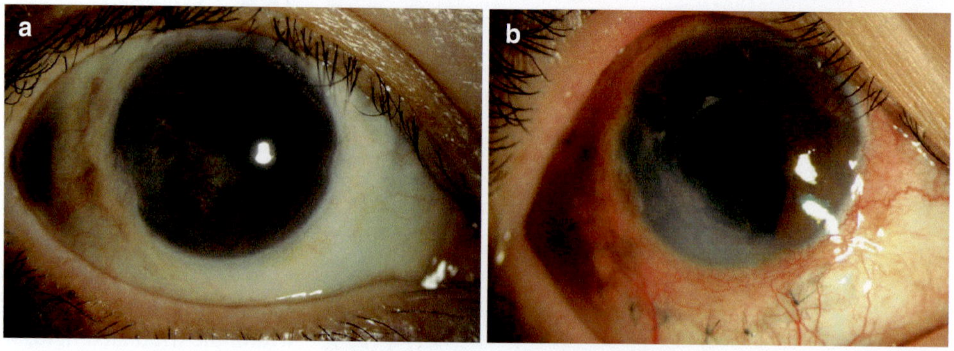

Fig. 15.13 Corneal opacification after excision of a large iris cyst (**a**) preoperative appearance, (**b**) postoperative appearance. Removal of the cyst required lamellar internal keratectomy where the cyst was adherent to the cornea. (From: Damato, B. Clinical Atlas of Ocular Oncology. Springer. 2022, with permission)

threaten to cause problems; once conjunctival ulceration occurs, the offending marker must be removed urgently.

Corneal endothelial damage during excision of a large iris tumor can be followed by corneal edema and opacification (Fig. 15.13).

After enucleation, the orbital implant can ulcerate the overlying conjunctiva, especially after chemotherapy in patients with retinoblastoma (Fig. 15.14). Measures to prevent this include placement of the orbital implant posteriorly in the orbit, meticulous closure of Tenon's capsule without tension, and suturing the rectus muscles together anterior to the implant [27]. Some authors consider porous implants to have a higher extrusion rate than nonporous implants [28]. Many techniques have been described for treating this complication, which are beyond the scope of this chapter.

Pyogenic granuloma can occur after enucleation and other procedures and must be differentiated from recurrent tumor [29].

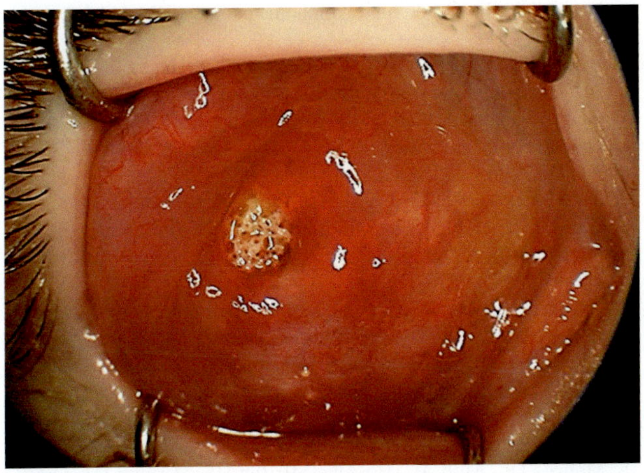

Fig. 15.14 Extruding hydroxyapatite orbital implant after enucleation for retinoblastoma

15.10 Systemic Therapy

Many systemic anticancer drugs can cause ocular surface disorders, which may be seen in patients with intraocular tumors such as metastasis, melanoma, and lymphoma.

15.10.1 Immune Checkpoint Inhibitors

T-lymphocytes attack foreign antigens without causing autoimmune disease because they are regulated by cytotoxic T-lymphocyte antigen-4 (CTLA-4) and programmed death protein 1 (PD-1). Such suppression, however, also prevents the T-cells from attacking cancer cells. Immune checkpoint inhibitors are monoclonal antibodies that bind to CTLA-4 and PD-1 on the T-lymphocytes, activating these immune cells so that they attack cancer cells. Some immune checkpoint inhibitors activate T-lymphocytes differently, by binding to programmed death ligand-1 (PD-L1), which is expressed by cancer cells and which interacts with PD-1 on T-lymphocytes to suppress these cells. However, as well as attacking cancer cells, the activated T-lymphocytes also attack normal cells to cause autoimmune disease, which affects many parts of the body, including the cornea and conjunctiva. Side effects of immune checkpoint inhibitors therefore include dry eye, conjunctivitis, conjunctival ulceration, keratitis, corneal ulceration, and corneal perforation [30–33]. Patients with intraocular tumors such as metastases and uveal melanoma may develop these side effects if they are receiving immune checkpoint inhibitors. These conditions are managed with ocular lubricants, topical steroids, bandage contact lenses, and corneal gluing for perforations, if possible, without stopping the anticancer therapy.

15.10.2 Other Agents

There are many other anticancer drugs that cause a wide variety of side effects affecting the ocular surface, and these have recently been reviewed by Vitiello et al. [34]. For example, epidermal growth factor receptor inhibitors, such as cetuximab, erlotinib, afatinib, and gefitinib, can cause conjunctivitis, dry eye, corneal erosions, superficial punctate keratopathy, corneal ulceration, and perforation [34]. Osimertinib can cause vortex keratopathy by suppressing corneal epithelial cell migration [35]. Trastuzumab, a human epidermal growth factor 2 inhibitor, can cause corneal infiltrates and ulceration [36]. Tamoxifen can cause asymptomatic subepithelial corneal deposits [37]. Ibrutinib, a Bruton's tyrosine kinase inhibitor, may cause dry eye, redness, and subconjunctival hemorrhage in patients receiving this drug for central nervous system and vitreoretinal lymphoma [38]. Crizotinib, a kinase inhibitor, recently reported to induce regression of uveal melanoma, can cause persistent chemosis [39, 40]. Apart from these novel agents, ocular surface side effects can occur in patients receiving chemotherapy with agents such as carboplatin, chlorambucil, methotrexate, vincristine, cyclophosphamide, and many others.

15.11 Conclusion

Anyone treating intraocular tumors must be aware of any side effects and complications that can occur so that such morbidity can be prevented, diagnosed, and treated successfully.

References

1. Schiffman RM, Christianson MD, Jacobsen G, Hirsch JD, Reis BL. Reliability and validity of the Ocular Surface Disease Index. Arch Ophthalmol. 2000;118(5):615–21.
2. Bron AJ, Evans VE, Smith JA. Grading of corneal and conjunctival staining in the context of other dry eye tests. Cornea. 2003;22(7):640–50.
3. Woo YJ, Ko J, Ji YW, Kim TI, Yoon JS. Meibomian gland dysfunction associated with periocular radiotherapy. Cornea. 2017;36(12):1486–91.
4. Kim SE, Yang HJ, Yang SW. Effects of radiation therapy on the meibomian glands and dry eye in patients with ocular adnexal mucosa-associated lymphoid tissue lymphoma. BMC Ophthalmol. 2020;20(1):24.
5. Jabbarli L, Guberina M, Biewald E, Flühs D, Guberina N, Le Guin CHD, et al. Scleral necrosis after brachytherapy for uveal melanoma: analysis of risk factors. Clin Experiment Ophthalmol. 2021;49(4):357–67.
6. Kaliki S, Shields CL, Rojanaporn D, Badal J, Devisetty L, Emrich J, et al. Scleral necrosis after plaque radiotherapy of uveal melanoma: a case-control study. Ophthalmology. 2013;120:1004.

7. Tsimpida M, Hungerford J, Arora A, Cohen V. Plaque radiotherapy treatment with ruthenium-106 for iris malignant melanoma. Eye (Lond). 2011;25(12):1607–11.
8. Shields CL, Naseripour M, Shields JA, Freire J, Cater J. Custom-designed plaque radiotherapy for nonresectable iris melanoma in 38 patients: tumor control and ocular complications. Am J Ophthalmol. 2003;135(5):648–56.
9. Eibenberger K, Heimann H, Gatchalian L, Kacperek A, Hussain R. Side effects of proton beam radiotherapy treatment on iris melanoma. Ophthalmology. 2023;130(9):958–65.
10. Versura P, Giannaccare G, Pellegrini M, Sebastiani S, Campos EC. Neurotrophic keratitis: current challenges and future prospects. Eye Brain. 2018;10:37–45.
11. Konstantinidis L, Roberts D, Errington RD, Kacperek A, Heimann H, Damato B. Transpalpebral proton beam radiotherapy of choroidal melanoma. Br J Ophthalmol. 2015;99(2):232–5.
12. Singh AD, Dupps WJ Jr, Biscotti CV, Suh JH, Lathrop KL, Nairn JP, et al. Limbal stem cell preservation during proton beam irradiation for diffuse iris melanoma. Cornea. 2017;36(1):119–22.
13. Franco JJ, Liu KX, Ioakeim-Ioannidou M, Davila JR, Chen YL, Kim IK, et al. Low-dose proton radiotherapy for pediatric choroidal hemangioma: a case series. Pediatr Blood Cancer. 2022;69(12):e29925.
14. Schmelter V, Heidorn S, Muacevic A, Priglinger SG, Foerster P, Liegl R. Robotic assisted CyberKnife radiosurgery for the treatment of iris melanoma. Sci Rep. 2021;11(1):5685.
15. Akbaba S, Foerster R, Nicolay NH, Arians N, Bostel T, Debus J, et al. Linear accelerator-based stereotactic fractionated photon radiotherapy as an eye-conserving treatment for uveal melanoma. Radiat Oncol. 2018;13(1):140.
16. Rudoler SB, Corn BW, Shields CL, De Potter P, Hyslop T, Shields JA, et al. External beam irradiation for choroid metastases: identification of factors predisposing to long-term sequelae. Int J Radiat Oncol Biol Phys. 1997;38(2):251–6.
17. Aronow ME, Portell CA, Sweetenham JW, Singh AD. Uveal lymphoma: clinical features, diagnostic studies, treatment selection, and outcomes. Ophthalmology. 2014;121(1):334–41.
18. Kaburaki T, Taoka K. Diagnosis and management of vitreoretinal lymphoma: present and future treatment perspectives. Jpn J Ophthalmol. 2023;67(4):363–81.
19. Schilling H, Sauerwein W, Lommatzsch A, Friedrichs W, Brylak S, Bornfeld N, et al. Long-term results after low dose ocular irradiation for choroidal haemangiomas. Br J Ophthalmol. 1997;81(4):267–73.
20. Shelukar S, Fernandez C, Bas Z, Komarnicky L, Lally SE, Shields CL, et al. High local control and low ocular toxicity using ultra-low-dose “boom-boom” radiotherapy for indolent orbital lymphoma. Chin Clin Oncol. 2022;11(6):44.
21. Habot-Wilner Z, Frenkel S, Pe'er J. Efficacy and safety of intravitreal methotrexate for vitreo-retinal lymphoma—20 years of experience. Br J Haematol. 2021;194(1):92–100.
22. Jeong Y, Ryu JS, Park UC, Oh JY. Corneal epithelial toxicity after intravitreal methotrexate injection for vitreoretinal lymphoma: clinical and in vitro studies. J Clin Med. 2020;9(8)
23. Zhou X, Zhou X, Shi H, Lai J, Wang Q, Li Y, et al. Reduced frequency of intravitreal methotrexate injection lowers the risk of keratopathy in vitreoretinal lymphoma patients. BMC Ophthalmol. 2020;20(1):189.
24. Jubran RF, Villablanca JG, Krailo M, Piao J, Huang L, Murphree AL, et al. A single-arm study of systemic and sub-Tenon chemotherapy for groups C and D intraocular retinoblastoma: a Children's Oncology Group study (ARET 0231). Pediatr Blood Cancer. 2020;67(9):e28502.
25. Mulvihill A, Budning A, Jay V, Vandenhoven C, Heon E, Gallie BL, et al. Ocular motility changes after subtenon carboplatin chemotherapy for retinoblastoma. Arch Ophthalmol. 2003;121(8):1120–4.
26. Tessler HH, Urist MJ. Corneal dellen in the limbal approach to rectus muscle surgery. Br J Ophthalmol. 1975;59(7):377–9.
27. Lang P, Kim JW, McGovern K, Reid MW, Subramanian K, Murphree AL, et al. Porous orbital implant after enucleation in retinoblastoma patients: indications and complications. Orbit. 2018;37(6):438–43.
28. Mourits DL, Moll AC, Bosscha MI, Tan HS, Hartong DT. Orbital implants in retinoblastoma patients: 23 years of experience and a review of the literature. Acta Ophthalmol. 2016;94(2):165–74.
29. Iordanidou V, De Potter P. Porous polyethylene orbital implant in the pediatric population. Am J Ophthalmol. 2004;138(3):425–9.
30. Dalvin LA, Shields CL, Orloff M, Sato T, Shields JA. Checkpoint inhibitor immune therapy: systemic indications and ophthalmic side effects. Retina. 2018;38(6):1063–78.
31. Parker JS, Feagin W, Wang C, Heersink M, Parker JS. Corneal ulceration associated with Nivolumab use. Am J Ophthalmol Case Rep. 2019;14:26–7.
32. Aschauer J, Donner R, Lammer J, Schmidinger G. Bilateral corneal perforation in Ipilimumab/Nivolumab—associated peripheral ulcerative keratitis. Am J Ophthalmol Case Rep. 2022;28:101686.
33. Kuhar B, Bailey J, Aeum J. Association of conjunctival ulceration with pembrolizumab. JAMA Ophthalmol. 2024;142:389.
34. Vitiello L, Lixi F, Coco G, Giannaccare G. Ocular surface side effects of novel anticancer drugs. Cancers (Basel). 2024;16(2):344.
35. Chia PL, John T. Vortex keratopathy presumed secondary to AZD9291. J Thorac Oncol. 2015;10(12):1807–8.
36. Orlandi A, Fasciani R, Cassano A, Agresta A, Calegari MA, Caporossi A, et al. Trastuzumab-induced corneal ulceration: successful no-drug treatment of a “blind” side effect in a case report. BMC Cancer. 2015;15:973.
37. Noureddin BN, Seoud M, Bashshur Z, Salem Z, Shamseddin A, Khalil A. Ocular toxicity in low-dose tamoxifen: a prospective study. Eye (Lond). 1999;13(Pt 6):729–33.
38. Kunkler AL, Binkley EM, Mantopoulos D, Hendershot AJ, Ohr MP, Kendra KL, et al. Known and novel ocular toxicities of biologics, targeted agents, and traditional chemotherapeutics. Graefes Arch Clin Exp Ophthalmol. 2019;257(8):1771–81.
39. Hiong A, O'Day R, Fog LS, McKay D, McKenzie J, Ameratunga M, et al. Globe salvage and vision preservation by neoadjuvant darovasertib and crizotinib in uveal melanoma. Ophthalmol Retina. 2023; https://doi.org/10.1016/j.oret.2023.10.009.
40. Das J, Das N. Chronic conjunctival chemosis-a new ocular side effect of crizotinib. Ophthalmic Plast Reconstr Surg. 2021;37(1):e18–21.

Conjunctival Tumors: Systemic Associations

16

Nasrine Anais El Salloukh, Arun D. Singh, and Elias I. Traboulsi

Abbreviations

AL	Light chain
CHRPE	Congenital hypertrophy of the retinal pigment epithelium
GS	Goldenhar syndrome
MEN	Multiple endocrine neoplasia
OAV	Oculoauriculovertebral dysplasia
OAVS	Oculoauriculovertebral spectrum
PJS	Peutz–Jeghers syndrome
PS	Proteus syndrome
TTR	Transthyretin
XP	Xeroderma pigmentosum

16.1 Carney Complex

Carney complex is characterized by cutaneous pigmentary abnormalities, myxomas, endocrine tumors, and schwannomas [1]. Benign conjunctival and caruncular pigmentation may be present in about one-fourth of cases [2]. Similar pigmentation of the skin is also present on the lips and genital mucosa (Table 16.1) [3].

N. A. El Salloukh · E. I. Traboulsi (✉)
Department of Pediatric Ophthalmology and Strabismus, Center for Genetic Eye Diseases, Cole Eye Institute (i-32), Cleveland Clinic, Cleveland, OH, USA
e-mail: traboue@ccf.org

A. D. Singh
Department of Ophthalmic Oncology, Cole Eye Institute, Cleveland Clinic, Cleveland, OH, USA

© The Author(s), under exclusive license to Springer Nature Switzerland AG 2024
J. Pe'er et al. (eds.), *Clinical Ophthalmic Oncology*, https://doi.org/10.1007/978-3-031-72443-5_16

Table 16.1 Conjunctival tumors that are markers of syndromic association

Pattern		Entity	Conjunctival features	Associated features	Locus/gene
Pigmentation		Carney complex	Conjunctival pigmentation	Spotty mucocutaneous pigmentation	17q
				Schwannoma	
				Endocrine overactivity	*PRKAR1A* gene chromosome 2
				Testicular tumor	
		Peutz–Jeghers syndrome	Conjunctival pigmentation	Mucocutaneous pigmentation	19p13.3
				Gastrointestinal polyposis	*STK11*
Benign tumors	Dermoid	Organoid nevus syndrome	Epibulbar dermoid	Cutaneous sebaceous nevus	Sporadic
			Coloboma		
		Goldenhar syndrome	Epibulbar dermoid	Preauricular appendages	Sporadic
				Pretragal fistula	
				Vertebral anomalies	
		Proteus	Epibulbar dermoid	Connective tissue nevi	Sporadic
			Strabismus	Lipoma	
			Orbital exostoses	Vascular malformations	
				Epidermal nevi	
	Neuroma	MEN 2B	Conjunctival neuroma	Thickened corneal nerves	10q11.2
				Mucocutaneous neuroma	*RET* proto-oncogene
				Endocrine tumor	
Malignant tumors		Xeroderma pigmentosum	Conjunctival xerosis	Skin atrophy with pigmentary changes	Variable
			Keratitis	Neurological abnormalities	
			Ocular surface neoplasms		
Amyloidosis			Conjunctival nodule	Variable	Sporadic
			Conjunctival hemorrhage		Familial

MEN multiple endocrine neoplasia

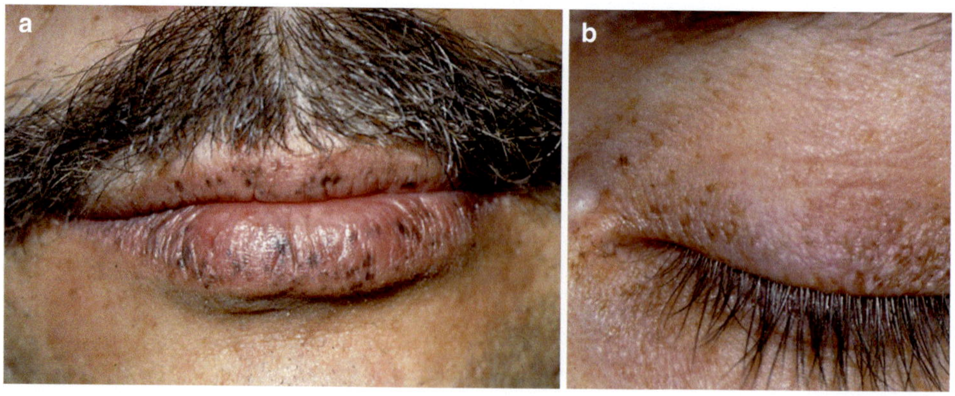

Fig. 16.1 Pigmentation of lips (**a**) and eyelid (**b**) in a patient with Peutz–Jeghers syndrome

16.2 Peutz–Jeghers Syndrome

Peutz–Jeghers syndrome (PJS) refers to the association of gastrointestinal hamartomatous polyposis and mucocutaneous pigmentation [4]. Peutz–Jeghers syndrome is inherited in an autosomal dominant fashion and results from mutations of *STK11* (also known as LKB1), a tumor suppressor gene on chromosome 19p13.3 in about 70–90% of patients [5, 6, 72]. Many missense mutations and deletions occur throughout the whole *LKB1* gene without any particular genotype/phenotype correlation [6].

Congenital hypertrophy of the retinal pigment epithelium (CHRPE)-like lesions of the fundus that are characteristic of patients with familial adenomatous polyposis (Gardner syndrome) do not occur in Peutz–Jeghers syndrome [7]. However, pigmented spots of the eyelids and conjunctiva have been observed (Fig. 16.1) [8].

The three clinical features of PJS are mucocutaneous melanin hyperpigmentation, multiple distinctive intestinal hamartomatous polyps, and a dominant inheritance of the condition with a positive family history [6]. Hamartomatous polyps are noncancerous tumors that occur mainly in the

Table 16.2 Peutz–Jeghers syndrome diagnostic criteria

Positive family history of PJS	Any number of histologically confirmed PJS polyps, or characteristic, prominent, mucocutaneous pigmentation
Negative family history of PJS	≥3 histologically confirmed PJS polyps, or any number of histologically confirmed PJS polyps and characteristic pigmentation

PJS Peutz–Jeghers syndrome

small bowel. Dysplastic transformation of a PJS polyp is very rare [6].

The pigmentation appears usually around the lips, eyes, hands, or feet, forming smooth melanin deposits in a round or oval shape, and fades with advancing age [6]. Perioral pigmentation is pathognomonic, particularly if it occurs across the vermilion border of the lips. Oral mucosa and fingertips are also commonly affected. About 50% of patients develop a wide variety of cancers such as breast, colorectal, and pancreatic cancers in adulthood among which colorectal cancer is the most common [9]. An overexpression of COX-2 has been reported in polyps and cancers related to PJS [10].

Diagnostic criteria were suggested by Van Lier et al. (Table 16.2) [11]. The European Society for Pediatric Gastroenterology Hepatology and Nutrition position paper provide a guide for diagnosis, assessment, and management of PJS in children and adolescent [73]. An annual physical examination with a complete blood count to detect iron-deficiency anemia because of occult bleeding from GI tract polyps or cancer is important, and a baseline endoscopic screening of the gastrointestinal tract is usually initiated around the age of 8 years [10].

16.3 Sebaceous Nevus Syndrome

Sebaceous nevus syndrome (of Jadassohn), also known as Schimmelpenning–Feuerstein–Mims syndrome, is a distinct clinical disorder within the spectrum of epidermal nevus syndrome (of Solomon) characterized by cutaneous sebaceous nevus and extracutaneous manifestations [12]. Up to 95% of patients have heterozygous mutations in *HRAS*, with the mutation c.37G > C (p.Gly13Arg) accounting for the majority of cases; most other cases result from mutations in *KRAS* (c.35G > A or c.35G > T) [13]. The *HRAS* and *KRAS* mutations are found in lesional keratinocytes only, confirming a mosaic RASopathy [13].

The classic triad is one of facial lesions, seizures, and mental retardation [14]. Ocular involvement is observed in about 40% of cases with epibulbar choristomas and coloboma of the eyelid being most common. Posterior segment tumors have included chondroid choristomas (intrascleral cartilage) with ossification [14–16]. The limbal choristomas can be simple or complex and usually are dermoid or lipodermoid in nature. Other ocular manifestations reported are strabismus and optic disc abnormalities (coloboma and hypoplasia) [74]. The *HRAS* and *KRAS* mutations lead to the activation of MAPK and PI3K-Akt signaling and cellular proliferation, which are associated with many cancers, providing an explanation for the high incidence of secondary tumors in approximately 25% of cases [13]. Trichoblastomas and syringocystadenoma papilliferum are the most common benign tumors, while malignant tumors occur in <1% [13].

16.4 Goldenhar Syndrome and the Oculoauriculovertebral Spectrum

Goldenhar described a triad of epibulbar dermoids, preauricular appendages, and pretragal fistula [17]. The etiology of Goldenhar syndrome (GS) has yet to be elucidated, but it has been suggested that a vascular insult and/or neural crest abnormality during embryogenesis could account for this syndrome [18]. Since then, the spectrum of manifestations has expanded to include vertebral anomalies and is also called oculoauriculovertebral dysplasia (OAV) [19].

Currently, GS is included in the oculoauriculovertebral spectrum (OAVS) that encompasses different overlapping diagnoses such as hemifacial microsomia, first and second branchial arches syndrome, otomandibular dysostosis, facioauriculovertebral syndrome, and Goldenhar syndrome, all representing a phenotypic continuum of the same entity [20].

Most cases occur sporadically, but exceptional cases with autosomal dominant and recessive inheritance patterns have also been reported [21]. Rooryck et al. identified 12% of familial cases in a cohort of 95 patients [22]. A more recent study described that up to 45% of relatives of probands with OAVS do have minor OAVS manifestations [23]. Environmental causes have also been suggested, particularly twinning, assisted reproductive techniques, and maternal pre-pregnancy diabetes [24, 25]. Hence, the phenotype is probably affected by other genetic and nongenetic factors, in line with an oligogenic or even a multifactorial etiology [20].

Epibulbar dermoid is a necessary diagnostic feature of Goldenhar syndrome (Fig. 16.2). The epibulbar dermoids are almost always located near the limbus in the inferotemporal quadrants. Secondary irregular astigmatism and anisometropic amblyopia may also be present, but no association with central corneal lesions was found [26]. Dermolipomas are typically in the subconjunctival plane and appear as a yellow soft mass in the superotemporal quadrant. In an observational case series of 55 patients with eyelid coloboma, 13 (45%) were due to GS [27]. Other associated anomalies include Duane syndrome [28], caruncular anomalies [29], and lacrimal system agenesis [76]. Involvement of the globe itself manifesting as microphthalmia [30], bilateral cataracts [31], exudative vitelliform maculopathy [32], or bilateral retinal detachment [75] is rare.

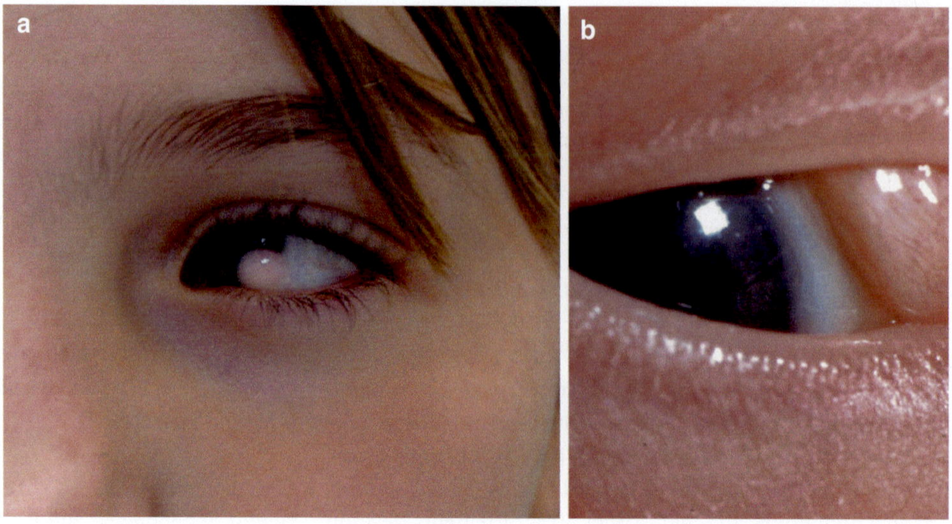

Fig. 16.2 Epibulbar dermoids in Goldenhar syndrome. Limbal (**a**) and extralimbal (**b**)

Rooijers et al. classified the ocular anomalies into four categories as follows [77]:

Type I: Anatomical anomalies usually not impairing vision like lid coloboma, lipodermoid, orbital dystopia, lacrimal stenosis, epicanthus, and telecanthus.
Type II: Anatomical anomalies likely to impair vision like epibulbar dermoid, microphthalmos, anophthalmos, exposure keratopathy, cataract, fundal coloboma, and optic nerve hypoplasia.
Type III: Motility disorders like esotropia, exotropia, Duane syndrome, abducens nerve anomaly, and ptosis.
Type IV: Refractive errors like astigmatism, anisometropia, myopia, and hyperopia.

A study of 51 patients with OAVS showed that the most common systemic manifestations were ear abnormalities in 92%, hearing loss in 85%, and hemifacial microsomia in 90% of patients [20]. Ocular anomalies were present in 29% of patients, while vertebral anomalies were confirmed in 20% of cases [20].

In addition to ophthalmic, ear, and vertebral anomalies, about 50% of cases have other malformations such as micrognathia, macrostomia, cleft lip and palate, developmental defects of the heart and brain, and urogenital or limb abnormalities [20, 23, 78]. There is a statistically significant association of GS with the VATER anomaly (vertebral defects, anal atresia, tracheoesophageal fistula with esophageal atresia, and radial dysplasia) and CHARGE syndrome (coloboma, heart anomaly, choanal atresia, retardation, genital and ear anomalies) [33].

Due to the variable phenotypic expressivity and the overlap with other conditions, it has been difficult to reach a consensus regarding the minimum diagnostic criteria for OAVS, but it has been proposed that they should include microtia or hemifacial microsomia, together with milder malformations and an associated family history of OAV [20].

All OAVS patients should be referred for audiology screening, ophthalmic examination, and x-rays of the spine, ideally anteroposterior and lateral views of the whole spine.

16.5 Proteus Syndrome

Proteus syndrome is a severe and highly variable disorder characterized by asymmetric and disproportionate overgrowth of body parts and hamartomas, along with a susceptibility to tumors [34]. Proteus syndrome was first recognized as a specific entity in 1979 and named after the Greek god Proteus, as he could change his shape or form, emphasizing the varied manifestations of the syndrome [35].

Proteus syndrome is inherited in a sporadic fashion as it is due to mutations that are lethal unless they occur in a mosaic fashion [36]. It does not seem to recur in families but does appear in discordant monozygotic twins, suggesting a somatic mutation that is lethal when constitutive [34]. More recent studies have supported a role for the *AKT1* c.49G → A variant in the pathogenesis of Proteus syndrome [34].

The systemic manifestations of Proteus syndrome are usually present at birth, progress during childhood, and are almost always asymmetric [37]. The disorder primarily manifests as postnatal overgrowth, with irregular, distorting, and quickly progressive overgrowth that can include many tissues, although the bone, connective tissue, and fat are the most involved tissues, but the central nervous system, spleen, thymus, colon, and other tissues could be interested too [37]. Connective tissue nevi are pathognomonic; other features include lipoma (92%), vascular malformations (88%), and epidermal nevi (67%) [38].

Ophthalmic involvement is common in Proteus syndrome. Epibulbar and eyelid dermoids, strabismus, nystagmus, high myopia, orbital exostoses, and posterior segment hamartoma are most observed [39]. Strabismus and nystagmus may be a consequence of low vision or severe congenital malfunction of the neuroretinal network. Retinal abnormalities typically accompany high myopia, and retinal detachment may occur when there is lattice degeneration. Cataracts can be the consequence of retinal detachment [39]. A complete list of published ophthalmic findings is given in Table 16.3 [39].

Due to its varied manifestations, the diagnosis of Proteus syndrome is frequently missed. A critical review of published cases revealed that only 47% of cases met the diagnostic criteria [40]; for this reason, a more recent list of diagnostic criteria has been proposed (Table 16.4) [39]. Individuals with significant clinical features but who do not meet the diagnostic criteria are labeled as having Proteus-like syndrome. The differential diagnosis of Proteus syndrome includes neurofibromatosis type 1, Klippel–Trenaunay–Weber syndrome, Maffucci's syndrome, Ollier's disease, Bannayan–Riley–Ruvalcaba syndrome, CLOVES syndrome, and hemihyperplasia.

Table 16.3 Ocular manifestations of Proteus syndrome

Strabismus
Nystagmus
High myopia
Retinal pigmentary abnormalities
Retinal detachment
Cataract
Posterior segment hamartomas
Epibulbar tumor
Eyelid hamartomas
Eyelid ptosis
Retinal coloboma
Glaucoma
Pale optic disk
Anisocoria
Heterochromia iridis

Table 16.4 Revised diagnostic criteria for Proteus syndrome

Must have all the general criteria and various specific criteria		
General criteria	All of the following: Mosaic distribution of lesions Sporadic occurrence Progressive course	
Specific criteria	Category A	Cerebriform connective tissue nevus
	Two from category B	Linear epidermal nevus Asymmetric, disproportionate overgrowth Specific tumors before second decade (bilateral ovarian cystadenoma or parotid monomorphic adenoma)
	Three from category C	Dysregulated adipose tissue Vascular malformations Lung cysts Facial phenotype

The management is challenging, due to the postnatal overgrowth. Furthermore, patients with PS have an increased risk of premature death, commonly caused by deep venous thrombosis and pulmonary embolism [41, 79].

Miransertib, an AKT1 inhibitor, has been recently studied as a treatment for Proteus syndrome [80].

16.6 Multiple Endocrine Neoplasia Type 2B

Multiple endocrine neoplasia (MEN) is a condition characterized by a genetic predisposition to develop benign and malignant tumors of various endocrine glands. Based upon the pattern of glandular involvement, MEN is classified as type 1 and type 2. MEN type 2 is comprised of three subtypes: familial medullary thyroid carcinoma, MEN 2A, and MEN 2B. MEN 2B, also called mucosal neuroma syndrome or Wagenmann–Froboese syndrome, is the only MEN subgroup that is of ophthalmic interest because of its association with mucosal neuromas and corneal abnormalities [42].

MEN 2B is inherited as an autosomal dominant trait, but about half the cases are due to de novo mutations, with more than 95% of cases resulting from a point mutation in the *RET* gene [43].

A comprehensive review of a large number of published cases of MEN 2B revealed that common ophthalmic manifestations include prominent corneal nerves (100%), eyelid neuroma or thickening (88%), subconjunctival neuroma (79%), and dry eyes (48%) (Fig. 16.3) [44, 45]. It has also been shown to be associated with glaucoma [81].The presence of prominent corneal nerves in an otherwise normal cornea should lead to investigations to exclude MEN 2B [46]. Other infrequent causes of prominent corneal nerves such as neurofibromatosis, leprosy, and congenital ichthyosis should also be considered in the differential diagnosis [46]. However, none of these conditions are associated with perilimbal neuromas or alacrima [47]. Histopathologic studies of the cornea have shown that prominent corneal nerves are axonal bundles of nonmyelinated nerves in association with Schwann cells [48].

A clinical diagnosis of MEN 2B is suspected in the presence of marfanoid body habitus, mucosal neuromas of the lips and tongue, prominent corneal nerves, and medullary thyroid carcinoma [42]. As medullary thyroid carcinoma tends to be aggressive, early prophylactic thyroidectomy is recommended [49]. Patients may also have chronic constipation and colonic cramping due to megacolon disorder [49]. About half of patients with MEN 2B also develop pheochromocytoma, while involvement of the parathyroid gland is rare. It remains elusive whether vascular anomalies are related to MEN type 2B [47].

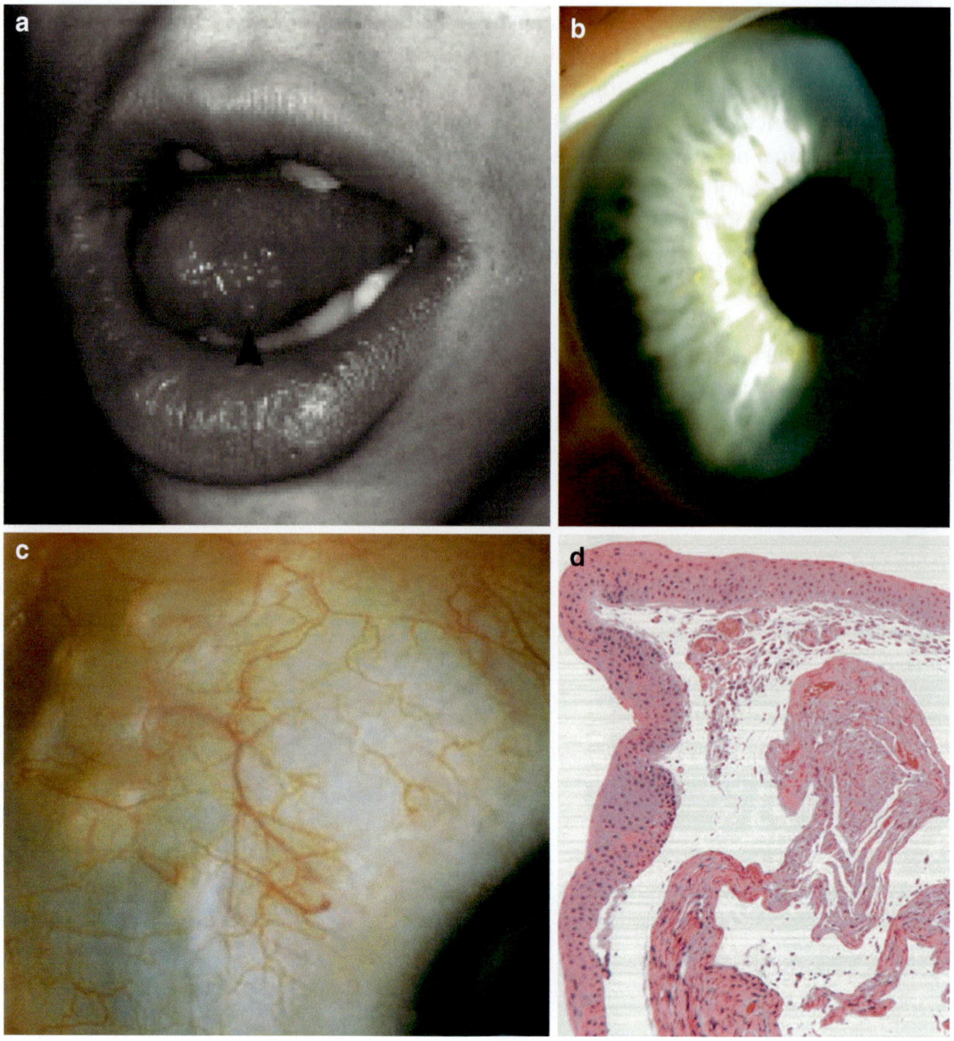

Fig. 16.3 Characteristic features of MEN 2B syndrome. Submucosal lip and tongue neuroma (**a**, arrow). Prominent corneal nerves (**b**). Plexiform subconjunctival neuroma (**c**). Histopathologic section of the conjunctiva shows thickened abnormal nerves in the substantia propria (**d**). ((**a**) Reprinted from Jacobs and Hawes [44]. With permission from Wolters Kluwer Health, Inc. (**c**) Reprinted from Eter et al. [45]. With permission from Springer Nature)

16.7 Xeroderma Pigmentosum

Xeroderma pigmentosum (XP) refers to a group of genetic disorders characterized by extreme sensitivity to sunlight and a constellation of cutaneous, ophthalmic, and neurological findings [50]. The estimated incidence of XP in the United States, Japan, and Western Europe is 1 in 250,000, 1 in 22,000, and 1 in 500,000, respectively [51].

XP is inherited as an autosomal recessive trait with full penetrance. There are eight known XP complementation groups (XP-A to XP-G and XP-V), which correspond to the eight genes that are implicated in this condition [51]. The proteins encoded by the *XPA* to *XPG* genes are involved in nucleotide excision repair of DNA damaged by UV light. The eighth gene (*POLH*) codes for a special polymerase used to replicate damaged DNA [52]. XP-C, E, and V patients have normal sunburn reactions for skin type and do not develop manifest neurodegeneration leading to later diagnosis and photoprotection and consequently an earlier age of onset of first skin cancer [51]. XP-A, B, D, F, and G have severe and exaggerated sunburn reactions on minimal sun exposure and suffer neurodegeneration making for earlier diagnosis and photo-protection and subsequently less skin cancers [51]. XP-C are particularly susceptible to ocular problems compared to other groups [82].

Ophthalmic complications are present in about 20–90% of cases, probably due to high exposure of the eye to UVR, as well as the role the eye has within the neurological system, which underscores the importance of regular ophthalmic examinations of XP patients [51, 52]. Eyelid skin atrophy with pigmentary changes and loss of lashes is common. Similar changes of the conjunctiva such as xerosis and pigmentation also occur (Fig. 16.4). Corneal complications include keratitis, pterygium, vascularization, corneal ulceration, and limbal stem cell deficiency [83]. Most significant is the predisposition to develop multiple eyelid and ocular surface neoplasms including basal cell carcinoma, squamous cell carcinoma, and melanoma [52]. Patients in groups XP-C, E, and V had significantly more ocular surface abnormalities, but a lower association with pupillary abnor-

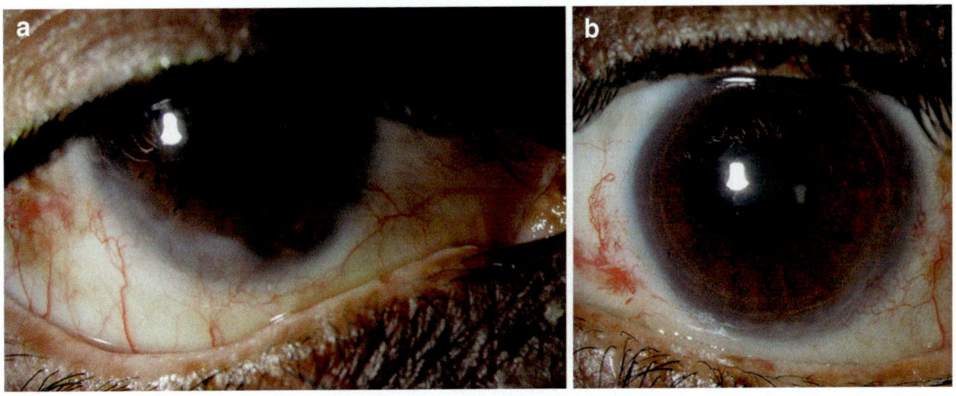

Fig. 16.4 Xeroderma pigmentosum with bilateral corneal and conjunctival squamous neoplasia (**a** right eye; **b** left eye)

Table 16.5 Ocular signs and symptoms in xeroderma pigmentosum

Ectropion or lagophthalmos
Periocular cancers
Photophobia
Conjunctival injection
Conjunctival corkscrew vessels
Interpalpebral melanosis regardless of skin pigmentation
Pterygium
Pinguecula
Corneal scar or neovascularization
Superficial punctate keratopathy
Ocular surface cancer
Sluggish pupils
Strabismus
Abnormal extraocular movement
Lens abnormality
Retinal abnormality

mality [49]. One case of iris melanoma has been reported [53]. The posterior segment is rarely affected, but there have been reported cases of optic atrophy, retinal degeneration, and mild macular edema, all secondary to neurodegeneration [54]. A complete list of ocular signs and symptoms in XP is given in Table 16.5.

Lim et al. reported that, in their study, 6% of patients initially presented to ophthalmologists with ocular surface signs related to XP and, before any formal diagnosis of XP had been made, underpinning the role of ophthalmologists in the diagnosis of this group of disorders [51]. Examinations facilitate the detection and treatment of any eye pathology as well as eyelid and ocular surface tumors. Some of the most important areas of management include the treatment of dry eyes, watery eyes, lagophthalmos, ectropion, pterygia, ocular surface cancers, eyelid cancers, strabismus, and double vision. In addition, ophthalmologists play a fundamental role in advising and facilitating adequate ophthalmic UVR protection. The gold standard for this is a full-face visor, which is 100% protective of ultraviolet A and ultraviolet B waves [51].

The cutaneous findings are the defining features of this entity [48]. A tendency to sunburn is evident in early childhood and may be the earliest sign of XP. This is followed by freckling in sun-exposed areas. These changes eventually progress to parchment-like dry pigmented skin and hence the name xeroderma pigmentosum [50]. There is a 1000-fold increased risk of developing cutaneous cancers such as squamous cell carcinoma, basal cell carcinoma, and melanoma [50]. Tumors tend to be multifocal and occur at a median age of less than 10 years. If protected from sunlight at an early life, the debilitating cutaneous changes can be almost completely avoided.

Neurological abnormalities, present in about 20% of cases, include the absence of deep tendon reflexes due to axonal loss and demyelination, progressive hearing loss, and ataxia [50].

16.8 Amyloidosis

Amyloidosis refers to the extracellular deposition of insoluble proteinaceous material called amyloid. Amyloid deposits exhibit characteristic staining reaction to iodine and Congo red stain (birefringence) [55]. From a clinical standpoint, amyloidosis can be classified into systemic forms, in which there is a multisystem involvement due to underlying neoplastic, inflammatory, genetic, iatrogenic, or idiopathic causes, or localized forms where amyloid deposits in isolated organs without evidence of systemic involvement; the latter forms are associated with aging and diabetes [56]. Another classification system is based on the nature of the fibril-forming proteins such as immunoglobulin light chains (AL), serum amyloid A (the most common form of systemic amyloidosis), and transthyretin [56].

Inherited forms of amyloidosis (familial amyloidosis) result from inherited protein mutations. The most common protein involved is transthyretin (TTR), also called prealbumin that functions as transport protein for both thyroxine and vitamin A [57]. Over 100 *TTR* point mutations have been reported in the literature with differing phenotypes [58]. TTR is synthesized mainly in the liver but also in the choroid plexuses of the brain and in retinal pigment epithelial cells;

in fact, almost 25% of patients with *TTR* mutations have ophthalmic involvement [59]. Much less commonly, abnormalities of several other proteins, including fibrinogen, ApoA1, ApoA2, lysozyme, gelsolin, and beta-2 microglobulin, have been known to cause a category classified as non-TTR amyloidosis [60].

Ophthalmic amyloidosis can affect the eyelids, conjunctiva, orbital tissues, cornea (lattice corneal dystrophy), and vitreous. Unilateral or bilateral eyelid involvement is frequent in systemic amyloidosis, in which clinical manifestations include recurrent purpura or periorbital bleeding because of a tendency for perivascular deposition of amyloid [61] and waxy nodules [62].

Conjunctival amyloidosis appears as a pale-yellow nodule associated with recurrent subconjunctival hemorrhage. In general, conjunctival amyloidosis tends to be localized, but association with systemic amyloidosis has also been reported. Orbital amyloidosis may involve the lacrimal gland, extraocular muscles, orbital fat, and lacrimal sac, mimicking inflammatory or lymphoproliferative disorders [63]. Deposition within the levator muscle may lead to a presentation of ptosis of unknown etiology. Glaucoma can be the result of amyloid deposition in the trabecular meshwork [64].

With rare exceptions, amyloid deposits in the vitreous are indicative of the familial neuropathic form of amyloidosis due to mutations in the transthyretin gene; this is a slowly progressive peripheral polyneuropathy with sparing of the central nervous system [57]. The vitreous deposits are grayish and cobweb-like and may be attached to the posterior surface of the lens as white dots resembling foot plates (pseudopodia lentis) [65]. The natural history of vitreous amyloidosis tends to involve floaters that progress, leading to visual impairment, which can be so significant that it leads to only light perception vision. Vision impairment can be reversed with vitrectomy, and some patients can have a complete restoration of vision [59, 66]. Similar white opacities may be observed in the retina over the arterioles and venules, which are otherwise clinically and angiographically normal, probably due to direct infiltration with amyloid, which has been described for oculoleptomeningeal amyloidosis [67]. Ando et al. found abnormal conjunctival vessels to be the most common ocular manifestation of TTR amyloidosis (75.5%), followed by pupillary abnormalities (43.2%), keratoconjunctivitis sicca (KCS) (40.5%), glaucoma (19.2%), and vitreous opacification (5.4%) [68].

Systemic amyloidosis can lead to ocular morbidity, such as involvement of the temporal artery, cornea, extraocular muscles, trabecular meshwork, and cranial nerves in AL amyloidosis or corneal dystrophy in gelsolin familial amyloidosis [60, 84].

The most common form of systemic amyloidosis is AL amyloidosis, which may be idiopathic in origin or associated with multiple myeloma. Amyloid A amyloidosis occurs most frequently as a complication of chronic inflammatory disease, and its disease course is dominated by renal dysfunction [69].

Familial amyloidosis most frequently results from mutations that lead to misfolding of the protein transthyretin. Manifestations vary depending on the individual TTR mutation [59]. Because of the hepatic production of TTR, mutations lead to systemic manifestations of familial amyloidosis that include peripheral neuropathy, autonomic neuropathy, and cardiomyopathy [59]. Vascular changes occur and can result in cardiac or pulmonary involvement; many patients with TTR amyloidosis have sleep-disordered breathing as well as cardiopulmonary amyloidosis [70].

Patients with systemic amyloidosis may present to the ophthalmologist for ocular symptoms before other systemic symptoms are apparent. Almost 7% of patients with systemic amyloidosis presented with ophthalmic signs and symptoms such as conjunctival masses, persistent subconjunctival hemorrhages, or diplopia related to infiltration of the extraocular muscles [60]. In addition, the vast majority of adnexal amyloidosis is AL type, necessitating systemic workup to exclude underlying lymphoproliferative disorder [71].

References

1. Carney JA, Gordon H, Carpenter PC. The complex of myxomas, spotty pigmentation, and endocrine overactivity. Medicine (Baltimore). 1985;64(4):270–83.
2. Kennedy RH, Waller RR, Carney JA. Ocular pigmented spots and eyelid myxomas. Am J Ophthalmol. 1987;104(5):533–8.
3. Rothenbuhler A, Stratakis CA. Clinical and molecular genetics of Carney complex. Best Pract Res Clin Endocrinol Metab. 2010;24(3):389–99.
4. Jeghers H, Mc KV, Katz KH. Generalized intestinal polyposis and melanin spots of the oral mucosa, lips and digits; a syndrome of diagnostic significance. N Engl J Med. 1949;241(26):1031–6.
5. Hearle N, Schumacher V, Menko FH. Frequency and spectrum of cancers in the Peutz-Jeghers syndrome. Clin Cancer Res. 2006;12(10):3209–15.
6. Ma H, Brosens LAA, Offerhaus GJA. Pathology and genetics of hereditary colorectal cancer. Pathology. 2018;50(1):49–59.
7. Traboulsi EI, Maumenee IH, Krush AJ. Pigmented ocular fundus lesions in the inherited gastrointestinal polyposis syndromes and in hereditary nonpolyposis colorectal cancer. Ophthalmology. 1988;95(7):964–9.
8. Traboulsi EI, Maumenee IH. Periocular pigmentation in the Peutz-Jeghers syndrome. Am J Ophthalmol. 1986;102(1):126–7.
9. Giardiello FM, Offerhaus JG. Phenotype and cancer risk of various polyposis syndromes. Eur J Cancer. 1995;31A(7–8):1085–7.
10. Beggs AD, Latchford AR, Vasen HF. Peutz-Jeghers syndrome: a systematic review and recommendations for management. Gut. 2010;59(7):975–86.
11. van Lier MG, Wagner A, Mathus-Vliegen EM. High cancer risk in Peutz-Jeghers syndrome: a systematic review and surveillance recommendations. Am J Gastroenterol. 2010;105(6):1258–64. author reply 65
12. Happle R. The group of epidermal nevus syndromes part I. Well defined phenotypes. J Am Acad Dermatol. 2010;63(1):1–22. quiz 3–4
13. Aslam A, Salam A, Griffiths CE, McGrath JA. Naevus sebaceus: a mosaic RASopathy. Clin Exp Dermatol. 2014;39(1):1–6.

14. Traboulsi EI, Zin A, Massicotte SJ. Posterior scleral choristoma in the organoid nevus syndrome (linear nevus sebaceus of Jadassohn). Ophthalmology. 1999;106(11):2126–30.
15. Shields JA, Shields CL, Eagle RC Jr. Ocular manifestations of the organoid nevus syndrome. Ophthalmology. 1997;104(3):549–57.
16. Echegaray JJ, Chen R, Bellerive C, Singh AD. Linear nevus sebaceous syndrome presenting as circumscribed choroidal hemangioma. Ophthalmic Genet. 2018;39(2):278–81.
17. Goldenhar M. Associations malformatives de l'oeil et de l'oreille: en particulier, le syndrome: dermoide epibulbaire-appendices auriculaires—fistula auris congenita et ses relations avec la dysostose mandibulo-faciale. J Genet Hum. 1952;1:243–82.
18. Golovine De S, Wu S, Hunter JV, Shearer WT. Goldenhar syndrome: a cause of secondary immunodeficiency? Allergy Asthma Clin Immunol. 2012;8:1–10.
19. Gorlin RJ, Jue KL, Jacobsen U, Goldschmidt E. Oculoauriculovertebral dysplasia. J Pediatr. 1963;63(991):999.
20. Beleza-Meireles A, Hart R, Clayton-Smith J. Oculo-auriculo-vertebral spectrum: clinical and molecular analysis of 51 patients. Eur J Med Genet. 2015;58(9):455–65.
21. Tasse C, Majewski F, Bohringer S. A family with autosomal dominant oculo-auriculo-vertebral spectrum. Clin Dysmorphol. 2007;16(1):1–7.
22. Rooryck C, Souakri N, Cailley D. Array-CGH analysis of a cohort of 86 patients with oculoauriculovertebral spectrum. Am J Med Genet A. 2010;152A(8):1984–9.
23. Rollnick BR, Kaye CI, Nagatoshi K. Oculoauriculovertebral dysplasia and variants: phenotypic characteristics of 294 patients. Am J Med Genet. 1987;26(2):361–75.
24. Beleza-Meireles A, Clayton-Smith J, Saraiva JM, Tassabehji M. Oculo-auriculo-vertebral spectrum: a review of the literature and genetic update. J Med Genet. 2014;51(10):635–45.
25. Barisic I, Odak L, Loane M. Prevalence, prenatal diagnosis and clinical features of oculo-auriculo-vertebral spectrum: a registry-based study in Europe. Eur J Hum Genet. 2014;22(8):1026–33.
26. Jakobiec FA, Pineda R, Rivera R. Epicorneal polypoidal lipodermoid: lack of association of central corneal lesions with goldenhar syndrome verified with a review of the literature. Surv Ophthalmol. 2010;55(1):78–84.
27. Smith HB, Verity DH, Collin JR. The incidence, embryology, and oculofacial abnormalities associated with eyelid colobomas. Eye (Lond). 2015;29(4):492–8.
28. Shrestha UD, Adhikari S. Goldenhar syndrome in association with Duane syndrome. JNMA J Nepal Med Assoc. 2012;52(185):33–5.
29. Nijhawan N, Morad Y, Seigel-Bartelt J, Levin AV. Caruncle abnormalities in the oculo-auriculo-vertebral spectrum. Am J Med Genet. 2002;113(4):320–5.
30. Margolis S, Aleksic S, Charles N. Retinal and optic nerve findings in Goldenhar-Gorlin syndrome. Ophthalmology. 1984;91(11):1327–33.
31. Shrestha UD, Adhikari S. Craniofacial Microsomia: Goldenhar syndrome in association with bilateral congenital cataract. Case Rep Ophthalmol Med. 2015;2015:435967.
32. Brue C, Mariotti C, Celani S. A case of Goldenhar syndrome associated with a new retinal presentation: exudative Vitelliform maculopathy. Case Rep Ophthalmol Med. 2015;2015:626027.
33. Kallen K, Robert E, Castilla EE. Relation between oculo-auriculo-vertebral (OAV) dysplasia and three other non-random associations of malformations (VATER, CHARGE, and OEIS). Am J Med Genet A. 2004;127(1):26–34.
34. Lindhurst MJ, Sapp JC, Teer JK. A mosaic activating mutation in AKT1 associated with the Proteus syndrome. N Engl J Med. 2011;365(7):611–9.
35. Wiedemann HR, Burgio GR, Aldenhoff P. The proteus syndrome. Partial gigantism of the hands and/or feet, nevi, hemihypertrophy, subcutaneous tumors, macrocephaly or other skull anomalies and possible accelerated growth and visceral affections. Eur J Pediatr. 1983;140(1):5–12.
36. Happle R. Lethal genes surviving by mosaicism: a possible explanation for sporadic birth defects involving the skin. J Am Acad Dermatol. 1987;16(4):899–906.
37. Biesecker LG, Happle R, Mulliken JB. Proteus syndrome: diagnostic criteria, differential diagnosis, and patient evaluation. Am J Med Genet. 1999;84(5):389–95.
38. Nguyen D, Turner JT, Olsen C. Cutaneous manifestations of proteus syndrome: correlations with general clinical severity. Arch Dermatol. 2004;140(8):947–53.
39. Becker De I, Gajda DJ, Gilbert-Barness E, Cohen MM Jr. Ocular manifestations in Proteus syndrome. Am J Med Genet. 2000;92(5):350–2.
40. Turner JT, Cohen MM Jr, Biesecker LG. Reassessment of the Proteus syndrome literature: application of diagnostic criteria to published cases. Am J Med Genet A. 2004;130(2):111–22.
41. Biesecker L. The challenges of Proteus syndrome: diagnosis and management. Eur J Hum Genet. 2006;14(11):1151–7.
42. Morrison PJ, Nevin NC. Multiple endocrine neoplasia type 2B (mucosal neuroma syndrome, Wagenmann-Froboese syndrome). J Med Genet. 1996;33(9):779–82.
43. Eng C, Smith DP, Mulligan LM. Point mutation within the tyrosine kinase domain of the RET proto-oncogene in multiple endocrine neoplasia type 2B and related sporadic tumours. Hum Mol Genet. 1994;3(2):237–41.
44. Jacobs JM, Hawes MJ. From eyelid bumps to thyroid lumps: report of a MEN type IIb family and review of the literature. Ophthalmic Plast Reconstr Surg. 2001;17(3):195–201.
45. Eter N, Klingmuller D, Hoppner W, Spitznas M. Typical ocular findings in a patient with multiple endocrine neoplasia type 2b syndrome. Graefes Arch Clin Exp Ophthalmol. 2001;239(5):391–4.
46. Robertson DM, Sizemore GW, Gordon H. Thickened corneal nerves as a manifestation of multiple endocrine neoplasia. Trans Sect Ophthalmol Am Acad Ophthalmol Otolaryngol. 1975;79(6):OP772–87.
47. Kreps EO, Herzeele Van I, Callewaert BL. Diagnosis of multiple endocrine neoplasia type 2B and management of its ocular features. Ophthalmic Genet. 2018;39(2):268–70.
48. Riley FC Jr, Robertson DM. Ocular histopathology in multiple endocrine neoplasia type 2b. Am J Ophthalmol. 1981;91(1):57–64.
49. Pacini F, Castagna MG, Cipri C, Schlumberger M. Medullary thyroid carcinoma. Clin Oncol (R Coll Radiol). 2010;22(6):475–85.
50. Kraemer KH, Lee MM, Scotto J. Xeroderma pigmentosum. Cutaneous, ocular, and neurologic abnormalities in 830 published cases. Arch Dermatol. 1987;123(2):241–50.
51. Lim R, Sethi M, Morley AMS. Ophthalmic manifestations of Xeroderma Pigmentosum: a perspective from the United Kingdom. Ophthalmology. 2017;124(11):1652–61.
52. Dollfus H, Porto F, Caussade P. Ocular manifestations in the inherited DNA repair disorders. Surv Ophthalmol. 2003;48(1):107–22.
53. Johnson MW, Skuta GL, Kincaid MC. Malignant melanoma of the iris in xeroderma pigmentosum. Arch Ophthalmol. 1989;107(3):402–7.
54. Ramkumar HL, Brooks BP, Cao X. Ophthalmic manifestations and histopathology of xeroderma pigmentosum: two clinicopathological cases and a review of the literature. Surv Ophthalmol. 2011;56(4):348–61.
55. Shields JA, Eagle RC, Shields CL. Systemic amyloidosis presenting as a mass of the conjunctival semilunar fold. Am J Ophthalmol. 2000;130(4):523–5.
56. Westermark P, Benson MD, Buxbaum JN. Amyloid: toward terminology clarification. Report from the Nomenclature Committee of the International Society of Amyloidosis. Amyloid. 2005;12(1):1–4.

57. Sandgren O. Ocular amyloidosis, with special reference to the hereditary forms with vitreous involvement. Surv Ophthalmol. 1995;40(3):173–96.
58. Benson MD, Kincaid JC. The molecular biology and clinical features of amyloid neuropathy. Muscle Nerve. 2007;36(4):411–23.
59. Reynolds MM, Veverka KK, Gertz MA. Ocular manifestations of familial transthyretin amyloidosis. Am J Ophthalmol. 2017;183:156–62.
60. Reynolds MM, Veverka KK, Gertz MA. Ocular manifestations of systemic amyloidosis. Retina. 2018;38(7):1371–6.
61. Landa G, Aloni E, Milshtein A. Eyelid bleeding and atypical amyloidosis. Am J Ophthalmol. 2004;138(3):495–6.
62. Al-Nuaimi D, Bhatt PR, Steeples L. Amyloidosis of the orbit and adnexae. Orbit. 2012;31(5):287–98.
63. Dinakaran S, Singh AD, Rennie IG. Orbital amyloidosis presenting as ptosis. Eye. 2005;19(1):110–2.
64. Shalchi Z, Taylor SR, Lightman S. The eye in haematological disease. Br J Hosp Med (Lond). 2011;72(12):691–7.
65. Hitchings RA, Tripathi RC. Vitreous opacities in primary amyloid disease. A clinical, histochemical, and ultrastructural report. Br J Ophthalmol. 1976;60(1):41–54.
66. Beirao NM, Matos E, Beirao I. Recurrence of vitreous amyloidosis and need of surgical reintervention in Portuguese patients with familial amyloidosis ATTR V30M. Retina. 2011;31(7):1373–7.
67. Savage DJ, Mango CA, Streeten BW. Amyloidosis of the vitreous. Fluorescein angiographic findings and association with neovascularization. Arch Ophthalmol. 1982;100(11):1776–9.
68. Ando E, Ando Y, Okamura R. Ocular manifestations of familial amyloidotic polyneuropathy type I: long-term follow up. Br J Ophthalmol. 1997;81(4):295–8.
69. Lachmann HJ, Goodman HJ, Gilbertson JA. Natural history and outcome in systemic AA amyloidosis. N Engl J Med. 2007;356(23):2361–71.
70. Bodez D, Guellich A, Kharoubi M. Prevalence, severity, and prognostic value of sleep apnea syndromes in cardiac amyloidosis. Sleep. 2016;39(7):1333–41.
71. Blandford AD, Yordi S, Kapoor S. Ocular adnexal amyloidosis: a mass spectrometric analysis. Am J Ophthalmol. 2018;193:28–32.
72. Julian D, John-Paul P, Anuradha P, Finlay M. An exploration of genotype-phenotype link between Peutz-Jeghers syndrome and STK11: a review. Familial Cancer. 2018;17(3):421–7. https://doi.org/10.1007/s10689-017-0037-3.
73. Andrew L, Shlomi C, Marcus A, Michele S, Jerome V, Richard D, Cecile T, Thomas A, Carol D, Warren H. Management of Peutz-Jeghers syndrome in children and adolescents: a position paper from the ESPGHAN Polyposis Working Group. J Pediatr Gastroenterol Nutr. 2019;68(3):442–52. https://doi.org/10.1097/MPG.0000000000002248.
74. Yan Y, Siyi Z, Henghua Z, Yixiong Z, Yao F. Ophthalmic manifestation and pathological features in a cohort of patients with linear nevus sebaceous syndrome and encephalocraniocutaneous lipomatosis. Front Pediatr. 2021;9 https://doi.org/10.3389/fped.2021.678296.
75. Phuntsho D, Muralidhar R, Brijesh T. Bilateral retinal detachment in Goldenhar syndrome. Indian J Ophthalmol. 2020;68(11):2585. https://doi.org/10.4103/ijo.IJO_401_20.
76. Tam MW, Boyle N. Goldenhar syndrome associated with lacrimal system agenesis: a case report. Am J Ophthalmol Case Rep. 2023;29:101766. https://doi.org/10.1016/j.ajoc.2022.101766.
77. Rooijers W, Caron CJJM, Loudon SE, Padwa BL, Dunaway DJ, Forrest CR, Koudstaal MJ. Ocular and adnexal anomalies in craniofacial microsomia: a systematic review. Int J Oral Maxillofacial Surg. 2020;49(9):1107–14. https://doi.org/10.1016/j.ijom.2020.03.003.
78. Katarzyna B, Aleksandra P, Piotr A. Goldenhar syndrome: current perspectives. World J Pediatr. 2017;13(5):405–15. https://doi.org/10.1007/s12519-017-0048-z.
79. Sapp Julie C, Lian H, Jean Z, Ashlyn G, Brian S, Dora F, Biesecker Leslie G. Quantifying survival in patients with Proteus syndrome. Genet Med. 2017;19(12):1376–9. https://doi.org/10.1038/gim.2017.65.
80. Keppler-Noreuil KM, Sapp JC, Lindhurst MJ, Darling TN, Jasmine B-A, Mohammadhadi B, Eva D, Ashlyn G, Jarosinski PF, Staci M, Neera N, Paul SM, Savage RE, Wolters PL, Brian S, Widemann BC, Biesecker LG. Pharmacodynamic study of miransertib in individuals with proteus syndrome. Am J Human Genet. 2019;104(3):484–91. https://doi.org/10.1016/j.ajhg.2019.01.015.
81. Chen CT, Okafor KC, Cavuoto KM, Dubovy SR, Karp CL. Pediatric multiple endocrine neoplasia type 2B: clinicopathological correlation of perilimbal mucosal neuromas and treatment of secondary open-angle glaucoma. Ocul Oncol Pathol. 2018;4(3):196–8. https://doi.org/10.1159/000484053.
82. Fassihi H, Sethi M, Fawcett H, Wing J, Chandler N, Mohammed S, Craythorne E, Morley AM, Lim R, Turner S, Henshaw T, Garrood I, Giunti P, Hedderly T, Abiona A, Naik H, Harrop G, McGibbon D, Jaspers NG, Botta E, Nardo T, Stefanini M, Young AR, Sarkany RP, Lehmann AR. Deep phenotyping of 89 xeroderma pigmentosum patients reveals unexpected heterogeneity dependent on the precise molecular defect. Proc Natl Acad Sci U S A. 2016;113:9. https://doi.org/10.1073/pnas.1519444113.
83. Majid M, Maliha M, Devon H, Carter P, Elayna B, Yasmyne R, Philip H. The multifold etiologies of limbal stem cell deficiency: a comprehensive review on the etiologies and additional treatment options for limbal stem cell deficiency. J Clin Med. 2023;12(13):4418. https://doi.org/10.3390/jcm12134418.
84. Reynolds MM, Veverka KK, Gertz MA, Angela D, Zeldenrust SR, Nelson L, Pulido JS. Ocular manifestations of systemic amyloidosis. Retina. 2018;38(7):1371–6. https://doi.org/10.1097/IAE.0000000000001901.

Index

© The Editor(s) (if applicable) and The Author(s), under exclusive license to Springer Nature Switzerland AG 2024
J. Pe'er et al. (eds.), *Clinical Ophthalmic Oncology*, https://doi.org/10.1007/978-3-031-72443-5

MIX
Papier aus verantwortungsvollen Quellen
Paper from responsible sources
FSC® C105338

If you have any concerns about our products,
you can contact us on
ProductSafety@springernature.com

In case Publisher is established outside the EU,
the EU authorized representative is:
Springer Nature Customer Service Center GmbH
Europaplatz 3, 69115 Heidelberg, Germany

Printed by Libri Plureos GmbH
in Hamburg, Germany